Adult Congenital Heart Disease

Editor

KAREN K. STOUT

CARDIOLOGY CLINICS

www.cardiology.theclinics.com

Consulting Editors
ROSARIO FREEMAN
JORDAN M. PRUTKIN
DAVID M. SHAVELLE
AUDREY H. WU

November 2015 • Volume 33 • Number 4

ELSEVIER

1600 John F. Kennedy Boulevard • Suite 1800 • Philadelphia, Pennsylvania, 19103-2899

http://www.theclinics.com

CARDIOLOGY CLINICS Volume 33, Number 4
November 2015 ISSN 0733-8651, ISBN-13: 978-0-323-41326-8

Editor: Lauren Boyle
Developmental Editor: Alison Swety

Cardiology Clinics (ISSN 0733-8651) is published quarterly by Elsevier Inc., 360 Park Avenue South, New York, NY 10010-1710. Months of issue are February, May, August, and November. Business and Editorial Offices: 1600 John F. Kennedy Blvd., Ste. 1800, Philadelphia, PA 19103-2899. Customer Service Office: 3251 Riverport Lane, Maryland Heights, MO 63043. Periodicals post-age paid at New York, NY and additional mailing offices. Subscription prices are $320.00 per year for US individuals, $530.00 per year for US institutions, $155.00 per year for US students and residents, $390.00 per year for Canadian individuals, $665.00 per year for Canadian institutions, $455.00 per year for international individuals, $665.00 per year for international institutions and $220.00 per year for Canadian and international students/residents. To receive student/resident rate, orders must be accompanied by name of affiliated institution, data of term, and the *signature* of program/residency coordinator on institution letterhead. Orders will be billed at individual rate until proof of status is received. Foreign air speed delivery is included in all *Clinics* subscription prices. All prices are subject to change without notice. **POSTMASTER:** Send address changes to *Cardiology Clinics*, Elsevier Health Sciences Division, Subscription Customer Service, 3251 Riverport Lane, Maryland Heights, MO 63043. **Customer Service: 1-800-654-2452 (U.S. and Canada); 314-447-8871 (outside U.S. and Canada). Fax: 314-447-8029. E-mail: journalscustomerservice-usa@ elsevier.com (for print support); journalsonlinesupport-usa@elsevier.com (for online support).**

Reprints. For copies of 100 or more, of articles in this publication, please contact the Commercial Reprints Department, Elsevier Inc., 360 Park Avenue South, New York, NY 10010-1710. Tel.: 212-633-3874; Fax: 212-633-3820; E-mail: reprints@elsevier.com.

Cardiology Clinics is also published in Spanish by McGraw-Hill Interamericana Editores S. A., P.O. Box 5-237, 06500, Mexico D. F., Mexico; in Portuguese by Reichmann and Alfonso Editores Rio de Janeiro, Brazil; and in Greek by Dimitrios P. Lagos, 8 Pondon Street, GR115-28 Ilissia, Greece.

Cardiology Clinics is covered in *MEDLINE/PubMed (Index Medicus), Excerpta Medica, The Cumulative Index to Nursing and Allied Health Literature* (CINAHL).

Contributors

EDITORIAL BOARD

ROSARIO FREEMAN, MD, MS, FACC
Associate Professor of Medicine; Director,
Coronary Care Unit; Director,
Echocardiography Laboratory, University of
Washington Medical Center, Seattle,
Washington

JORDAN M. PRUTKIN, MD, MHS, FHRS
Assistant Professor of Medicine, Division of
Cardiology/Electrophysiology, University of
Washington Medical Center, Seattle,
Washington

DAVID M. SHAVELLE, MD, FACC, FSCAI
Associate Professor, Keck School of Medicine;
Director, General Cardiovascular Fellowship
Program; Director, Cardiac Catheterization
Laboratory, Los Angeles County + USC
Medical Center; Division of Cardiovascular
Medicine, University of Southern California,
Los Angeles, California

AUDREY H. WU, MD
Assistant Professor, Internal Medicine,
University of Michigan, Ann Arbor, Michigan

EDITOR

KAREN K. STOUT, MD
Director, Adult Congenital Heart Disease
Program, Professor, Medicine/Pediatrics,
Division of Cardiology, Departments of
Medicine and Pediatrics, University of
Washington, Seattle, Washington

AUTHORS

AMI B. BHATT, MD, FACC
Director, Cardiovascular Disease and
Pregnancy Service; Adult Congenital Heart
Disease Program, Massachusetts General
Hospital Heart Center, Boston,
Massachusetts

CRAIG S. BROBERG, MD
Adult Congenital Heart Disease Program,
Knight Cardiovascular Institute, Oregon
Health and Science University, Portland,
Oregon

LUKE J. BURCHILL, MBBS, PhD
Adult Congenital Heart Disease Program,
Knight Cardiovascular Institute, Oregon
Health and Science University, Portland,
Oregon

STEPHEN C. COOK, MD, FACC
Department of Pediatrics, The Adult Congenital
Heart Disease Center, Heart Institute
Children's Hospital of Pittsburgh of UPMC,
Pittsburgh, Pennsylvania

JASON F. DEEN, MD
Assistant Professor of Pediatrics, Adjunct
Assistant Professor of Medicine, Adult
Congenital Heart Disease Service, Seattle
Children's Hospital, University of Washington,
Seattle, Washington

DOREEN DEFARIA YEH, MD, FACC
Director, Adult Congenital Heart Disease
Program; Cardiovascular Disease and
Pregnancy Service, Massachusetts General
Hospital Heart Center, Boston, Massachusetts

TACY E. DOWNING, MD
Division of Cardiology, The Children's Hospital of Philadelphia, Philadelphia, Pennsylvania

MICHELLE GURVITZ, MD, MS
Assistant Professor, Harvard Medical School; Department of Cardiology, Boston Children's Hospital; Department of Cardiology, Brigham and Women's Hospital, Boston, Massachusetts

CHRISTIANE HAEFFELE, MD, MPH
Division of Cardiovascular Medicine, Department of Medicine, Stanford University School of Medicine, Stanford, California

ANITHA S. JOHN, MD, PhD
Assistant Professor of Pediatrics, George Washington University; Director, Washington Adult Congenital Heart Program, Children's National Medical Center and MedStar Washington Hospital Center, Washington, DC

THOMAS K. JONES, MD
Professor of Pediatrics and Medicine, Director, Cardiac Catheterization Laboratories, Seattle Children's Hospital, University of Washington, Seattle, Washington

YULI Y. KIM, MD
Division of Cardiology, The Hospital of the University of Pennsylvania, Perelman School of Medicine at the University of Pennsylvania; Philadelphia Adult Congenital Heart Center, The Children's Hospital of Philadelphia, Perelman Center for Advanced Medicine, Penn Medicine, Philadelphia, Pennsylvania

ADRIENNE H. KOVACS, PhD
Associate Professor, Department of Psychiatry, Peter Munk Cardiac Centre, University Health Network, University of Toronto, Toronto, Ontario, Canada

ERIC V. KRIEGER, MD
Seattle Adult Congenital Heart Service, Division of Cardiology, Department of Medicine, University of Washington School of Medicine, Seattle, Washington

SAURABH KUMAR, BSc(Med)/MBBS, PhD
Arrhythmia Service, Cardiovascular Division, Brigham and Women's Hospital, Boston, Massachusetts

PETER J. LEARY, MD, MS
Pulmonary Vascular Disease Program, Division of Pulmonary and Critical Care Medicine, Department of Medicine, University of Washington School of Medicine, Seattle, Washington

LISA LEMOND, MD
Adult Congenital Heart Disease Program, Knight Cardiovascular Institute, Oregon Health and Science University, Portland, Oregon

GEORGE K. LUI, MD
Division of Cardiovascular Medicine, Department of Medicine; Division of Pediatric Cardiology, Department of Pediatrics, Stanford University School of Medicine, Stanford, California

TUAN MAI, MD
Adult Congenital Heart Disease Program, Knight Cardiovascular Institute, Oregon Health and Science University, Portland, Oregon

ARIANE J. MARELLI, MD, MPH, FRCPC, FACC, FAHA
Director, McGill Adult Unit for Congenital Heart Disease Excellence (MAUDE Unit), Associate Director of Research and Academic Affairs, Cardiology, McGill University Health Centre; Professor of Medicine, McGill University, Montreal, Quebec, Canada

EFRAT MAZOR DRAY, MD
McGill Adult Unit for Congenital Heart Disease Excellence (MAUDE Unit), McGill University Health Center, Montreal, Quebec, Canada

ASHOK MURALIDARAN, MD
Pediatric Cardiac Surgery, Doernbecher Children's Hospital, Oregon Health and Science University, Portland, Oregon

LAN NGUYEN, MD
Department of Cardiovascular Medicine, Heart and Vascular Institute, University of Pittsburgh, Pittsburgh, Pennsylvania

ALEXANDER R. OPOTOWSKY, MD, MPH
Boston Adult Congenital Heart and Pulmonary Hypertension Service, Department of Cardiology, Boston Children's Hospital and Brigham and Women's Hospital, Boston, Massachusetts

KERI SHAFER, MD
Instructor, Harvard Medical School;
Department of Cardiology, Boston Children's
Hospital; Department of Cardiology, Brigham
and Women's Hospital, Boston, Massachusetts

USHA B. TEDROW, MD, MSc
Arrhythmia Service, Cardiovascular Division,
Brigham and Women's Hospital, Boston,
Massachusetts

JOHN K. TRIEDMAN, MD
Department of Cardiology, Children's Hospital,
Boston, Boston, Massachusetts

ELISABETH M. UTENS, PhD
Associate Professor/Clinical Psychologist,
Department of Child and Adolescent
Psychiatry/Psychology, Erasmus Medical
Center-Sophia Children's Hospital, Rotterdam,
The Netherlands

KERI SHAFER, MD
Instructor, Harvard Medical School,
Department of Cardiology, Boston Children's
Hospital; Department of Cardiology, Brigham
and Women's Hospital, Boston, Massachusetts

USHA B. TEDROW, MD, MSc
Arrhythmia Service, Cardiovascular Division,
Brigham and Women's Hospital, Boston,
Massachusetts

JOHN K. TRIEDMAN, MD
Department of Cardiology, Children's Hospital,
Boston, Boston, Massachusetts

ELISABETH M. UTENS, PhD
Associate Professor/Clinical Psychologist,
Department of Child and Adolescent
Psychiatry/Psychology, Erasmus Medical
Center-Sophia Children's Hospital, Rotterdam,
The Netherlands

Contents

This article reviews the changing epidemiology of congenital heart disease, summarizing its impact on the demographics of the congenital heart disease population and the progress made in order to improve outcomes in this patient population. Birth prevalence of congenital heart disease can be modified by many factors. As a result of decreasing mortality and increasing survival in all forms of congenital heart disease, the median age of patients has increased and adults now compose two-thirds of patients with congenital heart disease. Disease burden and resulting health services utilization increase significantly across the lifespan. Bridging the gap between policy and quality of care can be improved by referral to specialized adult congenital heart disease centers and planning delivery of specialized services that are commensurate with population needs, program accreditation criteria, and certified training of designated workforce.

Intracardiac shunts are among the most common cardiac lesions seen in adult patients with congenital heart disease. Shunt lesions comprise much of the de novo congenital heart disease diagnosed in adults and engender a wide range of pathophysiologic consequences with a variety of treatment options. This article discusses the pathophysiology, clinical presentation, indications for intervention, late management issues, and pregnancy in adults with atrial septal defects, ventricular septal defects, and patent ductus arteriosus.

Coarctation of the aorta is a common congenital heart defect through which management has rapidly evolved over the last few decades. The role of transcatheter-based therapies is expanding and seems to be an effective treatment option for coarctation, especially in adults. Patients with prior coarctation repair are at risk of long-term complications related to prior surgeries and associated congenital heart defects, in particular, the risk of restenosis and aortic aneurysm development related to the timing and mode of prior intervention. This article outlines the evaluation and management of adults with unrepaired coarctation and patients after coarctation repair.

Repaired tetralogy of Fallot (TOF) is one of the most common diagnoses encountered when caring for adults with congenital heart disease. Although long-term survival after childhood TOF repair is excellent, morbidity is common and most patients require reintervention in adulthood. This review provides an overview of key surveillance and management issues for adults with TOF, including residual right ventricular outflow tract disease and timing of pulmonary valve replacement, arrhythmias and risk stratification, left-sided heart disease and heart failure, and pregnancy management.

Over the last 50 years, improved surgical techniques and progressive medical management have allowed patients with complete or dextro-transposition of the great arteries (D-TGA) to survive into adulthood. Older adult patients underwent an atrial switch procedure (Mustard or Senning operation), whereas the younger cohort of patients with TGA has undergone the arterial switch operation (ASO). The Mustard/Senning maintains the right ventricle as the systemic ventricle, whereas the more recently adopted ASO attempts to restore normal physiologic and anatomic relationships. Neither operation is without consequence and both require long term follow up.

The Fontan operation is a unique approach to create a circulation in series without 2 distinct pumping chambers. Although the approach has enabled many patients to live well into adulthood, the unique physiology results in many complications, cardiac and extracardiac. This review focuses on the pathophysiology of the failing Fontan and suggests possible treatment strategies. By understanding the physiology and interpreting patient data based on this understanding, an individualized treatment plan can be designed for this unique patient population.

Cardiac arrhythmias are a major source of morbidity and mortality in adults with congenital heart disease. A multidisciplinary approach in a center specializing in the care of adult congenital heart disease is most likely to have the expertise needed provide this care. Knowledge of the underlying anatomy, mechanism of arrhythmia, and potential management strategies is critical, as well as access and expertise in the use of advanced imaging and ablative technologies. Future challenges in management include refining the underlying mechanism and putative ablation targets for catheter ablation of atrial fibrillation, an arrhythmia rapidly rising in prevalence in this population.

In early stages, heart failure (HF) in adult congenital heart disease (ACHD) remains an elusive diagnosis. Many ACHD patients seem well-compensated owing to chronic physical and psychological adaptations. HF biomarkers and cardiopulmonary exercise tests are often markedly abnormal, although patients report stable health and good quality of life. Treatment differs from acquired HF. Evidence for effective drug therapy in ACHD-related HF is lacking. Residual ventricular, valvular, and vascular abnormalities contribute to HF pathophysiology, leading to an emphasis on nonpharmacologic treatment strategies. This article reviews emerging perspectives on nonpharmacologic treatment strategies, including catheter-based interventions, surgical correction, and palliative care.

Patients with adult congenital heart disease have an increased risk of developing pulmonary hypertension. There are several mechanisms of pulmonary hypertension in patients with adult congenital heart disease, and understanding them requires a systematic approach to define the patient's hemodynamics and physiology. This article reviews the updated classification of pulmonary hypertension in patients with adult congenital heart disease with a focus on pathophysiology, diagnostics, and the evaluation of pulmonary hypertension in special adult congenital heart disease populations.

Most women with known congenital heart disease can have successful pregnancy, labor, and delivery. Preconception assessment is essential in understanding anatomy, repairs, and current physiology, all of which can influence risk in pregnancy. With that foundation, a multidisciplinary cardio-obstetric team can predict and prepare for complications that may occur with superimposed hemodynamic changes of pregnancy. Individuals with Eisenmenger syndrome, pulmonary hypertension, cyanosis, significant left heart obstruction, ventricular dysfunction, or prior major cardiac event are at the highest risk for complications.

Most infants born with congenital heart disease (CHD) are now expected to reach adulthood. However, adults with CHD of moderate or great complexity remain at elevated risk of heart failure, arrhythmias, additional surgeries and interventional procedures, and premature mortality. This creates a need for lifelong specialized cardiac care and leads to 2 sets of potential challenges: (1) the transition from pediatric to adult care and (2) the psychosocial implications of coping with a chronic and often life-shortening medical condition. Many adolescents struggle with the transition to adult care, and mood and anxiety disorders are not uncommon in the adult setting.

Providing medical care for adults with congenital heart disease (CHD) is a complex endeavor requiring an understanding of all aspects of the health system. Adult patients with CHD often have multiple medical issues related to the underlying CHD, the sequelae of surgical or catheter interventions, and the addition of typical conditions of adulthood superimposed on the CHD. In this article, the authors first frame the assessment of quality in the health care system as a whole and then focus on CHD and the unique approach required in the care of the adult with CHD.

CARDIOLOGY CLINICS

THE CLINICS ARE AVAILABLE ONLINE!
Access your subscription at:
www.theclinics.com

Preface
Adult Congenital Heart Disease: The Coming Tide

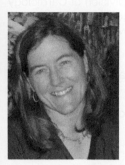

Karen K. Stout, MD
Editor

In the recent past, an adult with palliated or repaired congenital heart disease was something of a rarity. Patients with adult congenital heart disease (ACHD) were infrequently encountered in adult-oriented health care systems, and those who were seen most often had less complicated congenital heart disease like atrial septal defects or small ventricular septal defects. These abnormalities were relatively straightforward and were interesting intellectual additions to the more commonly encountered coronary artery disease and heart failure. Now, however, patients with ACHD are not only more commonly encountered, they have more complex heart disease, like tetralogy of Fallot, transposition of the great arteries, or palliated single ventricle and pose greater challenges in diagnosis and management.

What happened and why is all of this relevant to an adult cardiologist? Pediatric cardiology and pediatric cardiac surgery have been successful in diagnosing and treating all forms of congenital heart disease (CHD), including the most complex structural anomalies. While fewer than 10% of patients with complex CHD survived to adulthood 50 years ago, now over 90% are expected to survive due to effective diagnosis and treatment. This success results in not only more ACHD patients but also more ACHD patients with complex CHD. There are now estimated to be more adults than children with CHD in the United States, with over a million ACHD patients in the United States, growing by an estimated 50,000 people per year. Thus, adult cardiologists should expect to see more ACHD patients in all areas of the health care system.

Up to half the ACHD population have "simple" CHD, such as small shunts and isolated valve disease, but the other half have complex disease like tetralogy of Fallot, transposition of the great arteries, or single ventricles. Although they survive to adulthood, these patients are not cured, and many will have complications of their underlying disease or surgical repairs. The anatomy, physiology, and surgical repairs impart important differences between patients with ACHD and those patients with acquired heart disease. Complications such as arrhythmias, heart failure, and valvular dysfunction may not derive benefit from the usual treatment strategies for acquired heart disease, and those treatments may instead pose risk.

Concomitant with the increase in the patient population is growth in the resources available to care for these patients. ACHD was recognized as a subspecialty of both internal medicine and pediatric cardiology in 2012 and Accreditation Council for Graduate Medical Education ACHD fellowship accreditation began in 2015. There are ACHD curriculum requirements for both internal medicine and pediatric cardiology training, and the ACC/AHA Guidelines for the Care of Adults with Congenital Heart Disease were published in 2008 that are being revised for publication in 2015. Because there are relatively few ACHD cardiologists, there is variability in health care systems and many other generalists and specialists

Cardiol Clin 33 (2015) xiii–xiv
http://dx.doi.org/10.1016/j.ccl.2015.08.005
0733-8651/15/$ – see front matter © 2015 Published by Elsevier Inc.

needed, and it is important that all cardiologists are familiar with the key issues of ACHD patients. The goal of this issue of *Cardiology Clinics* is to discuss the current understanding of the most common issues in ACHD. We start with an overview of the changing demographics and then discuss the most commonly encountered lesions, move to a broader discussion of the overarching issues that these patients encounter, such as arrhythmias, heart failure, pulmonary hypertension, pregnancy, and psychosocial issues, and finish with a discussion of efforts to bring quality metrics to this diverse population. We hope that the articles in this issue provide information helpful to cardiologists and care providers both with and without experience in ACHD.

Karen K. Stout, MD
Adult Congenital Heart Disease Program
Division of Cardiology
Departments of Medicine and Pediatrics
University of Washington
1959 NE Pacific
Box 356422
Seattle, WA 98195, USA

E-mail address:
karenst@cardiology.washington.edu

Adult Congenital Heart Disease: Scope of the Problem

Efrat Mazor Dray, MD[a], Ariane J. Marelli, MD, MPH, FRCPC[b],*

KEYWORDS

- Adult • Congenital/epidemiology • Prevalence • Health services • Quality of care

KEY POINTS

- Birth prevalence of congenital heart disease (CHD) can be modified by many factors, including prenatal care, pregnancy termination and prevention, and changing sex distribution of the adult CHD population.
- As a result of decreasing mortality and increasing survival in all forms of CHD, the median age of patients has increased and adults now compose two-thirds of patients with CHD.
- Disease burden and resulting health services utilization increase significantly across the life span of the CHD population compared with the general population.
- Bridging the gap between policy and quality of care can be improved by referral to specialized adult CHD centers and planning delivery of specialized services that are commensurate with population needs, program accreditation criteria, and certified training of designated workforce.

INTRODUCTION

Congenital heart disease (CHD) lesions occur during embryonic development and consist of abnormal formations of the heart walls, valves or blood vessels. The adult congenital heart disease (ACHD) population is one of the fastest growing populations in cardiology. Contributing factors includes the improvement in CHD prenatal detection and treatment, novel surgical and interventional procedures, and the improvement in the organization of care. Echocardiography in clinical practice improves the ability to diagnose asymptomatic patients and patients with only mild lesions. These strides have resulted in rapidly changing demographics of those born with congenital lesions.

Previously almost exclusively in the domain of pediatric cardiology, care delivery needs to be continuous across pediatric and adult health care systems.

This article is divided in 3 parts. The authors first review the epidemiology of CHD summarizing the impact of the changing epidemiology on the demographics of the CHD population. Then they review the impact of changing demographics on this population's disease burden across the life span and the resulting increase in health services utilization (HSU). Finally, they examine the progress in how as a field we are beginning to bridge the gap between policy and quality in order to improve outcomes in this patient population.

Disclosures: The authors have no conflict of interest to disclose. Dr A.J. Marelli is a Clinical Scholar of the Fonds de Recherche Santé Québec whose research is supported by the Heart and Stroke Foundation of Canada and the Canadian Institute of Health Research, both of which are publically funded institutions.

[a] McGill Adult Unit for Congenital Heart Disease Excellence (MAUDE Unit), McGill University Health Center, 1001 Decarie Boulevard, Montréal, Quebec H4A 3J1, Canada; [b] McGill Adult Unit for Congenital Heart Disease Excellence (MAUDE Unit), Cardiology, McGill University Health Centre, McGill University, D055108, 1001 Decarie Boulevard, Montreal, Quebec H4A 3J1, Canada
* Corresponding author.
E-mail address: ariane.marelli@mcgill.ca

cardiology.theclinics.com

PREVALENCE OF CONGENITAL HEART DISEASE ACROSS THE LIFE SPAN
Incidence and Birth Prevalence of Congenital Heart Disease

The product of CHD incidence and survival determines the prevalence of CHD at all ages. Thus a clear understanding of the determinants of the incidence of CHD is important in understanding the challenges of measurement using empirical data. The exact incidence of CHD cannot be accurately measured because it would require tracking the number of new cases of CHD from conception in utero. Thus, the best proxy available to estimate the incidence of new cases of CHD born each year is *birth prevalence*.[1] Reported birth prevalence rates of CHD vary widely depending on the lesions included and geographic world region where they were measured. In the United States, data from the Centers for Disease Control and Prevention (CDC) from 1998 to 2005 identified using the Metropolitan Atlanta Congenital Defects Program, an overall prevalence of 8.14 per 1000 births in 398,140 births of which 3240 had CHD. The most common CHDs were muscular ventricular septal defect, perimembranous ventricular septal defect, and secundum atrial septal defect.[2] The prevalence of tetralogy of Fallot, the most common cyanotic CHD, was twice that of transposition of the great arteries. The European Surveillance of Congenital Anomalies (EUROCAT) database is a population-based surveillance system for CHD based on more than 16 European countries.[3] These registry data were based on cases including live births, late fetal death/stillbirths, as well as terminations of pregnancy for fetal anomaly. The reported total CHD prevalence based on 26,598 cases of CHD was 8.0 per 1000 births (ranging across the countries between 5.36 and 15.32 per 1000 births), and live birth prevalence was 7.2 per 1000 births.[3]

A worldwide overview was provided in a recent systematic review of birth prevalence for the 8 most common CHD lesions through 2010.[4] The reported birth prevalence of CHD increased to 9.1 per 1000 live births after 1995.[4] The birth prevalence among different geographic areas and World Bank income groups was statistically significant. The reported total CHD prevalence was higher in Asia (9.3 per 1000 live births) compared with all other continents, including Africa. High-income countries consistently had higher CHD birth prevalence (8.0 per 1000 live births) compared with lower-middle-income countries (6.9 per 1000 live births).[4] These variations likely reflect variations in infant health surveillance systems and the availability of early diagnostic tools. There were also significant geographic changes among the prevalence of the CHD subtypes. Asia reported more pulmonary outflow obstructions and lower rates of transposition of the great arteries at birth prevalence compared with the other continents.[4]

Factors that can modify prevalence of CHD at birth are numerous. Prenatal care and pregnancy prevention and termination impact both measures and biologically mediated pathways of birth prevalence rates of CHD. In reports from the EUROCAT registry, perinatal mortality was 0.25 per 1000 live births. Pregnancy termination for fetal anomaly after prenatal diagnosis varied widely ranging between less than 0.3 and 1.1 per 1000 births.[3] Other factors, including mandatory folate supplementation during pregnancy, may also modify birth rates of CHD, in particular decreasing the birth rate of severe CHD. This finding has been observed in Quebec and in other jurisdictions.[5]

Sex Differences in Congenital Heart Disease Distribution and Outcomes

Sex differences in the incidence of CHD are well described. Of the most common CHD lesions, atrial septal defects have a higher frequency in females, whereas conotruncal anomalies, such as transposition of the great arteries, are more common in males.[6] Consistent with the finding that female babies are less likely to have severe CHD, a large US population study, showed that more male children underwent CHD surgery and had high-risk procedures, although female infants who had high-risk procedures were at higher risk of death. In Canada in more than 45,000 adults with CHD, women accounted for 57% of patients, a proportion that was significantly higher than the predominance of females observed in the general population.[7] Using death registry data in 11,040 adults in the United States, a study from the CDC showed lower mortality rates in women with CHD compared with men.[8] Potential causes of a shift in demographics toward a predominance of females in the ACHD population include milder lesions in females and/or differences in outcomes in adults. A protective effect of sex was demonstrated on in-hospital mortality in women between 18 and 45 years of age.[9] In a large European survey of adults with CHD, men were more likely to die of CHD than women. Although women had a 33% higher risk for pulmonary hypertension, they also had a 47% lower risk for endocarditis, a 55% lower risk of cardioverter-defibrillator implant, and a lower risk of supraventricular arrhythmias compared with men.[10]

It is interesting to speculate how a larger proportion of surviving healthy girls with less severe lesions in addition to prevention and pregnancy termination of fetuses with severe lesions will interact to impact the birth prevalence of CHD from one generation to the next. A predominantly female ACHD population with less severe CHD may result in a higher number of CHD offspring. The effect will be further magnified if there exists potential sex differences in mortality during adult years. On the other hand, these trends may be offset by prevention of severe CHD and pregnancy termination in the context of the birth prevalence of CHD.[11] These observations suggest that future generations of predominantly female surviving patients with ACHD may have more offspring with CHD but that future generations of CHD births may have a decreasing prevalence of severe CHD.

Mortality and Survival Shifts in the Congenital Heart Disease Population

In the United States, *mortality of patients with CHD*, from 1979 through 1997, has been measured using statistics from the CDC. Almost half of all deaths from CHD occurred in infancy. The mortality from CHD decreased for all ages by 40% but particularly among children less than 5 years old.[12] Variations in mortality occur as a result of defect type, sex, age, and race. Using death certificates data in the United States from 1999 to 2006, annual CHD mortality rates by age at death, race-ethnicity, and sex were calculated for individuals 1 year of age or older. During this period, mortality resulting from CHD declined by 24% overall among all race-ethnicities studied. However, disparities persisted with rates that were consistently higher among non-Hispanic blacks compared with non-Hispanic whites. Infant mortality accounted for 48% of all CHD mortality; among those who survived the first year of life, 76.1% of deaths occurred during adulthood (≥18 years of age).[8] These findings underscore the need for more uniform access to care and continued surveillance as patients age.

Using the Quebec population-based database, temporal trends in all-cause mortality in patients with CHD across six 3-year intervals between the years 1987 and 2005 were characterized. Mortality was compared between 1987 to 1988 and 2004 to 2005. The study population included 8123 deaths over 1,008,835 patient-years of follow-up. In 1987 to 1988, the peak mortality was highest at infancy with a second peak later in adulthood. By 2004 to 2005, the overall mortality declined by 31% and the age distribution of death was no longer bimodal with a shift in mortality toward older age. Furthermore, for ages less than 65 years, the adjusted mortality rates declined in all age categories.[13]

Concurrent with decreasing mortality rates, *survival of the CHD population* has improved considerably.[14] A retrospective US population-based cohort study of infants born with CHD between 1979 and 2005 ascertained using the Metropolitan Atlanta Congenital Defects Program analyzed survival in critical CHD. Survival to adulthood remained significantly lower for those with critical versus noncritical CHD: 69% compared with 95%, respectively.[15] In Belgium, an analysis of survival trends by cohort and defect type was performed using administrative and clinical records of 7497 patients with CHD born between 1970 and 1992. Overall survival to 18 years of age for children born between 1990 and 1992 was nearly 90% corresponding to a significant improvement compared with previous decades. For this cohort, survival into adulthood for those with mild heart defects was 98%, whereas survival for those with moderate- and severe-complexity heart defects was 90% and 56%, respectively. Analyses by specific defect indicated that patients with a univentricular heart had poor survival rates, less than 50%.[16]

As a result of decreasing mortality and increasing survival in all forms of CHD, including severe CHD, the median age of patients with severe CHD has increased impressively from 11 years in 1985 to 17 years in 2000 and 25 years in 2010 (as illustrated in **Fig. 1**).[7,17] Care of adult patients with CHD, even those with severe

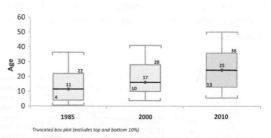

Truncated box plot (excludes top and bottom 10%)

Fig. 1. Median age of patients with severe CHD over time in 1985, 2000, and 2010. (*Data from* Marelli AJ, Mackie AS, Ionescu-Ittu R, et al. Congenital heart disease in the general population: changing prevalence and age distribution. Circulation 2007;115:163–72; and Marelli AJ, Ionescu-Ittu R, Mackie AS, et al. Lifetime prevalence of congenital heart disease in the general population from 2000 to 2010. Circulation 2014;130:749–56.)

CHD, falls squarely in the realm of adult cardiology.

Observations in North America and Europe are consistent for both mortality and survival. Despite great progress, these findings underscore work that lies ahead to meet the public health agenda as it relates to long-term follow-up, particularly in those with severe or critical CHD. These patients are largely young adults whose care can be improved during adulthood.

Prevalence and Population Size of Adult Congenital Heart Disease

Using Canadian longitudinal data from 1983 to 2010 and comprehensive population denominators, subjects with a CHD diagnosis were identified using the Quebec CHD database. From 1985 to 2000, the prevalence of CHD increased by 18% in children compared with 85% in adults.[7] Thus by the year 2000, the number of adults and children with CHD in Quebec had equalized.[7] From 2000 to 2010, the prevalence of CHD continued to increase, increasing by 11% in children compared with 57% in adults. Thus by 2010, the number of adults with CHD not only exceeded the number of children but adults also composed two-thirds of patients with CHD, for all CHD and for severe CHD (**Fig. 2**). The prevalence of severe CHD was 1.76 per 1000 children and 0.62 per 1000 adults.[17] These findings are consistent with a systematic review that estimated the prevalence of severe CHD in adults to be 0.93 per 1000.[18]

In an analysis done in conjunction with the CDC, empirical data from the Quebec CHD database in 2010 were used to generate age- and race-adjusted numbers of people living in the United States with CHD. It was estimated that by 2010, there were 2.4 million people living with CHD in the United States: 1.4 million adults and 1 million children, with 300,000 patients who had severe disease.

Fig. 3 illustrates the prevalence of CHD across the life span in infants, children, adults, and in geriatric patients in the same population using the Quebec CHD database.[7,17,19] This figure shows that 8 per 1000 patients have CHD at birth, consistent with the most often cited birth prevalence rate in the United States and elsewhere.[2,20] In children up to 18 years of age, 11 per 1000 children have CHD. The prevalence of CHD increases from infants to children because the ability to diagnose milder forms of CHD up to 18 years of age is possible with improved diagnostic tools, such as cardiac ultrasound. Six per 1000 adults have CHD, and nearly 4 per 1000 are more than 65 years of age. Ultimately, the absolute numbers of patients in each age group will be determined by the age distribution of the underlying population. In industrialized countries where adults outnumber children, there are now more adults than children with CHD despite the lower prevalence rate.

SPECIAL NEEDS AND THE IMPACT ON HEALTH SERVICES UTILIZATION
Disease Burden

The unique needs of this population center around life-long comorbidities.[21] Using the Quebec CHD database, the impact on morbidity and mortality of ongoing disease burden in those with atrial arrhythmias,[22] pulmonary hypertension,[23] infective endocarditis,[24] cardiovascular risk factors,[25] and the repeated need for interventions was documented.[26]

The impact on mortality remains a hard outcome targeted by clinicians, health services researchers, and administrators. The shift in mortality from infancy to adulthood[13] has resulted in a changing mode of death for patients with ACHD. Cardiovascular disease remains the main mode of death.[27,28] In a single-center cross-sectional study of 2600 patients of whom 199 died, the mean age

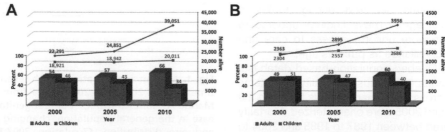

Fig. 2. (*A*) The number and proportions of adults and children in Quebec, Canada with all CHD over time in 2000, 2005, and 2010. (*B*) The number and proportions of adults and children in Quebec, Canada with severe CHD over time in 2000, 2005, and 2010. (*From* Marelli AJ, Ionescu-Ittu R, Mackie AS, et al. Lifetime prevalence of congenital heart disease in the general population from 2000 to 2010. Circulation 2014;130:753; with permission.)

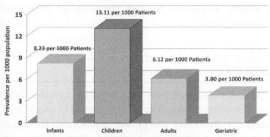

Fig. 3. Prevalence of CHD across the life span in infants, children, adults, and geriatric patients in Quebec, Canada. (*Data from* Marelli AJ, Mackie AS, Ionescu-Ittu R, et al. Congenital heart disease in the general population: changing prevalence and age distribution. Circulation 2007;115:163–72; and Afilalo J, Therrien J, Pilote L, et al. Geriatric congenital heart disease burden of disease and predictors of mortality. J Am Coll Cardiol 2011;58:1509–15.)

of death was 37 ±15 years. Patients with a univentricular heart, tricuspid atresia, and congenitally corrected transposition of the great arteries accounted for 75% of deaths. The most common mechanisms of death from cardiovascular causes were sudden death, heart failure, and arrhythmia. These mechanisms were followed by endocarditis, stroke, severe hemoptysis, and other bleeding events.[27] A study using the CONCOR (CONgenital CORvitia) registry in the Netherlands[29] analyzed deaths in 197 patients from 6933 patients with ACHD during a follow-up of 24,865 patient-years. The median age at death was 49 years. Of all deaths, 77% had a cardiovascular origin largely caused by chronic heart failure or sudden death. Predictors of mortality included age, male sex, CHD severity, number of interventions, and number of complications. Other predictors of all-cause mortality included endocarditis, supraventricular arrhythmias, ventricular arrhythmias, conduction disturbances, myocardial infarction, and pulmonary hypertension.[28]

Findings in patients beyond 60 years of age are interesting in that they reflect the similar impact of cardiovascular disease on mortality as in younger patients with ACHD, but they also highlight the effects of multisystem-acquired complications. In a single-center retrospective cohort study of an approximate 7000 patients from the Royal Brompton examining all-cause mortality stratified by age, the leading cause of death in patients greater than 60 years of age included multiorgan failure, cerebrovascular accident, and cancer. Significant independent predictors of all-cause mortality were coronary artery disease, heart failure, New York Heart Association (NYHA) functional class, and systemic ventricular function.[30] A study using the

Quebec CHD database reported dementia, gastrointestinal bleeding, and chronic kidney failure as important predictors of mortality in ACHD patients more than 65 years of age.[19] Thus in older patients with ACHD who tend to have milder forms of CHD, acquired cardiovascular and systemic disease superimposed on underlying congenital heart lesions is important and requires particular consideration. As younger patients with ACHD with severe and critical CHD age, the complexity of the care will only be magnified.

Impact on Health Services Utilization

Using the Quebec CHD database, significant increases in HSU across the life span is shown: during childhood with increasing readmission rates from 1990 to 2005,[31] during transition years with care gaps affecting 60% of all patients with CHD,[32] in adulthood with a 4-fold increase in hospitalization rates in patients with ACHD compared with the general population,[33] and into the geriatric years with comorbidity driving HSU.[19] Specifically documenting the frequency of HSU in the ACHD population, they showed that over a 5-year period between 1996 and 2000 in a population of 22,096 adults, 87% received outpatient care from specialists, 68% visited emergency departments, 51% were hospitalized, and 16% were admitted to critical care units, all of which were significantly higher than the age-adjusted general Quebec adult population for all patients with ACHD but even more so for those with severe CHD.[33,34]

Using data from the Nationwide Inpatient Sample from 1998 to 2005, the number of hospitalizations of patients with ACHD in the United States was observed to increase by 102%, with heart failure hospitalizations increasing by 82%.[35] Of approximately 84,000 hospitalizations of adults with CHD in the United States in 2007, 17,000 had a diagnosis of heart failure.[36] The overall mortality of patients with ACHD with heart failure was 4.1%, which was significantly greater than patients with ACHD without heart failure even after controlling for age and comorbidities.[36]

Using the CONCOR registry database, the extent and the characteristics of hospital admissions for patients with ACHD were followed from the year 2001 up until 2006.[29] Compared with the general Dutch population, the admission rate for patients with ACHD was 2 to 3 times higher among all age groups, with the highest admission rate in patients more than 40 years old. Most of the hospital admissions were for cardiovascular causes (61%). The most frequent cardiovascular admission diagnoses were arrhythmias (31%), followed by chest pain and heart failure.[37]

To better understand the diagnostic spectrum and resource utilization of the aging CHD population, a retrospective cohort study done at the Royal Brompton Hospital was performed in 375 patients aged 60 years and older and under active follow-up between January 2000 and March 2012. Most of the patient population consisted of patients with simple shunt lesions. Most were asymptomatic, with only 19% reporting symptoms that were compatible with NYHA class III or IV. Even so, the number of interventions per 100 patient-years was significantly higher in the elderly patient population (more than 60 years of age) compared with the younger age group (20–60 years of age). The number of hospitalization, the cumulative length of hospital stay, and the number of outpatient clinic visits was also significantly higher in this age group.[30]

Taken together, these findings suggest that HSU rates in the United States, Canada, and Europe where patients undergo surgical repair of CHD continue to be high compared with the general population. This finding is so not only for those with severe CHD who are young and for whom morbidity and mortality continue to center around cardiovascular complications of the underlying CHD but also for the aging CHD population whereby the disease burden is governed by acquired cardiovascular complications and systemic multiorgan systems disease.

BRIDGING THE POLICY TO QUALITY GAP

Policy matters because CHD is a life-span disease associated with high HSU and, therefore, high health care costs. Working with policy makers we can impact resource allocation increasing capacity in terms of structure and process elements of health care delivery that will allow us to shape quality of care moving forward, ultimately impacting outcomes. *Quality of care* matters because it gives us the opportunity to achieve desired health outcomes. The purpose of improving quality is to provide health services that increase the likelihood of desired outcomes in a manner that is consistent with current professional knowledge.[38] As a field, we have begun to make strides in terms of addressing knowledge gaps that will start to address the policy-to-quality gap. In the last 5 years, we have shown that specialized ACHD care beneficially impacts mortality; we have renewed clinical practice guidelines with more rigor in the analysis of current professional knowledge; we have developed quality measures related to the implementation of these guidelines; we have created board certification for ACHD specialists; and we have

become engaged in the process of program accreditation.

Impact of Specialized Adult Congenital Heart Disease Care on Mortality

The authors have now demonstrated that ACHD care matters. Analyzing the impact of ACHD care on mortality using the Quebec CHD database, the authors have shown that policy can impact quality. In 1998, the Canadian Cardiovascular Society published a document on ACHD care, the appendix of which included a list of ACHD specialized care across Canada to which patients should be referred. Three of these were in Quebec.[39] Thus using the Quebec CHD database, the impact of accelerated referral to specialized ACHD centers in Quebec was examined by examining outcomes in 7000 to 8000 patients yearly from 1990 to 2005 and comparing those referred with those not referred to specialized ACHD centers.[40] In a time-series analysis, Mylotte and colleagues[40] showed that mortality of the ACHD population began to decrease significantly after the onset of accelerated referrals to specialized ACHD centers consistent with policy recommendations of the published guidelines (**Fig. 4**). Moreover, in a matched case-control analysis for the death outcome, the impact of exposure to an ACHD specialized center care on the mortality outcome was examined. Not surprisingly, older age, male sex, CHD disease severity, and comorbidity were all strong predictors of mortality. However, exposure to a referral center conferred a protective effect, decreasing the odds of death even after adjustment for all confounder variables.[40]

Planning Specialized Care of Patients with Adult Congenital Heart Disease

The data cited earlier support the recommendations in the United States,[41] Canada,[42] and Europe[43] that patients with ACHD should be referred to ACHD specialized centers with follow-up planned in conjunction with other cardiologists and primary care providers. These centers should ideally offer the entire spectrum of ACHD, pediatric cardiology, and congenital heart surgery. Multidisciplinary teams with defined referral pathways should also be available. With the advancing age of the ACHD population, invasive CHD procedures should be performed by or in partnership with ACHD experts. Additionally, the increasing burden of arrhythmias in the ACHD population necessitates access to electrophysiologists specializing in ACHD.[44]

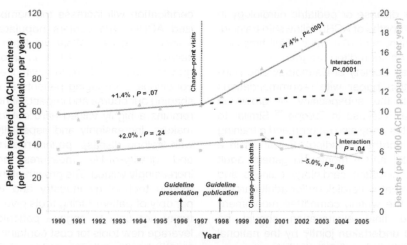

Fig. 4. Time-series analysis: referral to specialized ACHD centers and mortality of patients with ACHD. Time-series analysis illustrating observed specialized ACHD center referral (*black line*) and ACHD mortality (*gray line*) per 1000 ACHD population per year, between 1990 and 2005. The dashed lines indicate expected trends after the change points identified by Poisson regression, and the black or gray lines represent the observed trends. (*From* Mylotte D, Pilote L, Ionescu-Ittu R, et al. Specialized adult congenital heart disease care: the impact of policy on mortality. Circulation 2014;129:1807; with permission.)

Estimates regarding the needed number of specialist ACHD centers on a population level will vary depending on access to health care in the local environment. Access is a complex construct that is driven not only by individual and population needs but also by health insurance, geographic, socioeconomic, and health systems variables. Using population data applicable to industrialized countries, the authors have generated estimates on number of centers needed per population in the millions depending on different models of access. In the first scenario, if regional ACHD centers target only patients with severe CHD, an approximate 1 center for every 10 million adult inhabitants is required. If regional ACHD centers target all patients with moderate and severe CHD or 50% of the ACHD population, an estimated number of 1 center per 2 to 3 million adult population would be needed.[45] In Canada, the ratio of specialized ACHD centers is 1 per 3 to 7 million depending on the region and the extent of services offered.[46] Even so, in 2010, less than one-third of patients with ACHD expected to be alive were being actively followed in these centers.[46] These findings in a country where there exists universal health insurance in a publically funded health care system underscore the challenges of adequate delivery of specialized services and the need for advocacy and policy intended to improve the quality of health services delivered. The authors estimated that the United States will require at least 150 ACHD centers to care for the 50% of the ACHD population with moderate and severe forms of CHD.[45]

Delivering Specialized Adult Congenital Heart Disease Care

The United States has taken the lead in the development of an accreditation process and criteria for US ACHD clinics in collaboration with the patient advocacy within the Adult Congenital Heart Association. This effort is remarkable not only in the scope of its intent but also for its forward thinking partnership with patients to insure that efforts and outcomes are patient centered. The Adult Congenital Heart Association is building a roadmap of standards based on expert consensus with an emphasis on collaboration with the intent of strengthening the network of specialized ACHD care programs.[47]

To address the gap in health care providers to populate ACHD specialized care centers with adequately trained physician and caregivers, a collaboration between the American Board of Pediatrics and the American Board of Internal Medicine has led to the creation of a subspecialty certification in ACHD, with the first qualifying examination scheduled for 2015.[47] To support this effort, the Accreditation Council for Graduate Medical Education agreed in 2013 to accredit fellowship programs in the subspecialty of ACHD.[47] The training pathway involves completion of the training required for certification in cardiovascular disease or pediatric cardiology in addition to 24 months of ACHD fellowship training, including a minimum of 18 months of full-time clinical training in an accredited program.[48]

The European Society of Cardiology also published a position paper with recommendations for training in the subspecialty of grown-up congenital heart disease in Europe.[49] Similar to the United States, they also recommend a training period of 24 months, including 18 months in a specialist center and 6 months in general adult cardiology for pediatric cardiology trainees and 6 months in pediatric cardiology for adult cardiology trainees. The writing committee recommended that the final examination should be organized and undertaken jointly by the national societies of adult and pediatric cardiology.

Importantly ACHD specialized centers should be located in an environment with academic links that promote research and innovation so that we may as a field insure training not only the next generation of clinicians but also clinician scientists and researchers with translational capabilities.[49]

SUMMARY AND FUTURE DIRECTIONS

The prevalence of CHD on a population level is determined by birth prevalence of CHD and survival of CHD across the life span. With substantial improvement in survival, the prevalence of CHD in adults continues to increase. Two-thirds of the entire CHD population is now composed of adults, including those with severe CHD. With mortality shifts away from infants and toward adults, the landscape of comorbidity is changing. Although cardiac complications of the CHD lesion continues to account for substantial morbidity and mortality in young adults with severe CHD, as the population ages, acquired cardiovascular complications and multisystem disease are becoming increasingly important in aging adults with CHD. Special needs in the management of arrhythmias, heart failure, pulmonary hypertension, endocarditis, heart failure, and interventional procedures have been identified. Improving the quality of care can be attained through referral to specialized centers, training, and well-designed research in ACHD. Lifelong disease burden results in increasing HSU and costs across the lifespan with care gaps and high hospitalization rates in adults. The importance of policy is in setting the stage for delivering improved quality of care in a health economic environment of cost containment. Our field is making strides in providing the evidence needed to provide the underpinning of policy and in putting in place standards for improving access to high-quality care. Program accreditation and specialty

certification will increase the number of specialized ACHD care centers populated by ACHD-trained caregivers. What we learn about health services delivery in CHD is informative to a growing number of children with life span chronic conditions.[50] Engaging patients in our journey is shaping our course and impact. Although mortality remains a highly valued hard outcome for policy makers, increasingly and especially for patients with lifelong disease, patient-reported outcomes and quality-of-life measures are becoming increasingly valued. The growth of the health information technology industry and the increasing panoply of patient-facing tools gives us an opportunity not only to engage patients but also to leverage new tools for cost containment, improvement in health wellness, and novel ways to access big data to improve the quality of care.

REFERENCES

1. Marelli A. The future of adult congenital care symposium: changing demographics of congenital heart disease. Prog Pediatr Cardiol 2012;34:85–90.
2. Reller MD, Strickland MJ, Riehle-Colarusso T, et al. Prevalence of congenital heart defects in metropolitan Atlanta, 1998-2005. J Pediatr 2008;153:807–13.
3. Dolk H, Loane M, Garne E. Congenital heart defects in Europe: prevalence and perinatal mortality, 2000 to 2005. Circulation 2011;123:841–9.
4. van der Linde D, Konings EE, Slager MA, et al. Birth prevalence of congenital heart disease worldwide: a systematic review and meta-analysis. J Am Coll Cardiol 2011;58:2241–7.
5. Ionescu-Ittu R, Marelli AJ, Mackie AS, et al. Prevalence of severe congenital heart disease after folic acid fortification of grain products: time trend analysis in Quebec, Canada. BMJ 2009;338:1673–83.
6. Fyler DC. Report of the New England regional infant cardiac program. Pediatrics 1980;65:375–461.
7. Marelli AJ, Mackie AS, Ionescu-Ittu R, et al. Congenital heart disease in the general population: changing prevalence and age distribution. Circulation 2007;115:163–72.
8. Gilboa SM, Salemi JL, Nembhard WN, et al. Mortality resulting from congenital heart disease among children and adults in the United States, 1999 to 2006. Circulation 2010;122:2254–63.
9. Zomer AC, Ionescu-Ittu R, Vaartjes I, et al. Sex differences in hospital mortality in adults with congenital heart disease: the impact of reproductive health. J Am Coll Cardiol 2013;62:58–67.
10. Verheugt CL, Uiterwaal CS, van der Velde ET, et al. Gender and outcome in adult congenital heart disease. Circulation 2008;118:26–32.

11. Germanakis I, Sifakis S. The impact of fetal echocardiography on the prevalence of live-born congenital heart disease. Pediatr Cardiol 2006;27:465–72.

12. Boneva RS, Botto LD, Moore CA, et al. Mortality associated with congenital heart defects in the United States: trends and racial disparities, 1979-1997. Circulation 2001;103:2376–81.

13. Khairy P, Ionescu-Ittu R, Mackie AS, et al. Changing mortality in congenital heart disease. J Am Coll Cardiol 2010;56:1149–57.

14. Greutmann M, Tobler D, Biaggi P, et al. Echocardiography for assessment of regional and global right ventricular systolic function in adults with repaired tetralogy of Fallot. Int J Cardiol 2010;157:53–8.

15. Oster ME, Lee KA, Honein MA, et al. Temporal trends in survival among infants with critical congenital heart defects. Pediatrics 2013;131:e1502–8.

16. Moons P, Bovijn L, Budts W, et al. Temporal trends in survival to adulthood among patients born with congenital heart disease from 1970 to 1992 in Belgium. Circulation 2010;122:2264–72.

17. Marelli AJ, Ionescu-Ittu R, Mackie AS, et al. Lifetime prevalence of congenital heart disease in the general population from 2000 to 2010. Circulation 2014;130:749–56.

18. van der Bom T, Bouma BJ, Meijboom FJ, et al. The prevalence of adult congenital heart disease, results from a systematic review and evidence based calculation. Am Heart J 2012;164:568–75.

19. Afilalo J, Therrien J, Pilote L, et al. Geriatric congenital heart disease burden of disease and predictors of mortality. J Am Coll Cardiol 2011;58:1509–15.

20. Hoffman JI, Kaplan S. The incidence of congenital heart disease. J Am Coll Cardiol 2002;39:1890–900.

21. Marelli A, Beauchesne L, Mital S, et al. Canadian cardiovascular society 2009 consensus conference on the management of adults with congenital heart disease: introduction. Can J Cardiol 2010;26:e65–9.

22. Bouchardy J, Therrien J, Pilote L, et al. Atrial arrhythmias in adults with congenital heart disease. Circulation 2009;120:1679–86.

23. Lowe BS, Therrien J, Ionescu-Ittu R, et al. Diagnosis of pulmonary hypertension in the congenital heart disease adult population impact on outcomes. J Am Coll Cardiol 2011;58:538–46.

24. Rushani D, Kaufman JS, Ionescu-Ittu R, et al. Infective endocarditis in children with congenital heart disease: cumulative incidence and predictors. Circulation 2013;128:1412–9.

25. Roifman I, Therrien J, Ionescu-Ittu R, et al. Coarctation of the aorta and coronary artery disease: fact or fiction? Circulation 2012;126:16–21.

26. Ionescu-Ittu R, Mackie AS, Abrahamowicz M, et al. Valvular operations in patients with congenital heart disease: increasing rates from 1988 to 2005. Ann Thorac Surg 2010;90:1563–9.

27. Oechslin EN, Harrison DA, Connelly MS, et al. Mode of death in adults with congenital heart disease. Am J Cardiol 2000;86:1111–6.

28. Verheugt CL, Uiterwaal CS, van der Velde ET, et al. Mortality in adult congenital heart disease. Eur Heart J 2010;31:1220–9.

29. van der Velde ET, Vriend JW, Mannens MM, et al. CONCOR, an initiative towards a national registry and DNA-bank of patients with congenital heart disease in the Netherlands: rationale, design, and first results. Eur J Epidemiol 2005;20:549–57.

30. Tutarel O, Kempny A, Alonso-Gonzalez R, et al. Congenital heart disease beyond the age of 60: emergence of a new population with high resource utilization, high morbidity, and high mortality. Eur Heart J 2014;35:725–32.

31. Mackie AS, Ionescu-Ittu R, Pilote L, et al. Hospital readmissions in children with congenital heart disease: a population-based study. Am Heart J 2008;155:577–84.

32. Mackie AS, Ionescu-Ittu R, Therrien J, et al. Children and adults with congenital heart disease lost to follow-up: who and when? Circulation 2009;120:302–9.

33. Mackie AS, Pilote L, Ionescu-Ittu R, et al. Healthcare resource utilization in adults with congenital heart disease: a population-based study. Am J Cardiol 2007;33:839–43.

34. Marelli AJ, Gurvitz M. From numbers to guidelines. Prog Cardiovasc Dis 2011;53:239–46.

35. Opotowsky AR, Siddiqi OK, Webb GD. Trends in hospitalizations for adults with congenital heart disease in the U.S. J Am Coll Cardiol 2009;54:460–7.

36. Rodriguez FH 3rd, Marelli AJ. The epidemiology of heart failure in adults with congenital heart disease. Heart Failure Clin 2014;10:1–7.

37. Verheugt CL, Uiterwaal CS, van der Velde ET, et al. The emerging burden of hospital admissions of adults with congenital heart disease. Heart 2010;96:872–8.

38. Blumenthal D. Part 1: quality of care–what is it? N Engl J Med 1996;335:891–4.

39. Connelly M, Webb G, Somerville J, et al. Canadian consensus conference on adult congenital heart disease 1996. Can J Cardiol 1998;14:395–452.

40. Mylotte D, Pilote L, Ionescu-Ittu R, et al. Specialized adult congenital heart disease care: the impact of policy on mortality. Circulation 2014;129:1804–12.

41. Warnes CA, Williams RG, Bashore TM, et al. ACC/AHA 2008 guidelines for the management of adults with congenital heart disease: executive summary: a report of the American College of Cardiology/American Heart Association Task Force on Practice Guidelines (writing committee to develop guidelines for the management of adults with congenital heart disease). Circulation 2008;118:2395–451.

42. Silversides CK, Marelli A, Beauchesne L, et al. Canadian Cardiovascular Society 2009 consensus conference on the management of adults with congenital heart disease: executive summary. Can J Cardiol 2010;26:143–50.

43. Baumgartner H, Bonhoeffer P, De Groot NM, et al. Esc guidelines for the management of grown-up congenital heart disease (new version 2010). Eur Heart J 2010;31:2915–57.

44. Khairy P, Van Hare GF, Balaji S, et al. PACES/HRS expert consensus statement on the recognition and management of arrhythmias in adult congenital heart disease: developed in partnership between the Pediatric and Congenital Electrophysiology Society (PACES) and the Heart Rhythm Society (HRS). Endorsed by the governing bodies of PACES, HRS, the American College of Cardiology (ACC), the American Heart Association (AHA), the European Heart Rhythm Association (EHRA), the Canadian Heart Rhythm Society (CHRS), and the International Society for Adult Congenital Heart Disease (ISACHD). Heart Rhythm 2014;11:e102–65.

45. Marelli AJ, Therrien J, Mackie AS, et al. Planning the specialized care of adult congenital heart disease patients: from numbers to guidelines; an epidemiologic approach. Am Heart J 2009;157:1–8.

46. Beauchesne LM, Therrien J, Alvarez N, et al. Structure and process measures of quality of care in adult congenital heart disease patients: a pan-Canadian study. Int J Cardiol 2010;157:70–4.

47. Webb G, Landzberg MJ, Daniels CJ. Specialized adult congenital heart care saves lives. Circulation 2014;129:1795–6.

48. Avila P, Mercier LA, Dore A, et al. Adult congenital heart disease: a growing epidemic. Can J Cardiol 2014;30:S410–9.

49. Baumgartner H, Budts W, Chessa M, et al. Recommendations for organization of care for adults with congenital heart disease and for training in the subspecialty of 'grown-up congenital heart disease' in Europe: a position paper of the Working Group on Grown-up Congenital Heart Disease of the European Society of Cardiology. Eur Heart J 2014;35:686–90.

50. Van Cleave J, Gortmaker SL, Perrin JM. Dynamics of obesity and chronic health conditions among children and youth. JAMA 2010;303:623–30.

Shunt Lesions

Jason F. Deen, MD[a],*, Thomas K. Jones, MD[b]

KEYWORDS

- Adult congenital heart disease • Intracardiac shunt • Septal defects • Pregnancy

KEY POINTS

- Atrial septal defects are a common primary diagnosis in adults.
- Ventricular septal defects are usually treated in childhood, although hemodynamically insignificant isolated lesions may be seen in adulthood and warrant routine surveillance.
- Percutaneous closure of a patent ductus arteriosus is the treatment of choice in adulthood.
- Shunt-related Eisenmenger physiology is an absolute contraindication to pregnancy.

INTRODUCTION

Intracardiac shunts are among the most common cardiac lesions seen in adult patients with congenital heart disease, and indeed typify congenital heart disease for many medical providers. Shunt lesions comprise much of the de novo congenital heart disease diagnosed in adults and engender a wide range of pathophysiologic consequences with a variety of treatment options.

In the normal heart, septation of the right-sided and left-sided cardiac chambers separates the pulmonary circulation from the systemic circulation. Although the 2 circulations are contiguous, they can also be thought of as occurring in parallel. The right atrium collects deoxygenated blood from the systemic veins and the right ventricle delivers blood to the pulmonary circulation. Simultaneously, the left atrium collects oxygenated blood from the pulmonary veins and the left ventricle ejects blood to the systemic circulation. Shunting occurs as a consequence of a connection between the pulmonary and systemic circulations, either at the atrial, ventricular, or great vessel level, resulting in an atrial septal defect (ASD), ventricular septal defect (VSD), or patent ductus arteriosus (PDA), respectively. Differences in ventricular

compliance and vascular resistance of the 2 circulations result in left-to-right shunting, which allows oxygenated blood to be recirculated through the pulmonary circulation. If the shunt volume is significant, this inefficient recirculation of blood causes an excessive volume load on the ventricles and transmits a combination of volume and pressure to the pulmonary vascular bed.

Quantification of the ratio of pulmonary blood flow (Qp) to systemic blood flow (Qs) is useful to estimate the net shunt volume. In most patients, the volume of shunted blood is directly proportional to the symptoms experienced. A Qp/Qs ratio of 1:1 is normal and indicates a balanced circulation without shunting. A Qp/Qs ratio greater than 1 indicates a left-to-right shunt with excessive pulmonary blood flow. A Qp/Qs ratio of less than 1 indicates a right-to-left shunt and may indicate a long-standing intracardiac shunt with Eisenmenger physiology.

ATRIAL SEPTAL DEFECT

The atrial septum develops from both the growth and subsequent partial resorption of the septum primum and septum secundum as the septum attaches to the crux of the heart as well as an

No relevant disclosures (J.F. Deen); Dr T.K. Jones receives research grant support and consulting fees from St. Jude Medical and W.L. Gore and Assoc., Inc.

[a] Adult Congenital Heart Disease Service, Seattle Children's Hospital, University of Washington, 4800 Sand Point Way Northeast, RC.2.820, Heart Center, Seattle, WA 98105, USA; [b] Cardiac Catheterization Laboratories, Seattle Children's Hospital, University of Washington, 4800 Sand Point Way Northeast, RC.2.820, Heart Center, Seattle, WA 98105, USA
* Corresponding author.
E-mail address: Jason.deen@seattlechildrens.org

cardiology.theclinics.com

incorporation of the fetal sinus venosus into the nascent posterior right atrium. Developmental abnormalities in this process result in a communication between the right and left atria through the septum itself, an ASD. There are several types of ASDs; the most common of these are the secundum type (which results from excessive resorption of the septum primum), the primum type (a deficiency of the endocardial cushions of the cardiac crux), and the sinus venosus type (which results from a medial incorporation of the fetal sinus venosus). ASDs are among the most common congenital heart lesions, occurring in 1.64 per 1000 live births.[1] Although many are diagnosed and treated in childhood, a significant number of ASDs are diagnosed in adulthood, accounting for 25% to 30% of newly diagnosed congenital heart lesions (**Fig. 1**).[2]

Pathophysiology

Flow through a communication in the atrial septum occurs throughout the cardiac cycle, although predominantly in diastole when the atrioventricular valves are open. Direction of flow depends on the differential compliance of the ventricles, which, in turn, is largely determined by ventricular afterload. In the normal heart, the left ventricle is subjected to systemic pressures that far exceed the pressure seen by the right ventricle. As a consequence of this increased myocardial work, the

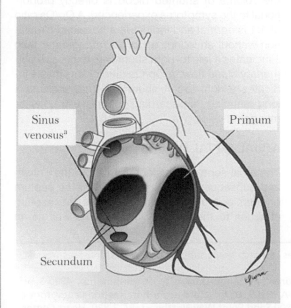

Fig. 1. Anatomy of atrial septal defects seen from the right atrium. [a]Both superior and inferior sinus venosus defects are shown. (*Adapted from* Vasquez AF, Lasala JM. Atrial septal defect closure. Cardiol Clin 2013;31(3):385–400; with permission.)

left ventricle becomes hypertrophied and the right ventricular wall thins. The result of this difference in ventricular compliance is a left-to-right atrial shunt with filling of the more compliant right ventricle. Factors that decrease right ventricular compliance (pulmonary artery obstruction, increased pulmonary vascular resistance, and pulmonary venous obstruction) may equalize the ability of the right and left ventricles to fill, thereby leading to bidirectional shunting. Severe right ventricular noncompliance caused by hypoplasia or infarction may result in predominantly right-to-left shunting at the atrium. The size of the ASD is also a determinant of shunt flow and may restrict volume by virtue of the resistance of the ASD itself despite the differences in ventricular compliance.

Clinical Presentation

Although infants and children may present with activity intolerance and heart failure, this is a rare occurrence; most young patients with an ASD are asymptomatic and present with a cardiac murmur. Adult patients are more likely to manifest symptoms from an atrial level shunt because shunt flow through an ASD is age dependent. A young infant's right ventricle is relatively noncompliant as a result of increased pulmonary vascular resistance experienced during fetal life and there may be minimal atrial shunting in young infants. As a consequence of the normal decrease in pulmonary vascular resistance in infancy and childhood, the right ventricle becomes more compliant with a resultant left-to-right shunt. Furthermore, as part of the typical aging process, the left ventricle becomes the dominant ventricle and its compliance decreases. As adults age, therefore, atrial shunts are augmented by normal physiologic changes of the ventricles.[3]

Most patients with clinically important ASDs will develop symptoms, although it is difficult to predict when these symptoms will arise. Most commonly, adult patients will complain of progressive activity intolerance with dyspnea on exertion. Occasionally, they will present with palpitations caused by new-onset atrial dysrhythmia as a consequence of atrial myocardial stretch. Rarely, paradoxic embolus will occur in the setting of transiently increased right ventricular pressure as with Valsalva maneuver.

Pulmonary vascular disease with subsequent pulmonary arterial hypertension occurs in patients with ASDs with a prevalence noted between 6% and 35%.[4–6] Patients with unrepaired ASDs and pulmonary arterial hypertension usually present with activity limitations and atrial dysrhythmias, although they may have classic right ventricular systolic failure (peripheral edema and impaired cardiac output) in advanced situations. Patients may be cyanotic from a right-to-left atrial shunt (Eisenmenger physiology). Despite reports of the high prevalence of pulmonary arterial hypertension in patients with ASDs, little is known about the specific risk factors associated with the development of pulmonary vascular occlusive disease.

Indications for Intervention

Given the known morbidity associated with ASDs, there is a general consensus that hemodynamically significant ASDs with and without symptoms should be closed either by surgical or percutaneous techniques.[7] An ASD is considered hemodynamically significant if there is demonstrable right-sided cardiac volume overload as shown by right ventricular enlargement on echocardiography or MRI. In addition, ASD closure should be considered in the setting of paradoxic embolism, with orthodeoxia-platypnea or in the presence of symptoms from effort-related hypoxia.

Severe irreversible pulmonary arterial hypertension (pulmonary vascular resistance >2/3 systemic vascular resistance without left-to-right atrial shunting) is a contraindication to ASD closure.[7] However, in patients with increased pulmonary vascular resistance but with vasoreactivity demonstrated by pulmonary vasodilator therapy or balloon, occlusion of the defect closure of the ASD may be considered.

Studies suggest closure of an ASD should take place before 24 years of age to maximize the mortality benefit from intervention; in patients repaired before 40 years of age, the occurrence or persistence of atrial dysrhythmias, which may develop in older individuals after late primary repair, is minimized.[8,9]

Surgical closure has long been considered the gold standard approach to treatment of ASDs. It is still the treatment of choice for certain types of ASDs, including primum ASDs and sinus venosus defects, or if antiarrhythmic surgery is offered concurrently. However, with uncomplicated secundum ASDs with favorable morphology, percutaneous ASD closure has surpassed surgery as the treatment of choice with a minimal (<1%) risk of major complications and a high success rate.[10] This procedure is undertaken with transesophageal or intracardiac echocardiography guidance. Antiplatelet therapy with acetylsalicylic acid as well as endocarditis prophylaxis is routinely prescribed for 6 months after the procedure (**Fig. 2**).

Early and intermediate postprocedure results are excellent for both surgical and percutaneous closure of ASDs with high rates of success with few major complications.[10] Symptoms experienced before ASD closure lessen and subside, and patients have an improvement in functional class and activity tolerance.[11,12] The risk of pulmonary arterial hypertension is attenuated. Furthermore, there is evidence that these clinical improvements along with favorable cardiac remodeling may occur earlier with percutaneous ASD closure.[13,14]

Percutaneous ASD closure also carries unique risks compared with surgical closure. These include an increased risk of atrial dysrhythmia caused by atrial inflammation and device embolization, both of which occur in the early postprocedure period.[15,16] Few embolized devices require surgical removal as they can be removed percutaneously. Device erosion is a rare but potentially serious complication with most occurring within 72 hours of device implantation.[17] The incidence of device erosion has significantly decreased recently due proper to device sizing.

Late Management Issues

All patients after ASD closure carry a significant dysrhythmic potential, including atrial tachyarrhythmia and bradyarrythmia, hence follow-up

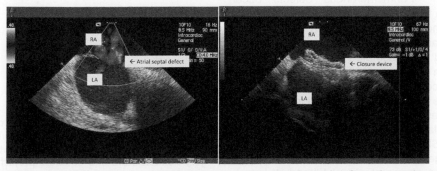

Fig. 2. Intracardiac echocardiogram of a patient with a secundum atrial septal defect who underwent percutaneous device closure. LA, left atrium; RA, right atrium.

should include regular electrocardiogram surveillance and event recording when indicated. This seems to be particularly true after surgical repair of ASDs in older individuals.[8,9] In addition, patients with increased pulmonary arterial pressure or ventricular dysfunction at time of repair should have regular follow-up with echocardiographic surveillance to monitor for signs of ongoing pulmonary arterial hypertension or worsening ventricular function, respectively. Insignificant residual ASDs are commonly seen after percutaneous closure with spontaneous resolution within 1 year. Larger residual defects are most commonly caused by surgical patch dehiscence and should be assessed for hemodynamic significance.

Pregnancy

Pregnancy is well tolerated in patients with repaired and unrepaired ASDs.[18] Close supervision is recommended for pregnant patients with unrepaired defects throughout pregnancy to identify dysrhythmia, paradoxic embolus, or heart failure in rare cases. Symptomatic secundum ASDs may be closed percutaneously during pregnancy. Women with significant pulmonary arterial hypertension should be advised against pregnancy because of high maternal and fetal risks.

VENTRICULAR SEPTAL DEFECT

The ventricular septum is made of several component septa originating from the muscular walls of the ventricle, the endocardial cushions, and the conus cordis. These fuse at the membranous septum under the septal leaflet of the tricuspid valve and separate the right and left ventricles. Abnormal fusion of these components or persistence of fetal myocardial channels (as is the case for defects in the muscular septum) gives rise to communications between the right and left ventricle, a VSD. VSDs are the most common congenital heart lesion encountered in children and account for more than 20% of all cardiac malformations.[19] Perimembranous defects occur adjacent to the membranous septum and are the most common type of significant VSD, accounting for more than 80% of all VSDs. Muscular VSDs are the second most common type and may occur singly or in multiples. Other types of VSDs are rare and occur in the outlet septum (common in Asians), the inlet septum (common in Down syndrome), or as a result of malalignment of the conal and muscular septa (as with tetralogy of Fallot). In addition, VSDs are commonly seen in concert with other congenital heart malformations. Although encountered commonly in childhood, the incidence of isolated VSDs seen in adults is less

common. Moderate or large VSDs may cause significant heart failure symptoms in infants and are therefore closed when clinically indicated in early life. Smaller VSDs have a high rate of spontaneous closure in childhood, although they may persist into adulthood if the indication for closure was not met (**Fig. 3**).

Pathophysiology

Flow across a VSD occurs in systole only, with the directionality and volume of the shunt related to comparative ventricular afterload. This is usually determined by differences in systemic vascular resistance and pulmonary vascular resistance, although restriction to flow may occur at the ventricular outflow tracts or VSD itself. In the normal heart, with an isolated large VSD, flow is unfettered and results in left-to-right shunting as a result of low pulmonary vascular resistance. Small VSDs may restrict significant flow across the defect despite a low pulmonary vascular resistance. In contrast, in a situation of increased pulmonary vascular resistance, shunting may be minimal if the pulmonary resistance is equivalent to systemic vascular resistance or may result in right-to-left shunting with suprasystemic pulmonary resistance regardless of defect size.

Left-to-right ventricular level shunting is at the expense of cardiac output. To compensate for this, left ventricular end-diastolic volume is increased so that the volume of blood ejected from the left ventricle meets systemic perfusion demands with a proportion of the ejection fraction shunted to the pulmonary vasculature. This leads

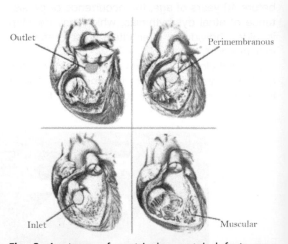

Fig. 3. Anatomy of ventricular septal defects seen from the right ventricle. (*Adapted from* Jacobs JP, Burke RP, Quintessenza JA, et al. Congenital heart surgery nomenclature and database project: ventricular septal defect. Ann Thorac Surg 2000;69(3 Supp 1):25–35; with permission.)

to significant left ventricular overload and may lead to left atrial hypertension, causing pulmonary venous congestion and resulting in symptomatic left heart failure with volume retention and dyspnea. In addition to shunt volume, hemodynamically significant VSDs also relate pressure from the left ventricle to the pulmonary vasculature. This occurs in the absence of pressure restriction at the right ventricular outflow tract or the VSD. This combination of a volume and pressure load on the pulmonary vasculature speeds the development of pulmonary vascular disease with subsequent Eisenmenger physiology.

Clinical Presentation

The natural history of VSDs is such that patients with hemodynamically significant VSDs present in infancy. As pulmonary vascular resistance decreases normally during the first few weeks of life, ventricular shunt flow worsens and infants manifest congestive heart failure symptoms with increased work of breathing and feeding intolerance with eventual failure to thrive.

Indications for Intervention

Although medical management strategies are used in efforts to allow somatic growth of the child to minimize surgical complications, the indication and timing of intervention is dictated by the severity of symptoms. Furthermore, closure is indicated with signs of left ventricular volume overload via echocardiography.

If no intervention is performed on a hemodynamically significant VSD and the infant survives, they will develop pulmonary vascular disease after the age of 2 years that will progress to Eisenmenger physiology with eventual right-to-left shunting through the ventricular defect. This is heralded by improvement in congestive heart failure symptoms as the pulmonary vascular resistance increases, which lessens left-to-right ventricular shunting. Closure of the VSD after Eisenmenger physiology is established is contraindicated because of excessive morbidity and mortality from right ventricular failure and impaired cardiac output.[20]

Inherently small ventricular shunts do not cause symptoms, and the infants grow and develop normally. Both perimembranous and muscular VSDs may become smaller over time, usually as a result of myocardial growth or restriction of shunt flow by an adjacent structure, such as a tricuspid valve septal leaflet. Small perimembranous and muscular VSDs may close spontaneously, whereas inlet and outlet VSDs do not become smaller and do not close spontaneously.

The natural history of significant VSDs is proved by the time a patient reaches adulthood, therefore there are few indications for intervention in adults. These patients will have pulmonary arterial hypertension and cyanosis with mortality and morbidity defined by their Eisenmenger physiology.[7] Adult patients with small hemodynamically insignificant VSDs require ongoing surveillance for the following special circumstances. Occasionally small VSDs (usually perimembranous and outlet types as they are adjacent to the left ventricular outflow tract) may cause deformation of an aortic valve leaflet with progressive aortic valve insufficiency. Closure of the VSD is indicated when the aortic insufficiency progresses beyond a mild degree.[21,22] Significant right ventricular outflow tract obstruction may be seen if a high velocity left-to-right shunt causes muscle bundle hypertrophy at the site of impact with the right ventricular myocardium (double-chambered right ventricle). The VSD in this case should be closed concurrently with a muscle bundle resection. Surgical closure should be considered if there is recurrent endocarditis believed to be caused by ventricular shunt flow.[23]

Surgical repair remains the gold standard for treating VSDs and is associated with excellent long-term survival with minimal complications when performed in childhood.[24] Furthermore, surgical closure of VSDs in adults is associated with low mortality and morbidity.[25] Although surgery is the treatment of choice for most types of VSDs, including perimembranous and inlet and outlet types, percutaneous VSD closure has gained prominence with certain hemodynamic states, particularly with apical muscular VSDs and spontaneous ventricular septal rupture after myocardial infarction.[26] First described in 1988 with subsequent development of a dedicated VSD occluder device, percutaneous VSD closure has a high rate of success although its regular use has been hampered by a high incidence (>10%) of postprocedural complications, including device embolization, hypotension, adjacent valve dysfunction, and conduction abnormalities.[27–30]

Late Management Issues

Adult patients with remote VSD closure may have a slightly decreased life expectancy, particularly if pulmonary hypertension is present after repair.[31] Conduction abnormalities may arise late after VSD repair, so regular electrocardiographic monitoring is necessary.[31] Residual defects may be present and are an indication for endocarditis prophylaxis; occasionally residual defects require repeat closure, therefore they should be assessed for hemodynamic significance. Patients with small VSDs should be monitored for aortic valve dysfunction and right ventricular outflow tract obstruction as described earlier. Eisenmenger physiology as a result of a large unrepaired VSD portends a poor prognosis.[32]

Pregnancy

Pregnancy is well tolerated in patients with re-paired VSDs and small to moderate VSDs.[18] Patients with hemodynamically important left-to-right ventricular shunts usually do not experience worsening of the shunt as systemic vascular resistance is decreased in pregnancy, although they should be monitored closely for signs of ventricular dysfunction or dysrhythmia. Eisenmenger physiology poses a significant risk of maternal and fetal mortality hence patients should be counseled against pregnancy.[33]

PATENT DUCTUS ARTERIOSUS

The PDA is a remnant of the fetal circulation and connects the pulmonary artery and the aorta. Critical in utero, the ductus arteriosus accepts the fetal cardiac output from the right ventricle, allowing bypass of the high-resistance pulmonary vascular bed. This flow is directed to the descending aorta and back to the placenta. Soon after birth, the PDA normally closes spontaneously, leaving a residual ligamentous structure. Persistence of the vessel (and its corresponding flow of blood) is considered a congenital malformation and is a direct connection between the pulmonary and systemic circulations. In the normal heart, a left-sided ductus arteriosus is associated with a left aortic arch. In more rare arrangements, such as a left ductus arteriosus and right aortic arch, formation of a vascular ring occurs. Presence of a PDA is common with other congenital heart lesions. Indeed, certain complex congenital lesions may rely on the PDA to support the pulmonary or systemic circulation soon after birth (ie, ductal-dependent pulmonary or systemic circulation, respectively) and patency of the ductus arteriosus is maintained with prostaglandin use until surgical palliation is performed. Isolated PDAs are discussed in the remainder of the article because they are the most common form seen in adults, with an incidence estimated at 1 in every 500 births (**Fig. 4**).[34]

Pathophysiology

As with the VSD, the magnitude and direction of the PDA shunt defines the subsequent hemodynamic effect and depends primarily on both the

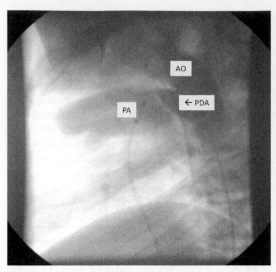

Fig. 4. Aortic angiogram in the lateral projection demonstrating a patent ductus arteriosus. AO, aorta; PA, pulmonary artery; PDA, patent ductus arteriosus.

size of the PDA as well as the relative difference between the pulmonary and systemic vascular resistance. In the setting of a hemodynamically significant PDA with low pulmonary vascular resistance, left-to-right shunting results in pulmonary overcirculation and left ventricular volume overload. This results in a left ventricular end-diastolic volume increase to augment cardiac output so that systemic perfusion is maintained despite shunt loss, which in turn causes left atrial hypertension, pulmonary venous congestion, and eventual left heart failure symptomatology. Like the VSD, a PDA may relate systemic pressure along with the volume load to the pulmonary vasculature, leading to the development of pulmonary vascular disease and pulmonary arterial hypertension. Eisenmenger physiology develops as pulmonary vascular resistance increases above systemic vascular resistance with a resultant right-to-left shunt. A distinction from a VSD is that a PDA is an extracardiac structure, hence its flow is not constrained by the cardiac cycle, allowing for a continuous flow of blood from the aorta to the pulmonary artery. With unrestrictive shunts, this continuation of diastolic flow may lower systemic diastolic blood pressure and compromise coronary or mesenteric perfusion. In additional, PDAs carry a known, although rare, risk of both endarteritis and aneurysm formation.

Clinical Presentation

The presentation of the PDA depends on the size of the shunt itself, which also informs management.[35] Silent PDAs and hemodynamically insignificant PDAs are not audible by physical examination and are diagnosed incidentally with cardiac imaging. Small PDAs are also clinically insignificant, although they are detected by the presence of a continuous cardiac murmur. Small PDAs are not associated with left ventricular overload or pulmonary hypertension. Rarely seen in adults, moderate PDAs are associated with prominent peripheral pulses as a result of low systemic diastolic pressure and produce a continuous cardiac murmur. Some degree of left ventricular dilation is present with varying degrees of increased pulmonary arterial pressure, which usually reverses with correction of the shunt. In the adult, large PDAs are associated with pulmonary hypertension and Eisenmenger physiology. Right-to-left ductal shunting may be evident with differential cyanosis (lower oxygen saturation in the lower extremities) and clubbing in the feet caused by the PDA connection to the aorta distal to the head and neck vessels.

Indications for Intervention

Although PDA presence alone does not meet the criteria for intervention when silent, endarteritis associated with a silent PDA should indicate closure. The small PDA detected on cardiac examination is routinely referred for closure because of the risk of endarteritis, albeit low. Hemodynamically significant PDAs associated with left heart volume loading and increased pulmonary arterial pressure in the setting of pulmonary vasoreactivity should also be referred for closure, although they warrant increased surveillance after the procedure to monitor for persistent pulmonary hypertension. Irreversible severe pulmonary hypertension is a contraindication to PDA closure and those patients should be referred for care by a pulmonary arterial hypertension specialist.[35]

Percutaneous PDA closure has largely supplanted surgical ligation and closure is achieved using a variety of devices.[36–38] Percutaneous closure should be planned for concurrently with a diagnostic cardiac catheterization. Closure is successful in 95% of patients at 1 year after device implantation.[37,38] Surgical closure is now routinely reserved for PDAs with unfavorable anatomy or those deemed too large to be closed percutaneously.[35]

Late Management Issues

Endocarditis prophylaxis is recommended for 6 months following PDA device closure. These patients may also benefit from infrequent periodic cardiology evaluation to monitor for recanalization of the duct. Persisting sequelae from a hemodynamically significant PDA, such as atrial fibrillation and ventricular dysfunction, should prompt regular cardiology follow-up. Patients with pulmonary arterial hypertension and Eisenmenger physiology have a poor prognosis and should be cared for in specialized centers.

Pregnancy

Pregnancy is well tolerated in patients with repaired and unrepaired PDAs, although patients with hemodynamically significant PDAs may find that left heart failure symptoms or atrial dysrhythmia are exacerbated by the later stages of pregnancy. Pregnancy in women with pulmonary arterial hypertension and/or Eisenmenger physiology is not advised because of high maternal and fetal mortality.[33]

REFERENCES

1. van der Linde D, Konings EM, Slager MA, et al. Birth prevalence of congenital heart disease worldwide: a systematic review and meta-analysis. J Am Coll Cardiol 2011;58(21):2241–7.
2. Lindsey JB, Hillis LD. Clinical update: atrial septal defects in adults. Lancet 2007;133:229–34.
3. Booth DC, Wisenbaugh T, Smith M, et al. Left ventricular distensibility and passive elastic stiffness in atrial septal defect. J Am Coll Cardiol 1988;12:1231–6.
4. Steele PM, Fuster V, Cohen M, et al. Isolated atrial septal defect with pulmonary vascular obstructive disease—long-term follow-up and prediction of outcome after surgical correction. Circulation 1987; 76:1037–42.
5. Vogel M, Berger F, Kramer A, et al. Incidence of secondary pulmonary hypertension in adults with atrial septal or sinus venosus defects. Heart 1999;82:30–3.
6. Engelfriet PM, Duffels MG, Moller T, et al. Pulmonary arterial hypertension in adults born with a heart septal defect: the Euro Heart Survey on adult congenital heart disease. Heart 2007;93:682–7.
7. Warnes CA, Williams RG, Bashore TM, et al. ACC/AHA 2008 guidelines for the management of adults with congenital heart disease: executive summary: a report of the American College of Cardiology/American Heart Association Task Force on Practice Guidelines (writing committee to develop guidelines for the management of adults with congenital heart disease). Circulation 2008;118(23):2395–451.
8. Murphy JG, Gersh BJ, McGoon MD, et al. Long-term outcome after surgical repair of isolated atrial septal defect: follow-up at 27–32 years. N Engl J Med 1990;323:1645–50.
9. Gatzoulis MA, Freeman MA, Siu SC, et al. Atrial arrhythmia after surgical closure of atrial septal defects in adults. N Engl J Med 1999;340:839–46.

10. Du ZD, Hijazi ZM, Kleinman CS, et al. Comparison between transcatheter and surgical closure of secundum atrial septal defect in children and adults: results of a multicenter nonrandomized trial. J Am Coll Cardiol 2002;39:1836–44.

11. Attie F, Rosas M, Granados N, et al. Surgical treatment for secundum atrial septal defects in patients >40 years old: a randomized clinical trial. J Am Coll Cardiol 2001;38:2035–42.

12. Brochu MC, Baril JF, Dore A, et al. Improvement in exercise capacity in asymptomatic and mildly symptomatic adults after atrial septal defect percutaneous closure. Circulation 2002;106: 1821–6.

13. Veldtman GR, Razack V, Siu S, et al. Right ventricular form and function after percutaneous atrial septal defect device closure. J Am Coll Cardiol 2001;37: 2108–13.

14. Salehian O, Horlick E, Schwerzmann M, et al. Improvements in cardiac form and function after transcatheter closure of secundum atrial septal defects. J Am Coll Cardiol 2005;45:499–504.

15. Spies C, Khandelwal A, Timmermanns I, et al. Incidence of atrial fibrillation following transcatheter closure of atrial septal defects in adults. Am J Cardiol 2008;102:902–6.

16. Levi DS, Moore JW. Embolization and retrieval of the Amplatzer septal occluder. Catheter Cardiovasc Interv 2004;61:543–7.

17. Amin Z, Hijazi ZM, Bass JL. Erosion of Amplatzer septal occluder device after closure of secundum atrial septal defects: review of registry of complications and recommendations to minimize future risk. Catheter Cardiovasc Interv 2004;63:496–502.

18. Uebing A, Steer PJ, Yentis SM, et al. Pregnancy and congenital heart disease. BMJ 2006;332:401–6.

19. Hoffman JI, Kaplan S. The incidence of congenital heart disease. J Am Coll Cardiol 2002;39(12):1890–900.

20. Fuster V, Brandenberg RO, McGoon DC, et al. Clinical approach and management of congenital heart disease in the adolescent and adult. Cardiovasc Clin 1980;10:161–97.

21. Moreno-Cabral RJ, Mamiya RT, Nakamura FF, et al. Ventricular septal defects and aortic insufficiency. Surgical treatment. J Thorac Cardiovasc Surg 1977;73:358–65.

22. Trusler GA, Williams WG, Smallhorn JF, et al. Late results after repair of aortic insufficiency associated with ventricular septal defect. J Thorac Cardiovasc Surg 1992;103:276–81.

23. Li W, Somerville J. Infective endocarditis in the grown up congenital heart (GUCH) population. Eur Heart J 1998;19:166–73.

24. Meijboom F, Szatmari A, Utens E, et al. Long-term follow-up after surgical closure of ventricular septal defect in infancy and childhood. J Am Coll Cardiol 1994;24(5):1358–64.

25. Mongeon FP, Burkhart HM, Ammash NM, et al. Indications and outcomes of surgical closure of ventricular septal defect in adults. JACC Cardiovasc Interv 2010;3(3):290–7.

26. Landzberg MJ, Lock JE. Transcatheter management of ventricular septal rupture after myocardial infarction. Semin Thorac Cardiovasc Surg 1998;10(2):128–32.

27. Lock JE, Block PC, McKay RG, et al. Transcatheter closure of ventricular septal defects. Circulation 1988;78:361–8.

28. Hijazi ZM, Hakim F, Haweleh A, et al. Catheter closure of perimembranous ventricular septal defects using the new Amplatzer membranous VSD occluder: initial clinical experience. Catheter Cardiovasc Interv 2002;56:508–15.

29. Holzer R, Balzer D, Cao QL, et al, Amplatzer Muscular Ventricular Septal Defect Investigators. Device closure of muscular ventricular septal defects using the Amplatzer muscular ventricular septal defect occluder: immediate and mid-term results of a U.S. registry. J Am Coll Cardiol 2004;43(7):1257–63.

30. Butera G, Carminati M, Chessa M, et al. Transcatheter closure of perimembranous ventricular septal defects: early and long-term results. J Am Coll Cardiol 2007;50(12):1189–95.

31. Roos-Hesselink JW, Meijboom FJ, Spitaels SE, et al. Outcome of patients after surgical closure of ventricular septal defect at young age: longitudinal follow-up of 22–34 years. Eur Heart J 2004; 25(12):1057–62.

32. Kidd L, Driscoll DJ, Gersony WM, et al. Second natural history study of congenital heart defects. Results of treatment of patients with ventricular septal defects. Circulation 1993;87(2 Suppl I):I38–151.

33. Daliento L, Somerville J, Presbitero P, et al. Eisenmenger syndrome. Factors relating to deterioration and death. Eur Heart J 1998;19(12):1845–55.

34. Lloyd TR, Beekman RH III. Clinically silent patent ductus arteriosus [Letter]. Am Heart J 1994;127:1664–5.

35. Silversides CK, Dore A, Poirier N, et al. Canadian Cardiovascular Society 2009 Consensus Conference on the management of adults with congenital heart disease: shunt lesions. Can J Cardiol 2010; 26(3):e70–9.

36. Cambier PA, Kirby WC, Wortham DC, et al. Percutaneous closure of small (<2.5 mm) patent ductus arteriosus using coil embolization. Am J Cardiol 1992; 69:815–8.

37. Masura J, Walsh KP, Thanopoulos B, et al. Catheter closure of moderate- to large-sized patent ductus arteriosus using the new Amplatzer duct occluder: immediate and short-term results. J Am Coll Cardiol 1998;31:878–82.

38. Faella HJ, Hijazi ZM. Closure of the patent ductus arteriosus with the Amplatzer PDA device: immediate results of the international clinical trial. Catheter Cardiovasc Interv 2000;51:50–4.

Coarctation of the Aorta
Strategies for Improving Outcomes

Lan Nguyen, MD[a], Stephen C. Cook, MD[b],*

KEYWORDS

- Congenital heart disease • Aortic coarctation • Bicuspid aortic valve • Cardiac surgery • Stent
- Aneurysm • Aorta • Treatment outcome

KEY POINTS

- Coarctation of the aorta is defined by a discrete narrowing of the aorta.
- Transcatheter systolic coarctation gradient ≥20 mm Hg is an indication for intervention with treatment choice guided by patient age and anatomy of obstruction.
- Follow-up imaging should be tailored to early identification of recoarctation/aneurysm with directed intervention.
- Hypertension is common in the aging patient with coarctation despite successful repair.
- Lifelong routine evaluation by cardiology specialists with expertise in adult congenital heart disease is required to identify late-onset complications.

INTRODUCTION

Coarctation of the aorta (CoA) is a common congenital heart defect (CHD) found in approximately 1 per 2900 live births[1–3] and is the seventh most common type of CHD.[4] Still, this is likely an underestimate, because the diagnosis may be delayed, even in the pediatric population.[4,5] In simple terms, coarctation is characterized by discrete narrowing of the thoracic aorta adjacent to the ligamentum arteriosum. Importantly, discrete coarctation is an aortopathy that lies within a spectrum of arch abnormalities ranging from discrete narrowing to a long segment of arch hypoplasia. The prognosis of untreated coarctation was extremely poor during the presurgical era with median survival age of 31 years and a quarter of patients dying before the age of 20 years.[6] Since the first surgical repair of aortic coarctation performed in the 1940s, treatment of coarctation has dramatically changed. Overall, survival into adulthood is now expected. However, these patients continue to require lifelong follow-up for management of associated problems including arterial hypertension, atherosclerotic disease, recoarctation, and aneurysm formation.

CAUSE AND PATHOGENESIS OF COARCTATION

Histologic examination of localized aortic coarctation lesions has demonstrated the presence of a tissue ridge extending from the posterior aortic wall and protruding into aortic lumen. This ridge consists of ductal tissue with in-folding of the aortic media.[6] In older patients, aortic intimal proliferation also contributes to the narrowing at the site of coarctation.[7] The cause of discrete aortic coarctation remains unclear, but is likely multifactorial. Prenatal environmental exposures have been associated with CoA and other left-sided lesions.[8] However, there is a growing body of literature that suggests a genetic basis for development of these lesions. Case series have described

The authors have nothing to disclose.
a Department of Cardiovascular Medicine, Heart and Vascular Institute, University of Pittsburgh, Scaife Hall S560.1, 200 Lothrop Street, Pittsburgh, PA 15213, USA; b Department of Pediatrics, The Adult Congenital Heart Disease Center, Heart Institute Children's Hospital of Pittsburgh of UPMC, 4401 Penn Avenue, Pittsburgh, PA 15224, USA
* Corresponding author.
E-mail address: stephen.cook@chp.edu

Cardiol Clin 33 (2015) 521–530
http://dx.doi.org/10.1016/j.ccl.2015.07.011
0733-8651/15/$ – see front matter © 2015 Elsevier Inc. All rights reserved.

clustering of coarctation cases in families. Evaluation of families with an index case of left ventricular outflow tract abnormalities of aortic valve stenosis, CoA, or hypoplastic left heart syndrome suggest a strong genetic influence, with an estimated sibling recurrence risk of greater than 30-fold.[9] Recently, mutations in the NOTCH1 gene have been identified in individuals with left ventricular outflow tract malformation, including coarctation.[10] In particular, the NOTCH1 variant R1279H seems to be more common in individuals with aortic coarctation.[11] NOTCH1 mutations have also been shown to contribute to abnormal epithelial-to-mesenchymal transition in endothelial cells, which is an important step in the development of the left ventricular outflow tract. Mechanical models have suggested that abnormalities of blood flow, defective endothelial cell migration, and excessive deposition of aortic duct tissue at the aortic isthmus can result in coarctation. Furthermore, embryonic studies in zebrafish have highlighted the importance of intracardiac hemodynamics in epigenetic control of distal chamber development.[12]

ASSOCIATED CONGENITAL HEART LESIONS

Although CoA can be an isolated CHD, it is also commonly found in other congenital syndromes and cardiovascular anomalies. Thus, deliberate investigation for the presence of coarctation should be made in these patients. The most common cardiovascular malformation associated with CoA is bicuspid aortic valve (BAV). Prior autopsy examination showed 46% of patients with CoA have congenital BAV.[13] More modern studies in patients with repaired coarctation found similar results with up to 45% to 62% prevalence of BAV.[14–16] The coincidence of BAV and CoA is difficult to determine, because BAV is very common and not everyone is screened for the presence of coarctation. In a study of 102 patients with BAV diagnosed by computed tomography (CT) imaging, 22% of patients either had prior coarctation repair, or were found to have CoA.[17] The coexistence of BAV and coarctation is important to consider, because it places the patient at a higher risk of aortic complications.[18] In a study following 341 patients with BAV over a median of 7 years, patients with bicuspid valve in the presence of coarctation had 7.5 times increased risk of ascending aortic complications, most commonly dilation of the ascending aorta.[19] The same group also found that among patients with aortic coarctation, the presence of a BAV was an independent risk factor for the development of aortic wall complications.[16]

Turner syndrome has a strong association with CoA. In a study of 132 girls diagnosed with aortic coarctation who subsequently underwent karyotyping, Turner syndrome was diagnosed in 5.3%.[20] CoA is found in 18% of patients with Turner syndrome.[21] Williams syndrome, a congenital and multisystem genetic disorder, has been associated with supravalvular aortic stenosis. Aortic arch abnormalities, including coarctation, are present in 10% of patients with Williams syndrome.[22] Coarctation can also be present in congenital cardiovascular anomalies involving multiple left-sided lesions, including Shone syndrome and hypoplastic left heart syndrome.

NONCARDIAC ASSOCIATIONS

The link between intracranial aneurysms and CoA was described well before the surgical era, accounting for 5% deaths in patients with aortic coarctation on autopsy review.[23] In the modern era, with the availability of brain MRI the reported prevalence of intracranial aneurysms in patients with CoA is approximately 10%,[24] which is five times more common than the average population (**Fig. 1**). In one study, hypertension was more common in the population of coarctation patients with

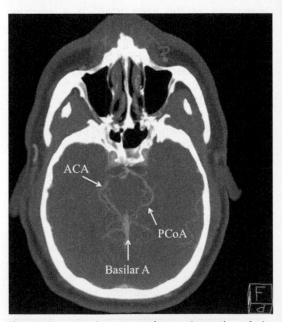

Fig. 1. Computed tomography angiography of the head showing normal anatomy of the circle of Willis without cerebral artery aneurysm in a 36 year old with coarctation of the aorta. Given that hypertension may play a role in the growth of intracranial aneurysm, these patients should be monitored and treated if indicated. ACA, anterior cerebral artery; basilar A, basilar artery; PCoA, posterior communicating artery.

intracranial aneurysms.[24] Most of the aneurysms described are small, and therefore have a low risk of spontaneous rupture. Currently the benefits of routine screening for intracranial aneurysms in coarctation remain unclear.

CLINICAL PRESENTATION

The clinical presentation of coarctation differs significantly in pediatric patients in comparison with adults. Although infants with severe coarctation may present with signs and symptoms of heart failure and cardiogenic shock as the ductus closes, most adults with unrepaired coarctation are generally asymptomatic. A common presentation of coarctation is systemic arterial hypertension. In young adults presenting with severe upper extremity hypertension, coarctation should be excluded. Patients presenting with severe hypertension may experience symptoms including angina, headache, epistaxis, and heart failure.

On physical examination, femoral arterial pulses are diminished and usually delayed. Rarely, claudication may be reported because of lower extremity ischemia. Auscultation of the left sternal border may demonstrate a harsh systolic murmur with radiation to the back. An associated thrill may be palpable in the suprasternal notch. If left ventricular pressure or volume overload have developed, a left ventricular lift can be present. The finding of a continuous murmur may suggest the presence of arterial collaterals in those with long-standing unrepaired significant coarctation.[25] Arterial pulsations from collaterals to the intercostal and interscapular arteries can also be palpated. In patients with suspected coarctation, it is important to assess for systolic blood pressure discrepancy between upper and lower extremities. The upper extremity systolic blood pressure is usually 20 mm Hg higher than the lower extremities in patients with significant coarctation. In rare instances of coarctation patients with concomitant anomalous subclavian artery origin distal to the coarctation, systolic blood

pressure differences may not be detected between ipsilateral arm and legs.[25] Therefore, complete evaluation should involve measurement of blood pressure in all four extremities.

DIAGNOSTIC EVALUATION

The electrocardiogram of a patient with coarctation may be normal or demonstrate evidence of left ventricular hypertrophy from chronic left ventricular pressure overload. On chest radiograph, a "figure of three" sign formed by the aortic nob, the stenotic segment, and the dilated poststenotic segment of the aorta suggests CoA. The heart border can be normal or mildly enlarged. Inferior rib notching can also be seen in the third to eighth ribs bilaterally caused by the presence of dilated intercostal collateral arteries.

Among the noninvasive modalities to evaluate CoA, transthoracic echocardiography is the most accessible for the practicing physician. A comprehensive echocardiogram is recommended in the initial evaluation of a patient with repaired or suspected CoA. In addition to characterization of the coarctation itself, it is important to evaluate for evidence of left ventricular pressure or volume overload, left ventricular hypertrophy, size, and left ventricular systolic and diastolic dysfunction. Particular attention should be placed in identifying associated cardiac defects especially left-sided lesions. The morphology of the aortic valve, and evidence of subvalvular, valvular, and supravalvular aortic stenosis should be interrogated. The dimensions of the aortic root and ascending aorta can be followed serially to assess for associated aortopathy. Suprasternal windows are important to view the aortic arch from the long-axis view, in two-dimensional imaging and by color flow Doppler. Visualization of the aortic arch in the long axis may demonstrate a focal area of narrowing of the thoracic aorta distal to the takeoff of the left subclavian artery with associated flow turbulence on color flow Doppler (**Figs. 2** and **3**).

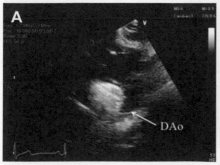 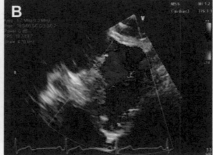

Fig. 2. Suprasternal notch view in a 50-year-old woman with known bicuspid aortic valve demonstrating narrowing of the proximal descending aorta (*A, arrow*) aided by color Doppler interrogation (*B*). DAo, descending aorta.

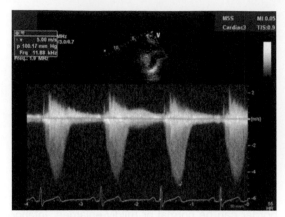

Fig. 3. Spectral Doppler interrogation demonstrates severe arch obstruction.

Doppler interrogation shows increased velocity across the site of coarctation. Typically, the modified Bernoulli equation can be used to calculate the peak instantaneous gradient across the coarctation. However, because patients with CoA may have multiple left-sided lesions (eg, stenotic, BAV, subaortic membrane) leading to an increased velocity before the CoA site, the expanded Bernoulli equation should be used to avoid overestimation of the peak gradient. Yet with long-standing coarctation, significant collaterals may have developed thereby reducing the peak systolic gradient across the site of stenosis. A saw-tooth pattern seen on continuous-wave Doppler reflects the persistent forward flow in

diastole because of diastolic run-off. Higher gradient across the coarctation and longer duration of diastolic forward flow in the thoracic aorta suggest more significant coarctation. Similarly, Doppler examination of the abdominal descending aorta provides useful information in the presence of significant coarctation. Here, Doppler demonstrates a continuous antegrade flow signal without evidence of flow reversal.

CARDIAC MRI

Cardiac MRI (cMRI) has become a valuable noninvasive modality to assess patients with unrepaired and repaired coarctation. In adults with suboptimal echocardiographic imaging window, cMRI can be used to characterize the aortic valve, aortic root, left ventricular size, and function. cMRI, along with gadolinium-enhanced magnetic resonance angiography, provides excellent resolution of cardiac anatomy and vascular structures (**Fig. 4**). Additionally, phase contrast flow analysis can be used to estimate flow and peak gradient through the coarctation.[26] Compared with echocardiography, cMRI demonstrates superior visualization of the aortic arch with precise characterization of the location and extent of coarctation, and assessment of the presence and extent of collateral vessels (**Fig. 5**). In the unrepaired patient, the measured minimum aortic cross-sectional area and heart rate–corrected deceleration time in the descending aorta can be used to predict a significant gradient by cardiac catheterization[27] and

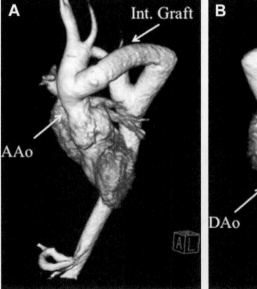
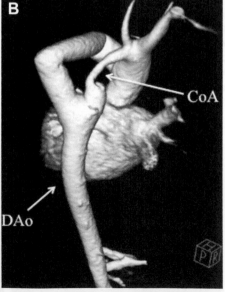

Fig. 4. Volume-rendered magnetic resonance angiographic reconstruction (*A*, anterior; *B*, posterior view) in a 35-year-old patient with coarctation of the aorta who underwent surgical repair with an interposition graft. AAo, ascending aorta; Int. Graft, interposition graft.

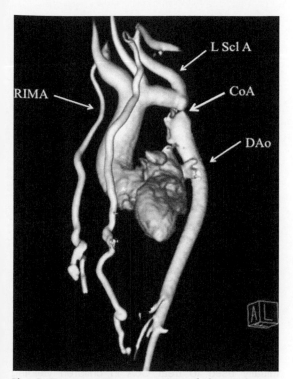

Fig. 5. Severe, native coarctation of the aorta in a 51-year-old patient presenting with severe hypertension refractory to antihypertensive therapy identified by contrast-enhanced magnetic resonance angiography. Dilated left and right internal mammary arteries suggest collateral circulation. L Scl A, left subclavian artery; RIMA, right internal mammary artery.

future need for intervention.[28] Compared with conventional echocardiography, cMRI provides exceptional visualization of the aortic arch and detection of postrepair complications including arch "kinking" and pseudoaneurysm.[29] Thoracic aortic magnetic resonance angiography also provides assessment of poststenotic dilation or aneurysmal formation at the site of a previous repair. Importantly, the lack of ionizing radiation provides an advantage of cMRI over CT, in the serial evaluation of late complications after repair. Recognizing the benefits of advanced cMRI and CT the 2008 American College of Cardiology/American Heart Association Guidelines for the Management of Adults with Congenital Heart Disease recommend that patients with coarctation have serial evaluation with CT or MRI at least every 5 years.

COMPUTED TOMOGRAPHY

Although cMRI is the preferred mode of serial follow-up for patients after coarctation repair, the use of cardiovascular CT may be considered in selected patients. In particular, cMRI in patients with transcatheter stents may have susceptibility artifact precluding accurate assessment of late complications associated with these interventions. With cMRI, metallic artifact can lead to difficulty in the assessment of vessel lumen patency, identifying restenosis, aneurysm, or stent fracture.[30] Use of CT obviates concerns about metallic artifact impairing accurate assessment (**Fig. 6**). Other advantages of cardiac CT over cMRI include improved image resolution, shorter scan time, and greater availability across different institutions. CT angiography is also used to assess concomitant coronary anomalies that may not be well visualized with cMRI. Patients with pacemakers or implantable cardioverter defibrillators that are not cMRI compatible may benefit from surveillance with cardiovascular CT. Similar to cMRI, cardiovascular CT can be performed to follow serial aortic dimensions. Small studies of patients postcoarctation repair have shown good correlation of aortic diameter

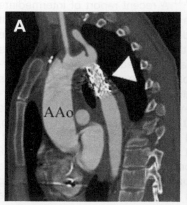
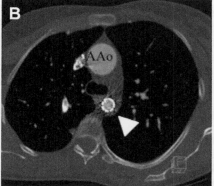
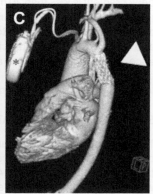

Fig. 6. (A–C) Computed tomography angiography of the aorta in the sagittal and axial planes demonstrates no evidence of in-stent stenosis (*arrowheads*) in a 38-year-old patient with history of native coarctation presenting after sudden cardiac arrest. Three-dimensional reconstruction displaying previously placed implantable cardioverter defibrillator (*asterisk*) and luminal surface of the Cheatham-Platinum covered stent.

measurements between helical CT and MRI. Still, considerable variations in measurements between these two modalities have been reported in the same patient, highlighting the importance of using one specific modality in serial assessment.[31] When using cardiovascular CT to assess the patient with repaired coarctation, adhering to radiation safety principles (as low as reasonably achievable) and minimizing radiation dose should be a regulatory requirement for all programs.

CARDIAC CATHETERIZATION

Cardiac catheterization remains essential in the management of patients with coarctation. However, because of recent advances in noninvasive imaging with cMRI and cardiovascular CT, cardiac catheterization is used more frequently in the setting of intervention than diagnosis. In those patients who are not suitable for transcatheter intervention, cardiac catheterization is performed to accurately assess the coarctation gradient, which is integral to determine need for intervention. In older patients with potential concomitant coronary artery disease (CAD) who require operative intervention for coarctation or aneurysm, coronary angiography should be performed before surgery.

INDICATIONS FOR INTERVENTION

In patients with a native CoA or recoarctation, a measured peak-to-peak gradient greater than or equal to 20 mm Hg by cardiac catheterization is an indication for intervention, either by transcatheter or surgical approach.[32] Patients with longstanding native coarctation who have developed significant collateral flow over time may have a lower measured gradient despite severe coarctation. Therefore, patients with extensive collaterals should undergo intervention even if the peak-to-peak gradient is less than 20 mm Hg.[32] The decision regarding transcatheter versus surgical intervention depends on a variety of factors including location and complexity of the coarctation, patient preference, and the availability of an interventionalist or cardiac surgeon capable of performing the intervention with a low rate of complication.

SURGICAL AND TRANSCATHETER THERAPIES

There have been major advances in the treatment of CoA since the first successful surgical repair by Craaford and Nylan in 1944. This was performed with resection of the narrowed segment and reattachment of the transected ends using a circumferential suture line or an end-to-end anastomosis.[33] This remains the most common type of surgical repair for children with critical coarctation.

The subclavian flap repair was introduced in the 1960s[34] as an alternative to the end-to-end anastomosis to avoid the circumferential sutures, and reducing the risk of future restenosis. Nonetheless, the rates of restenosis are similar between the two techniques,[35] because the subclavian flap technique leaves behind residual abnormal ductal and coarctation tissue.[34] The synthetic patch aortoplasty approach became popular when first introduced in the 1970s. This approach has since fallen out of favor because of high occurrence of late-term aneurysm formation.[36] Patients with a long segment of coarctation or arch hypoplasia not amenable to resection with an end-to-end anastomosis may require use of an interposition graft or extended end-to-end anastomosis.

In addition to the variety of surgical repairs for coarctation, transcatheter options are now available and are especially useful for adult patients with native coarctation or restenosis of a previous surgical repair. Transcatheter management is now preferred over surgical management in adult patients with discrete coarctation without associated arch hypoplasia.[37] Balloon angioplasty was initially used to treat CoA in children yielding acceptable results in reduction of aortic coarctation gradient.[38] However, midterm follow-up of these patients demonstrated a high rate of restenosis (>20%),[38] likely caused by elastic recoil of the aortic wall. Furthermore, acute complications have been described with balloon angioplasty[39] and subsequent aneurysm development.[40] Currently, balloon angioplasty alone is not recommended for treatment of significant aortic coarctation in adults. Instead, the treatment of choice to treat discrete aortic coarctation involves the use of intravascular stents. This can now be safely performed with a lower rate of complication and restenosis when compared with balloon angioplasty alone.[39,41] A recent report of intermediate outcomes from the Coarctation of the Aorta Stent Trial (COAST) demonstrated that placement of the Cheatham–Platinum bare-metal stent in patients older than the age of 8 years with native or recurrent coarctation can be performed in patients with appropriate anatomy for transcatheter intervention. At 2-year follow-up, 13% of patients required repeat catheterization for stent redilation, but none had need for surgical management. Although stent fractures were observed in 22% of patients, none had significant clinical adverse events. Development of aortic wall injury during catheterization or subsequent aneurysm at the site of stent placement was seen in 9% of patients who subsequently underwent placement of a covered stent.[42] Overall, the results are promising and suggest that transcatheter treatment of coarctation can be offered to adult patients with unrepaired CoA and recoarctation.

LONG-TERM COMPLICATIONS

Despite advancements in the treatment of CoA, patients remain at risk for a variety of long-term complications. Patients who have undergone coarctation repair are at a higher risk of death compared with the general population.[43] In one of the largest single-center studies of postsurgical coarctation repair, survivorship was 84% at 20 years and 72% at 30 years follow-up.[44] The most common mode of death was CAD, accounting for 37% of late deaths. Sudden death and heart failure were the next common causes of death in this population. Although early studies suggest an increased prevalence of death caused by CAD,[44] a more recent study demonstrated that coarctation in itself was not an independent risk factor for the development of premature CAD.[45] Cardiac risk factors predisposing to CAD were the same in those with CoA and the general population. These results suggest targeting traditional risk factors rather than untreatable vascular reactivity defects may lead to improved clinical outcomes in this population.

Patients with other cardiac defects in addition to CoA tend to have worse outcomes.[46] Reoperation in patients who have undergone primary repair is often related to associated cardiac defects rather than a direct complication from coarctation repair.[44,47] Aortic valve disease is the most common associated defect requiring surgical management in patients with coarctation who have undergone prior repair.

RECOARCTATION AND ANEURYSM DEVELOPMENT

Patients with repaired coarctation are at risk of late recoarctation and aneurysm development. The rate of recoarctation after surgical repair ranges between 3% and 15% in most studies.[34,44,48] Younger age at the time of surgery is associated with a higher risk of restenosis.[44,48,49] Although earlier studies suggest a high rate of restenosis in patients with end-to-end anastomosis, current reports suggest that an end-to-end anastomosis is comparable with other types of surgical repair.[50] It is difficult to compare long-term outcomes among various types of surgical repair because complication rates are also determined by patient's age at repair and the surgical experience of the operator.

The rate of aneurysm formation has been reported to be between 3% and 20%[44,49,51] in long-term studies of patients who have undergone coarctation repair. Patients repaired with synthetic patch technique are at higher risk of late-term aneurysm development.[52] With the development of cMRI, the prevalence of aneurysm identified by surveillance imaging approaches 46%[36] (Fig. 7). Patients with large aneurysm after coarctation repair often require surgical management with use of an interposition graft.[53] However, there have been several small case series of successful treatment of aneurysm using bare-metal and covered endovascular stents.[54–57] Long-term studies are needed to determine the safety and durability of interventional repairs. Currently, COAST II aims to evaluate the efficacy and safety of covered endovascular stents for treatment of coarctation with associated aortic wall injury, including aortic aneurysm and pseudoaneurysm.

MEDICAL MANAGEMENT OF SYSTOLIC ARTERIAL HYPERTENSION

Despite excellent early to midterm outcomes of adults with CoA, long-term morbidity remains, especially with respect to premature arterial hypertension. Numerous studies have demonstrated

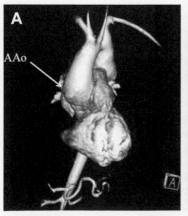
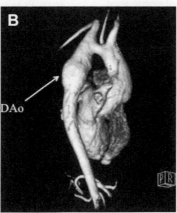

Fig. 7. Volume-rendered magnetic resonance angiographic reconstruction revealing ascending (*A, arrow*) and proximal descending aortic (*B, arrow*) aneurysms in a 25-year-old patient who underwent prior patch repair.

that hypertension is prevalent in patients with coarctation. Two studies by Wells and co-workers[58] and Bhat and colleagues[59] sought to evaluate the effect of coarctation repair on systolic blood pressure. In these studies, all patients had hypertension characterized by a systolic blood pressure greater than 140 mm Hg. Following coarctation repair, there was an improvement in systolic blood pressure in all patients and concomitant decrease in the use of antihypertensive medications. Still, systemic arterial hypertension remains in some patients despite coarctation repair. The prevalence of systemic arterial hypertension following coarctation repair ranges from 25% to 68%.[60] The mechanism of late-onset hypertension in repaired coarctation is unclear, although some have implicated the role of abnormal vascular compliance or impaired baroreceptor sensitivity.[60] Factors associated with higher prevalence of late hypertension include older age at time of repair[44] and older age at time of follow-up.[61] Children who underwent subclavian flap repair were found to have higher systolic blood pressure than those who underwent end-to-end anastomosis. Yet, it is unclear whether this trend continues into adulthood.[62]

There are limited data on the efficacy of different classes of antihypertensive medications in hypertensive patients after coarctation repair. A study of 128 young-adult patients with hypertension after coarctation repair reported better control of hypertension with candesartan over metoprolol with fewer side effects.[63] However, in a small crossover study of 18 adult patients, metoprolol was found to be more effective than candesartan at lowering systolic blood pressure.[64] The 2008 American College of Cardiology/American Heart Association Guidelines for the Management of Adults with Congenital Heart Disease recommend use of a β-blocker, angiotensin-converting enzyme inhibitor, or angiotensin II receptor blocker as first-line therapy, with a preference of one agent over another dependent on the presence of aortic root dilation or aortic regurgitation.[32]

SUMMARY

Patients with CoA who have undergone repair require lifelong surveillance. Because this type of CHD is associated with many long-term complications, collaborative management by cardiologists with expertise in adult CHD is recommended. Current guidelines on the management of adults with CHD recommend at least annual follow-up of patients after coarctation repair[32] to identify long-term complications including restenosis, aortic aneurysm, and systolic arterial hypertension. In

those patients with CoA with associated congenital cardiac defects, additional surveillance is required to identify late-onset complications specific to associated defects that may require additional medical and surgical therapies. Although echocardiography is a fundamental tool in the assessment of patients after coarctation repair, advanced imaging is often necessary for comprehensive evaluation. cMRI is the preferred imaging modality for repaired and unrepaired CoA. Alternatively, cardiovascular CT is best suited to evaluate patients with endovascular stents or those with contraindications to cMRI. Ultimately, multicenter research is needed to determine optimal mode of intervention, medical therapies, safety and efficacy of transcatheter-based therapies, and long-term outcomes in this growing patient population.

REFERENCES

1. Samanek M, Slavik Z, Zborilova B, et al. Prevalence, treatment, and outcome of heart disease in live-born children: a prospective analysis of 91,823 live-born children. Pediatr Cardiol 1989;10(4):205–11.
2. Grech V. Diagnostic and surgical trends, and epidemiology of coarctation of the aorta in a population-based study. Int J Cardiol 1999;68(2):197–202.
3. van der Linde D, Konings EE, Slager MA, et al. Birth prevalence of congenital heart disease worldwide: a systematic review and meta-analysis. J Am Coll Cardiol 2011;58(21):2241–7.
4. Hoffman JI, Kaplan S. The incidence of congenital heart disease. J Am Coll Cardiol 2002;39(12):1890–900.
5. Strafford MA, Griffiths SP, Gersony WM. Coarctation of the aorta: a study in delayed detection. Pediatrics 1982;69(2):159–63.
6. Campbell M. Natural history of coarctation of the aorta. Br Heart J 1970;32(5):633–40.
7. Elzenga NJ, Gittenberger-de Groot AC. Localised coarctation of the aorta. An age dependent spectrum. Br Heart J 1983;49(4):317–23.
8. Tikkanen J, Heinonen OP. Risk factors for coarctation of the aorta. Teratology 1993;47(6):565–72.
9. McBride KL, Pignatelli R, Lewin M, et al. Inheritance analysis of congenital left ventricular outflow tract obstruction malformations: segregation, multiplex relative risk, and heritability. Am J Med Genet A 2005;134A(2):180–6.
10. McBride KL, Riley MF, Zender GA, et al. NOTCH1 mutations in individuals with left ventricular outflow tract malformations reduce ligand-induced signaling. Hum Mol Genet 2008;17(18):2886–93.
11. Freylikhman O, Tatarinova T, Smolina N, et al. Variants in the NOTCH1 gene in patients with aortic coarctation. Congenit Heart Dis 2014;9(5):391–6.

12. Hove JR, Koster RW, Forouhar AS, et al. Intracardiac fluid forces are an essential epigenetic factor for embryonic cardiogenesis. Nature 2003;421(6919):172–7.

13. Becker AE, Becker MJ, Edwards JE. Anomalies associated with coarctation of aorta: particular reference to infancy. Circulation 1970;41(6):1067–75.

14. Roos-Hesselink JW, Scholzel BE, Heijdra RJ, et al. Aortic valve and aortic arch pathology after coarctation repair. Heart 2003;89(9):1074–7.

15. Kappetein AP, Gittenberger-de Groot AC, Zwinderman AH, et al. The neural crest as a possible pathogenetic factor in coarctation of the aorta and bicuspid aortic valve. J Thorac Cardiovasc Surg 1991;102(6):830–6.

16. Oliver JM, Gallego P, Gonzalez A, et al. Risk factors for aortic complications in adults with coarctation of the aorta. J Am Coll Cardiol 2004;44(8):1641–7.

17. Michalowska IM, Kruk M, Kwiatek P, et al. Aortic pathology in patients with bicuspid aortic valve assessed with computed tomography angiography. J Thorac Imaging 2014;29(2):113–7.

18. Braverman AC, Guven H, Beardslee MA, et al. The bicuspid aortic valve. Curr Probl Cardiol 2005; 30(9):470–522.

19. Oliver JM, Alonso-Gonzalez R, Gonzalez AE, et al. Risk of aortic root or ascending aorta complications in patients with bicuspid aortic valve with and without coarctation of the aorta. Am J Cardiol 2009;104(7):1001–6.

20. Wong SC, Burgess T, Cheung M, et al. The prevalence of turner syndrome in girls presenting with coarctation of the aorta. J Pediatr 2014;164(2):259–63.

21. Cramer JW, Bartz PJ, Simpson PM, et al. The spectrum of congenital heart disease and outcomes after surgical repair among children with Turner syndrome: a single-center review. Pediatr Cardiol 2014;35(2):253–60.

22. Pham PP, Moller JH, Hills C, et al. Cardiac catheterization and operative outcomes from a multicenter consortium for children with Williams syndrome. Pediatr Cardiol 2009;30(1):9–14.

23. Reifenstein GH, Levine SA, Gross RE. Coarctation of the aorta; a review of 104 autopsied cases of the adult type, 2 years of age or older. Am Heart J 1947;33(2):146–68.

24. Curtis SL, Bradley M, Wilde P, et al. Results of screening for intracranial aneurysms in patients with coarctation of the aorta. AJNR Am J Neuroradiol 2012;33(6):1182–6.

25. Moss AJ, Allen HD. Moss and Adams' heart disease in infants, children, and adolescents: including the fetus and young adult. 7th edition. Philadelphia: Wolters Kluwer Health/Lippincott Williams & Wilkins; 2008.

26. Shepherd B, Abbas A, McParland P, et al. MRI in adult patients with aortic coarctation: diagnosis and follow-up. Clin Radiol 2015;70(4):433–45.

27. Nielsen JC, Powell AJ, Gauvreau K, et al. Magnetic resonance imaging predictors of coarctation severity. Circulation 2005,111(5):622–8.

28. Muzzarelli S, Meadows AK, Ordovas KG, et al. Usefulness of cardiovascular magnetic resonance imaging to predict the need for intervention in patients with coarctation of the aorta. Am J Cardiol 2012; 109(6):861–5.

29. Didier D, Saint-Martin C, Lapierre C, et al. Coarctation of the aorta: pre and postoperative evaluation with MRI and MR angiography; correlation with echocardiography and surgery. Int J Cardiovasc Imaging 2006;22(3–4):457–75.

30. Rosenthal E, Bell A. Optimal imaging after coarctation stenting. Heart 2010;96(15):1169–71.

31. Hager A, Kaemmerer H, Hess J. Comparison of helical CT scanning and MRI in the follow-up of adults with coarctation of the aorta. Chest 2005;127(6): 2296.

32. Warnes CA, Williams RG, Bashore TM, et al. ACC/AHA 2008 guidelines for the management of adults with congenital heart disease: a report of the American College of Cardiology/American heart association Task Force on Practice guidelines (Writing Committee to Develop guidelines on the management of adults with congenital heart disease). Developed in Collaboration with the American Society of Echocardiography, Heart Rhythm Society, International Society for Adult Congenital Heart Disease, Society for Cardiovascular Angiography and Interventions, and Society of Thoracic Surgeons. J Am Coll Cardiol 2008;52(23):e143–263.

33. Backer CL, Paape K, Zales VR, et al. Coarctation of the aorta. Repair with polytetrafluoroethylene patch aortoplasty. Circulation 1995;92(9 Suppl): II132–136.

34. Adams EE, Davidson WR Jr, Swallow NA, et al. Long-term results of the subclavian flap repair for coarctation of the aorta in infants. World J Pediatr Congenit Heart Surg 2013;4(1):13–8.

35. Beekman RH, Rocchini AP, Behrendt DM, et al. Long-term outcome after repair of coarctation in infancy: subclavian angioplasty does not reduce the need for reoperation. J Am Coll Cardiol 1986;8(6): 1406–11.

36. Bogaert J, Gewillig M, Rademakers F, et al. Transverse arch hypoplasia predisposes to aneurysm formation at the repair site after patch angioplasty for coarctation of the aorta. J Am Coll Cardiol 1995; 26(2):521–7.

37. Cardoso G, Abecasis M, Anjos R, et al. Aortic coarctation repair in the adult. J Card Surg 2014;29(4): 512–8.

38. Rao PS, Galal O, Smith PA, et al. Five- to nine-year follow-up results of balloon angioplasty of native aortic coarctation in infants and children. J Am Coll Cardiol 1996;27(2):462–70.

39. Forbes TJ, Kim DW, Du W, et al. Comparison of surgical, stent, and balloon angioplasty treatment of native coarctation of the aorta: an observational study by the CCISC (Congenital Cardiovascular Interventional Study Consortium). J Am Coll Cardiol 2011;58(25):2664–74.

40. Cooper RS, Ritter SB, Rothe WB, et al. Angioplasty for coarctation of the aorta: long-term results. Circulation 1987;75(3):600–4.

41. Kische S, D'Ancona G, Stoeckicht Y, et al. Percutaneous treatment of adult isthmic aortic coarctation: acute and long-term clinical and imaging outcome with a self-expandable uncovered nitinol stent. Circ Cardiovasc Interv 2015;8(1):1–8.

42. Meadows J, Minahan M, McElhinney DB, et al, COAST Investigators. Intermediate Outcomes in the prospective, multicenter coarctation of the aorta stent trial (COAST). Circulation 2015; 131(19):1656–64.

43. Brown ML, Burkhart HM, Connolly HM, et al. Late outcomes of reintervention on the descending aorta after repair of aortic coarctation. Circulation 2010; 122(11 Suppl):S81–84.

44. Cohen M, Fuster V, Steele PM, et al. Coarctation of the aorta. Long-term follow-up and prediction of outcome after surgical correction. Circulation 1989; 80(4):840–5.

45. Roifman I, Therrien J, Ionescu-Ittu R, et al. Coarctation of the aorta and coronary artery disease: fact or fiction? Circulation 2012;126(1):16–21.

46. Ungerleider RM, Pasquali SK, Welke KF, et al. Contemporary patterns of surgery and outcomes for aortic coarctation: an analysis of the Society of Thoracic Surgeons Congenital Heart Surgery Database. J Thorac Cardiovasc Surg 2013;145(1):150–7 [discussion: 157–8].

47. Attenhofer Jost CH, Schaff HV, Connolly HM, et al. Spectrum of reoperations after repair of aortic coarctation: importance of an individualized approach because of coexistent cardiovascular disease. Mayo Clinic Proc 2002;77(7):646–53.

48. Pandey R, Jackson M, Ajab S, et al. Subclavian flap repair: review of 399 patients at median follow-up of fourteen years. Ann Thorac Surg 2006;81(4):1420–8.

49. Brown ML, Burkhart HM, Connolly HM, et al. Coarctation of the aorta: lifelong surveillance is mandatory following surgical repair. J Am Coll Cardiol 2013; 62(11):1020–5.

50. Cobanoglu A, Thyagarajan GK, Dobbs JL. Surgery for coarctation of the aorta in infants younger than 3 months: end-to-end repair versus subclavian flap angioplasty: is either operation better? Eur J Cardiothorac Surg 1998;14(1):19–25 [discussion: 25–6].

51. Jenkins NP, Ward C. Coarctation of the aorta: natural history and outcome after surgical treatment. QJM 1999;92(7):365–71.

52. von Kodolitsch Y, Aydin MA, Koschyk DH, et al. Predictors of aneurysmal formation after surgical correction of aortic coarctation. J Am Coll Cardiol 2002;39(4):617–24.

53. Jonas RA, DiNardo JA. Comprehensive surgical management of congenital heart disease. London; New York: Arnold; Distributed in the United States of America by Oxford University Press; 2004.

54. Hormann M, Pavlidis D, Brunkwall J, et al. Long-term results of endovascular aortic repair for thoracic pseudoaneurysms after previous surgical coarctation repair. Interact Cardiovasc Thorac Surg 2011; 13(4):401–4.

55. Ince H, Petzsch M, Rehders T, et al. Percutaneous endovascular repair of aneurysm after previous coarctation surgery. Circulation 2003;108(24): 2967–70.

56. Juszkat R, Perek B, Zabicki B, et al. Endovascular treatment of late thoracic aortic aneurysms after surgical repair of congenital aortic coarctation in childhood. PLoS One 2013;8(12):e83601.

57. Khavandi A, Bentham J, Marlais M, et al. Transcatheter and endovascular stent graft management of coarctation-related pseudoaneurysms. Heart 2013; 99(17):1275–81.

58. Wells WJ, Prendergast TW, Berdjis F, et al. Repair of coarctation of the aorta in adults: the fate of systolic hypertension. Ann Thorac Surg 1996;61(4):1168–71.

59. Bhat MA, Neelakandhan KS, Unnikrishnan M, et al. Fate of hypertension after repair of coarctation of the aorta in adults. Br J Surg 2001;88(4):536–8.

60. Canniffe C, Ou P, Walsh K, et al. Hypertension after repair of aortic coarctation: a systematic review. Int J Cardiol 2013;167(6):2456–61.

61. Hager A, Kanz S, Kaemmerer H, et al. Coarctation long-term assessment (COALA): significance of arterial hypertension in a cohort of 404 patients up to 27 years after surgical repair of isolated coarctation of the aorta, even in the absence of restenosis and prosthetic material. J Thorac Cardiovasc Surg 2007;134(3):738–45.

62. Kenny D, Polson JW, Martin RP, et al. Surgical approach for aortic coarctation influences arterial compliance and blood pressure control. Ann Thorac Surg 2010;90(2):600–4.

63. Giordano U, Cifra B, Giannico S, et al. Mid-term results, and therapeutic management, for patients suffering hypertension after surgical repair of aortic coarctation. Cardiol Young 2009;19(5):451–5.

64. Moltzer E, Mattace Raso FU, Karamermer Y, et al. Comparison of candesartan versus metoprolol for treatment of systemic hypertension after repaired aortic coarctation. Am J Cardiol 2010;105(2): 217–22.

Tetralogy of Fallot
General Principles of Management

Tacy E. Downing, MD[a], Yuli Y. Kim, MD[b,c],*

KEYWORDS

- Tetralogy of Fallot • Adults with congenital heart disease • Pulmonary regurgitation
- Pulmonary valve replacement • Arrhythmia • Pregnancy

KEY POINTS

- Tetralogy of Fallot (TOF) is one of the most common diagnoses encountered when caring for adults with congenital heart disease.
- Key issues for follow-up and surveillance include residual right ventricular outflow tract (RVOT) disease, right ventricular dilation or dysfunction, heart failure, and arrhythmia.
- Most adults with repaired TOF require pulmonary valve replacement (PVR). Indications for PVR are evolving, and transcatheter pulmonary valves (TPVs) have emerged as an alternative to surgery for some patients.
- Arrhythmias are prevalent in patients with repaired TOF, and sudden death does occur. Risk stratification is complex and often requires expert consultation.
- Pregnancy is generally well tolerated in women with uncomplicated repaired TOF; however, individual risk-stratification is indicated.

INTRODUCTION

TOF is the most common cyanotic congenital heart lesion, affecting 3% to 10% of all babies born with congenital heart disease.[1–3] Historically, it was the first complex cardiac lesion to be palliated surgically.[4] During the ensuing six decades, advances in surgical technique and perioperative management have resulted in excellent survival rates into adulthood. Assessment of life expectancy after TOF repair remains limited by the few patients currently in their sixth and seventh decade of life, but in several large series, the 30- to 40-year survival rate has been reported at 85% to 90%.[5–8] Morbidities such as arrhythmia and heart failure are common, however, and many patients require reintervention in adulthood. Postoperative TOF therefore requires lifelong care and is one of the most common diagnoses encountered by practitioners caring for adults with congenital heart disease.

ANATOMY AND INITIAL SURGICAL REPAIR

Developmentally, TOF occurs when the conal or infundibular portion of the ventricular septum is displaced anteriorly into the RVOT. This displacement produces (1) a large ventricular septal defect

Disclosures: The authors have nothing to disclose.
[a] Division of Cardiology, The Children's Hospital of Philadelphia, Suite 8NW90, 3400 Civic Center Boulevard, Philadelphia, PA 19104, USA; [b] Division of Cardiovascular Medicine, The Hospital of the University of Pennsylvania, Perelman School of Medicine at the University of Pennsylvania, 3400 Civic Center Boulevard, Philadelphia, PA 19104, USA; [c] Philadelphia Adult Congenital Heart Center, The Children's Hospital of Philadelphia, Perelman Center for Advanced Medicine, Penn Medicine, 3400 Civic Center Boulevard, 2nd Floor East Pavilion, Philadelphia, PA 19104, USA
* Corresponding author. Philadelphia Adult Congenital Heart Center, Perelman Center for Advanced Medicine, Penn Medicine, 3400 Civic Center Boulevard, 2nd Floor East Pavilion, Philadelphia, PA 19104.
E-mail address: Yuli.Kim@uphs.upenn.edu

Cardiol Clin 33 (2015) 531–541
http://dx.doi.org/10.1016/j.ccl.2015.07.002
0733-8651/15/$ – see front matter © 2015 Elsevier Inc. All rights reserved.

(VSD) and (2) obstruction to right ventricular outflow at the infundibular, valvar, or supravalvar levels (**Fig. 1**). The degree of RVOT obstruction is highly variable, ranging from very mild (the so-called pink tetralogy) to complete pulmonary valve atresia with diminutive or absent branch pulmonary arteries.

Surgical repair of TOF consists of VSD closure and relief of RVOT obstruction to the greatest extent possible. This is usually accomplished as a primary repair in infancy. In the era when neonatal cardiopulmonary bypass was not readily available, however, a staged approach was used. Patients requiring augmentation of their pulmonary blood flow in infancy received a systemic to pulmonary shunt, followed by complete repair at an older age. Today's adult congenital heart disease (ACHD) practitioner encounters both of these histories in clinical practice.

ANATOMIC SEQUELAE OF REPAIRED TETRALOGY OF FALLOT

Hemodynamically significant residual VSDs are uncommon in the adult with repaired TOF. By contrast, the vast majority of patients have residual RVOT disease. Patients whose RVOT obstruction was initially mild may have been treated with a surgical pulmonary valvotomy and augmentation of the infundibulum, thereby sparing the pulmonary valve annulus but leaving the potential for recurrent stenosis. Conversely, those with significant pulmonary annular hypoplasia typically require a transannular patch at the time of initial repair. This technique disrupts the valve architecture, providing good relief of obstruction but resulting in significant pulmonary regurgitation (PR).

Finally, in a minority of patients, a right ventricle (RV) to pulmonary artery conduit is required, either because of complete pulmonary valve atresia or aberrant coronary anatomy that precludes an incision in the infundibulum. These conduits are not durable and often develop hemodynamically significant stenosis and/or regurgitation after one to two decades (or less). Knowledge of the individual surgical history is critical to the care of the postoperative patient, and therefore, review of original operative notes is recommended whenever possible.

GENERAL PRINCIPLES OF OUTPATIENT SURVEILLANCE

The 2008 American College of Cardiology (ACC)/ American Heart Association (AHA) Guidelines for Management of Adults with Congenital Heart Disease propose a general framework for outpatient surveillance of the adult with repaired TOF.[7] Office visits with an ACHD physician are recommended at least annually, with a focus on identifying and managing the commonly encountered complications outlined in **Box 1**. Guidelines for frequency of imaging and testing are based on expert consensus, but a typical framework includes, at minimum, annual physical examination and electrocardiography with echocardiography as indicated.[9]

The physical examination is a useful starting point in elucidating residual anatomic lesions or associated conditions. Findings that may be encountered in patients with TOF are presented in **Table 1**. In patients with significant RVOT disease, careful attention to the jugular venous waveform is imperative to evaluate for volume overload

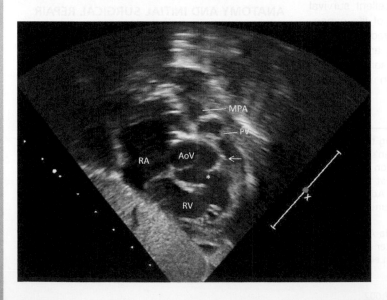

Fig. 1. Subcostal oblique view with anterior angulation demonstrating anteriorly malaligned conal septum (*arrow*) with resulting ventricular septal defect (*asterisk*) and hypoplastic pulmonary valve. AoV, aortic valve; MPA, main pulmonary artery; PV, pulmonary valve; RA, right atrium; RV, right ventricle.

Box 1
Common complications of postoperative tetralogy of Fallot

- Residual pulmonary regurgitation
- RV dilation and/or dysfunction
- Residual RVOT obstruction ± branch PA stenosis
- Arrhythmias and risk of sudden death
- Heart failure
- Aortic root dilation ± aortic regurgitation

Abbreviations: PA, pulmonary artery; RV, right ventricle; RVOT, right ventricular outflow tract.

or signs of elevated right atrial pressure. The electrocardiogram after TOF repair almost universally demonstrates right bundle branch block with variable QRS duration.

The utility of cardiac magnetic resonance imaging (CMR), Holter monitoring, and electrophysiology testing is discussed subsequently. Exercise testing may be used at intervals to quantify aerobic capacity. Although there are no formal

Table 1
Significance of common physical examination findings in repaired tetralogy of Fallot

Finding	Significance
Single S2	Absence of functional PV tissue
Loud or accentuated P2	Anterior location of PV (RV to PA conduit) Prior PV replacement Pulmonary hypertension
Systolic ejection murmur at LUSB	Residual RVOT obstruction Excess flow related to severe PR
Early diastolic murmur at LUSB	Pulmonary regurgitation
Holosystolic murmur at left sternal border	Tricuspid regurgitation Residual ventricular septal defect
Decreased or absent radial pulse Thoracotomy scar	History of Blalock-Taussig shunt
Facial dysmorphisms	22q11 deletion or other genetic syndrome

Abbreviations: LUSB, left upper sternal border; PA, pulmonary artery; PR, pulmonary regurgitation; PV, pulmonary valve; RV, right ventricle; RVOT, right ventricular outflow tract.

guidelines for frequency of exercise testing in repaired TOF, it can be useful when subjective symptoms are discordant with other objective data and potentially when indications for surgical intervention are borderline.

Choice of Imaging Modality

Surveillance imaging in TOF focuses on evaluation of the RVOT, pulmonary valve and branch pulmonary arteries, serial assessments of ventricular size and function, estimates of tricuspid regurgitation and RV pressure, and measurement of the aortic root (AoR). Poor acoustic windows may preclude detailed examination of right-sided structures by echocardiography, however, and it is rare to image the branch pulmonary arteries well in an adult. CMR has therefore emerged as a key imaging modality in the management of TOF and has the added benefit of providing important functional information.

The role of CMR in the assessment of TOF is beyond the scope of this article and is discussed in detail elsewhere.[10] CMR is considered the gold standard in quantitative assessment of right ventricular size and function and can provide flow measurements of pulmonary and tricuspid regurgitant fraction. Because clinical decisions often depend on an accurate assessment of RV volume, it is preferable for CMR to be performed at an experienced congenital center with a high volume of patients with TOF. There are no formal guidelines for frequency of CMR in the patient with repaired TOF, but a typical algorithm might include CMR every three to five years or when there is a substantial change in echo findings or symptoms.

MANAGEMENT OF RESIDUAL PULMONARY VALVE DYSFUNCTION

The surgical management of TOF has primarily focused on complete relief of RVOT obstruction, with the inevitable consequence of severe PR when a transannular patch technique is used. Most patients with significant PR are asymptomatic in early adult life, which undoubtedly contributed to decades of underappreciation of its hemodynamic importance.

In the 1990s, improved diagnostic techniques allowed the first correlations of severe PR with increased RV volume and reduced functional capacity in patients with TOF.[11] The advent of CMR as a reliable means of measuring RV volume then spurred numerous studies examining the potential beneficial effects of PVR. The idea emerged of a threshold value for RV size, beyond which PVR was less likely to result in RV reverse remodeling. The exact value of this threshold remains a matter of debate, but the most widely referenced studies propose 150 to 165 mL/m² right ventricular end-diastolic volume as the appropriate cutoff.[12–16] The general practice is to recommend PVR before the RV volume exceeds this value, thereby allowing the best chance of postoperative normalization. Although studies have primarily focused on CMR-derived RV volume as the predictive parameter, additional identified risk factors for poor surgical response include reduced RV ejection fraction and QRS duration greater than 180 milliseconds.[16,17]

Existing studies on timing of PVR have primarily used RV volume normalization as the postoperative outcome of interest. Whether that translates to other important clinical end points is not completely proven. An overview of selected recent studies is presented in **Table 2**. A prime example of the ambiguous effects of PVR relates to functional status. Although New York Heart Association functional class has universally been shown to improve after PVR, aerobic capacity fails to increase in the same patients when objectively assessed by exercise testing.[13,15,17,18] Studies of RV systolic function before and after PVR have also shown mixed results.[13,15,17–20] Although prolonged QRS duration has been shown to correlate with late adverse outcomes, its change after PVR has been variable.[13,17,18,21,22] No study has demonstrated that PVR affects long-term survival or the incidence of life-threatening arrhythmia,[23] although ascertainment of these outcomes is undoubtedly limited by follow-up time and their relative infrequency.

What is known is that patients with TOF with severe PR almost universally experience symptomatic improvement after PVR. In the asymptomatic patient, markedly increased RV volume and reduced RV ejection fraction may predict poor surgical response. A combination of these factors therefore serves as the basis of current recommendations for timing of PVR. ACC/AHA, European, and Canadian guidelines are summarized in **Box 2**.[7,24,25] It is important, however, to understand the heterogeneity of evidence on which these recommendations are based. There are no randomized trials of surgical versus medical management, and nearly all the recommendations are based on expert consensus or small retrospective studies.

A smaller percentage of patients with TOF have residual pulmonary stenosis (PS) as their dominant hemodynamic lesion; this is especially likely in patients who did not have a transannular patch at the time of initial repair or those with RV to pulmonary artery (PA) conduits. The indications for intervention in patients with TOF are similar to those with isolated valvar PS; PVR is suggested when there is at least moderate RVOT obstruction or greater than two-thirds systemic RV pressure.[7] Catheter-based valvuloplasty may be an alternative to surgery in anatomically appropriately patients.

Intervention is usually not required for mild RVOT obstruction. Some degree of PS may actually be protective against the adverse ventricular remodeling that occurs with longstanding PR, and there is an entire body of literature focusing on the subgroup of patients with TOF with mixed PR and PS.[26–31]

Surgical Versus Percutaneous Approach to Pulmonary Valve Replacement

The first TPV was implanted by Bonhoeffer and colleagues[32] in 2000, representing a promising advance toward less invasive management of residual RVOT disease. At present, the Melody TPV (Medtronic Inc., Minneapolis, MN, USA) is the only device specifically designed for use in the pulmonary position. It has been commercially available in Europe since 2006 and in the United States since 2010 and is indicated for patients

Table 2
Clinical response to pulmonary valve replacement—summary of recent evidence

Clinical Parameter	Studies Supporting Improvement After PVR (Reference Number)	Studies Supporting No Change After PVR (Reference Number)
NYHA class	13,15,17,18	—
RV systolic function	15,16,20	13,17–19
LV systolic function	15,16	13,17
Tricuspid regurgitation	17	13
Peak Vo₂	—	15,17,18
QRS duration	13,21,22	17,18

Includes studies with ≥50 patients published in 2005 or later.
Abbreviations: LV, left ventricle; NYHA, New York Heart Association; Vo₂, oxygen consumption.

Box 2
Current guidelines for pulmonary valve replacement in adults with repaired tetralogy of Fallot

ACC/AHA guidelines (2008)

1. PVR should be performed in adults with severe PR and symptoms or decreased exercise tolerance (class 1, LOE C)

2. In asymptomatic adults with severe PR and any of the following (class IIa, LOE C):

   - Moderate to severe RV dysfunction
   - Moderate to severe RV enlargement
   - Development of symptomatic or sustained atrial and/or ventricular arrhythmias
   - Moderate to severe TR

Canadian guidelines (2009)

The situations that may warrant PVR are as follows (class IIa, LOE C):

- Free PR associated with progressive or moderate to severe RV enlargement (RV end-diastolic volume of greater than 170 mL/m^2)
- Moderate to severe RV dysfunction
- Important TR, atrial or ventricular arrhythmias, or symptoms such as deteriorating exercise performance
- Residual pulmonary stenosis with RV pressures at least two-thirds systemic

European guidelines (2010)

1. PVR should be performed in symptomatic patients with severe PR and/or stenosis (RV systolic pressure >60 mm Hg, TR velocity >3.5 m/s) (class I, LOE C)

2. PVR should be considered in asymptomatic patients with severe PR and/or PS when at least 1 of the following criteria is present (class IIa, LOE C)

   - Decrease in objective exercise capacity
   - Progressive RV dilation
   - Progressive RV systolic dysfunction
   - Progressive TR (at least moderate)
   - RVOT obstruction with RV systolic pressure greater than 80 mm Hg (TR velocity >4.3 m/s)
   - Sustained atrial/ventricular arrhythmias

Abbreviations: LOE, level of evidence; TR, tricuspid regurgitation.

---

with dysfunctional RV to PA conduits 16 mm or more in original diameter. The Sapien valve (Edwards Lifesciences LLC, Irvine, CA, USA), originally designed for aortic deployment, is available for PVR in Europe and as part of an ongoing investigational trial in the United States (https://clinicaltrials.gov/ct2/show/NCT00676689).

Initial follow-up studies of the Melody valve have demonstrated good short-term technical results, with low procedural complication rates and greater than 90% success in relieving hemodynamically significant stenosis and/or regurgitation. Reductions in PR and RV volumes appear similar to surgical cohorts, although no randomized trials have directly compared the two approaches.[33–37] The first medium-term outcome study was recently published and showed a 95% freedom

from reintervention 5 years after Melody TPV implantation.[38]

The most significant long-term concern surrounding the Melody valve has been the potentially increased rate of bacterial endocarditis. Published studies have varied widely, but the incidence may be as high 10% to 15% in the medium term.[39,40] No direct comparisons with the surgical population have been performed. Emerging evidence suggests that the rate of endocarditis after surgical PVR depends significantly on the choice of prosthesis.[41] Further study of this issue is clearly warranted, and strict adherence to endocarditis prophylaxis (as indicated for surgical PVR) is recommended in patients after TPV implantation.

The primary limitation to widespread application of TPV is its restriction to use in patients with RV to

PA conduits. The vast majority of patients with repaired TOF do not have a conduit, and the native or patched RVOT is typically too large and irregularly shaped to accommodate the Melody valve. TPV implantation into the native RVOT has been reported,[42,43] but anatomically suitable candidates are rare and the procedure requires a high degree of technical skill. Widespread application of TPV therapy to the TOF population therefore depends on successful development of a device specific to the native reconstructed RVOT. The Medtronic native outflow device is available at a small number of centers as part of an early investigational trial (https://clinicaltrials.gov/ct2/show/NCT01762124); however, no such device is yet accessible to the general population.

ARRHYTHMIAS AND RISK OF SUDDEN DEATH

Despite the high success rate of surgical correction of TOF, late arrhythmias are prevalent and there is a small but not insignificant rate of sudden cardiac death (SCD). In a multicenter review of 556 adult patients with repaired TOF or pulmonary atresia, 43% either had a documented tachyarrhythmia or had received electrophysiologic intervention in the form of ablation or device implantation.[44]

The reported prevalence of atrial arrhythmias in patients with repaired TOF has ranged from 10% to 35% in cohorts of variable size and follow-up time. The most common is intra-atrial reentrant tachycardia (IART), followed by atrial fibrillation.[44–47] IART seems to be more prevalent in younger patients and those with right-sided anatomic residua, and atrial fibrillation in older patients and those with left-sided sequelae such as diminished left ventricular (LV) function.[44] Significant tricuspid regurgitation has been proposed as a predictor of atrial arrhythmias; however, this association has not been consistently reproducible.[44,45]

The most feared complication of SCD happens rarely, with a reported frequency of 1% to 3.5% in retrospective studies. Sustained ventricular tachycardia (VT) occurs at similar rates in short-term follow-up, although prevalence may be as high as 12% at 35 years after surgery.[45,48,49] Many investigators have attempted to identify risk factors for these life-threatening arrhythmias, but single-center series have been hampered by small cohort sizes and heterogeneous methodology in the setting of low event rates.[49–52]

Potential risk factors for SCD or sustained VT identified in recent studies are outlined in **Table 3**. Duration of the QRS complex greater than 180 milliseconds and LV dysfunction have consistently predicted adverse outcome. Symptomatic or inducible nonsustained VT is likely also a risk factor based on the predominance of evidence.[53–55] A newer finding is the association of atrial arrhythmias with SCD.[8,56] Many other clinical characteristics, such as RV pressure overload and RV systolic dysfunction, have been proposed as risk factors with inconsistent validation in the literature.[44,45,56] Despite the focus on residual PR and timing of PVR, no large study has clearly demonstrated that degree of PR or RV volume independently predict sudden death. Furthermore, the incidence of life-threatening arrhythmias does not clearly improve after PVR.[23]

There is no known association between SCD and premature ventricular beats, and the prognostic value of asymptomatic nonsustained VT remains unclear[45,53]; this calls into question the utility of surveillance Holter monitoring, and current guidelines make no definitive recommendation for or against screening the asymptomatic patient. If asymptomatic VT is identified, the optimal approach to management is not well defined. Some practitioners might opt for medical management, whereas others would pursue an electrophysiology study with programmed ventricular stimulation. There is insufficient evidence, however, to recommend routine invasive testing in low-risk patients.[57]

Implantable cardioverter-defibrillators are clearly indicated for secondary prevention in patients with prior SCD. As mentioned earlier, indications for primary prevention devices in this

Table 3	
Possible predictors of sustained VT or sudden cardiac death in repaired tetralogy of Fallot	
Likely Predictive	**Further Study Required**
QRS duration >180 ms	Asymptomatic NSVT
LV systolic or diastolic dysfunction	RV end-diastolic volume
Inducible VT at EPS	Degree of pulmonary regurgitation
Symptomatic NSVT	RV systolic dysfunction
History of atrial arrhythmia	RV hypertrophy or pressure overload

Abbreviations: EPS, electrophysiology study; NSVT, nonsustained ventricular tachycardia.

population are poorly defined and practice is variable. It is unlikely that any single parameter (e.g. QRS duration, degree of PR) is sufficiently discriminating, and the optimal approach may take the form of more complex risk modeling.[51] Such decisions should be undertaken in consultation with an electrophysiologist experienced in the care of patients with ACHD.

THE LEFT HEART IN TETRALOGY OF FALLOT
Aortic Root Dilation

Although much of the management of repaired TOF focuses on the RV and pulmonary valve, left heart pathology may occur as well. AoR dilation in particular is often observed, sometimes with associated aortic valve regurgitation. The pathophysiology of AoR dilation in TOF is incompletely understood, but histopathologic abnormalities of the aortic wall have been observed as early as infancy.[58] Fragmentation of elastic laminae and fibrosis are common, and abnormal aortic elasticity has been demonstrated in imaging studies,[59] suggesting an underlying aortopathy.

The reported prevalence of AoR dilation in TOF has ranged from 15% to 87% in single-center studies,[59,60] depending on the criteria used for definition and patient age. In a multicenter cross-sectional study of adults, mild enlargement of the AoR was common, but severe dilation was rare. Of 333 patients, 29% had an AoR diameter greater than 4 cm by echocardiography, but only 2% had greater than 5 cm. Only 4% of patients in that study had moderate or severe aortic regurgitation.[61] Only four cases of aortic dissection have ever been reported in patients with TOF. Three occurred in the context of massive AoR dilation to greater than 7 cm,[62] and the fourth was a limited dissection in a root measuring 5.5 cm.[63]

No clinical characteristics predisposing to root dilation or aortic regurgitation have been clearly identified. Early studies suggested male sex, pulmonary atresia, and longer time from palliation to primary repair as potential risk factors[60,64]; however, these findings could not be reproduced in a multicenter multivariate analysis.[61]

The current management strategy for dilated AoR in TOF is incompletely defined. ACC/AHA ACHD guidelines recommend serial imaging if root dilation is identified but do not specifically address indications for surgery.[7] Canadian guidelines apply the same standards to TOF as to other non–connective tissue disorder aortopathies and suggest surgical intervention at a root diameter of 5.5 cm.[25] There is no evidence specific to patients with TOF, however, and in the authors' center, patients are not routinely referred for aortic repair at this dimension in the absence of significant aortic regurgitation. Rapidly enlarging AoRs may represent a higher-risk subset, so acknowledging the lack of supporting data, most practitioners would consider surgery when the root dimension increases by more than 0.5 cm in one year.

Left Ventricular Dysfunction

LV dysfunction is observed in some adult patients with repaired TOF and is predictive of adverse outcomes such as sudden death even in the absence of additional risk factors such as coronary artery disease or ventricular arrhythmia. There has been limited investigation into this topic thus far, and the pathophysiology is not well understood. In one recent multicenter study, 14% of patients had mildly diminished LV systolic function and in 6% the function was moderately or severely decreased. Risk factors included longer duration of palliative shunt, RV dysfunction, and presence of arrhythmia.[65] Subsequent studies have confirmed the close relationship of RV and LV systolic function in these patients.[66]

HEART FAILURE IN TETRALOGY OF FALLOT

Clinically symptomatic heart failure is an increasingly recognized complication in adults with congenital heart disease. At least 14% of adults with TOF endorse New York Heart Association functional class 2 symptoms or higher.[67] Levels of biomarkers, such as brain natriuretic peptide, are elevated in patients with TOF and may have prognostic value.[68,69] The cause of heart failure is multifactorial, resulting from LV and/or RV systolic dysfunction, electrophysiologic abnormalities, residual structural disease, and acquired atherosclerotic disease. Clinical management is largely supportive, and there is little evidence to support conventional medical or device therapies in this population.

PREGNANCY AFTER TETRALOGY OF FALLOT REPAIR

The vast majority of women with repaired TOF express the desire to become pregnant.[70] Although pregnancy is generally well tolerated, there is an increased risk of maternal and offspring sequelae, and preconception counseling is indicated.

Pregnancy outcome studies have generally been limited to single-center retrospective reviews, but several themes do emerge. Maternal cardiac complications occur at a rate of 7% to 10%. Arrhythmia is the most common, occurring in 6% to 7%, followed by symptomatic heart failure in less than 2% to 3%. Serious offspring complications and premature birth are rare, although several series have demonstrated that the rate of small-for-gestational-age infants is increased. Iteration of congenital heart disease has been reported at 2% to 3%, higher than the approximately 1% incidence in the general population.[70–72] In a study specific to pregnant women with repaired TOF, the most important predictor of both maternal cardiac and offspring events was the use of cardiac medication before pregnancy.[70]

Severe PR seems to play a synergistic role with other risk factors. When present in isolation, it does not definitively confer risk; however, when other cardiac risk factors are present, the addition of severe PR substantially increases adverse outcomes.[73] One small series suggests that pregnancy may accelerate progression of RV dilation in patients with TOF. This effect was noted primarily in those women whose RV dilation was severe before pregnancy.[74] Clinically, the question frequently arises as to whether PVR should be pursued electively before pregnancy in the otherwise asymptomatic woman with severe PR. No guidelines exist, but in the authors' institution, this is not generally recommended if standard criteria for PVR are not met. This decision should be individualized, however, especially in the presence of other risk factors.

Labor and delivery plans must also be tailored to each woman, but for the typical patient with TOF, spontaneous labor and vaginal delivery are permissible in the absence of obstetric contraindication. Although there are no formal guidelines, it may be reasonable to recommend peripartum telemetry monitoring for those with a history of arrhythmia.

In summary, the asymptomatic woman with repaired TOF generally tolerates pregnancy well. Severe PR is not a contraindication but does increase the risk of adverse maternal outcome if other anatomic or hemodynamic lesions are present. When maternal cardiac events do occur, they typically consist of arrhythmia and/or heart failure, which generally respond to treatment and improve after delivery. Catastrophic events such as death, emergent surgery, or need for mechanical circulatory support are exceedingly rare.

SUMMARY

TOF is one of the most common diagnoses encountered when caring for adults with congenital heart disease. Long-term survival is excellent in the modern era, but morbidity is common. Most patients with a typical surgical history require PVR in adulthood, and indications and optimal timing for this are rapidly evolving. Arrhythmia, left heart disease, and pregnancy management are common associated issues that arise in this population, and heart failure is increasingly being recognized as a long-term sequela as these patients age. Although patients with repaired TOF do well overall, their management can be complex, and care at a dedicated ACHD center is recommended.

REFERENCES

1. Apitz C, Webb GD, Redington AN. Tetralogy of Fallot. Lancet 2009;374(9699):1462–71.
2. Hoffman JI. Incidence of congenital heart disease: I. Postnatal incidence. Pediatr Cardiol 1995;16(3): 103–13.
3. Kalra N, Klewer SE, Raasch H, et al. Update on tetralogy of Fallot for the adult cardiologist including a brief historical and surgical perspective. Congenit Heart Dis 2010;5(3):208–19.
4. Lillehei CW, Cohen M, Warden HE, et al. Direct vision intracardiac surgical correction of the tetralogy of Fallot, pentalogy of Fallot, and pulmonary atresia defects; report of first ten cases. Ann Surg 1955; 142(3):418–42.
5. Chiu SN, Wang JK, Chen HC, et al. Long-term survival and unnatural deaths of patients with repaired tetralogy of Fallot in an Asian cohort. Circ Cardiovasc Qual Outcomes 2012;5(1):120–5.
6. Bacha EA, Scheule AM, Zurakowski D, et al. Long-term results after early primary repair of tetralogy of Fallot. J Thorac Cardiovasc Surg 2001;122(1): 154–61.
7. Warnes CA, Williams RG, Bashore TM, et al. ACC/AHA 2008 guidelines for the management of adults with congenital heart disease: a report of the American College of Cardiology/American Heart Association Task Force on Practice Guidelines (Writing Committee to Develop Guidelines on the Management of Adults With Congenital Heart Disease). Developed in Collaboration with the American Society of Echocardiography, Heart Rhythm Society, International Society for Adult Congenital Heart Disease, Society for Cardiovascular Angiography and Interventions, and Society of Thoracic Surgeons. J Am Coll Cardiol 2008;52(23):e143–263.
8. Cuypers JA, Menting ME, Konings EE, et al. Unnatural history of tetralogy of Fallot: prospective follow-up of 40 years after surgical correction. Circulation 2014;130(22):1944–53.
9. Gurvitz M, Marelli A, Mangione-Smith R, et al. Building quality indicators to improve care for adults with congenital heart disease. J Am Coll Cardiol 2013; 62(23):2244–53.
10. Geva T. Repaired tetralogy of Fallot: the roles of cardiovascular magnetic resonance in evaluating

pathophysiology and for pulmonary valve replacement decision support. J Cardiovasc Magn Reson 2011;13:9.

11. Carvalho JS, Shinebourne EA, Busst C, et al. Exercise capacity after complete repair of tetralogy of Fallot: deleterious effects of residual pulmonary regurgitation. Br Heart J 1992;67(6):470–3.

12. Buechel ER, Dave HH, Kellenberger CJ, et al. Remodelling of the right ventricle after early pulmonary valve replacement in children with repaired tetralogy of Fallot: assessment by cardiovascular magnetic resonance. Eur Heart J 2005;26(24):2721–7.

13. Oosterhof T, van Straten A, Vliegen HW, et al. Preoperative thresholds for pulmonary valve replacement in patients with corrected tetralogy of Fallot using cardiovascular magnetic resonance. Circulation 2007;116(5):545–51.

14. Therrien J, Provost Y, Merchant N, et al. Optimal timing for pulmonary valve replacement in adults after tetralogy of Fallot repair. Am J Cardiol 2005; 95(6):779–82.

15. Frigiola A, Tsang V, Bull C, et al. Biventricular response after pulmonary valve replacement for right ventricular outflow tract dysfunction: is age a predictor of outcome? Circulation 2008;118(14 Suppl):S182–90.

16. Lee C, Kim YM, Lee CH, et al. Outcomes of pulmonary valve replacement in 170 patients with chronic pulmonary regurgitation after relief of right ventricular outflow tract obstruction: implications for optimal timing of pulmonary valve replacement. J Am Coll Cardiol 2012;60(11):1005–14.

17. Geva T, Gauvreau K, Powell AJ, et al. Randomized trial of pulmonary valve replacement with and without right ventricular remodeling surgery. Circulation 2010;122(11 Suppl):S201–8.

18. Gengsakul A, Harris L, Bradley TJ, et al. The impact of pulmonary valve replacement after tetralogy of Fallot repair: a matched comparison. Eur J Cardiothorac Surg 2007;32(3):462–8.

19. Graham TP Jr, Bernard Y, Arbogast P, et al. Outcome of pulmonary valve replacements in adults after tetralogy repair: a multi-institutional study. Congenit Heart Dis 2008;3(3):162–7.

20. Henkens IR, van Straten A, Schalij MJ, et al. Predicting outcome of pulmonary valve replacement in adult tetralogy of Fallot patients. Ann Thorac Surg 2007;83(3):907–11.

21. van Huysduynen BH, van Straten A, Swenne CA, et al. Reduction of QRS duration after pulmonary valve replacement in adult Fallot patients is related to reduction of right ventricular volume. Eur Heart J 2005;26(9):928–32.

22. Doughan AR, McConnell ME, Lyle TA, et al. Effects of pulmonary valve replacement on QRS duration and right ventricular cavity size late after repair of right ventricular outflow tract obstruction. Am J Cardiol 2005;95(12):1511–4.

23. Harrild DM, Berul CI, Cecchin F, et al. Pulmonary valve replacement in tetralogy of Fallot: impact on survival and ventricular tachycardia. Circulation 2009;119(3):445–51.

24. Baumgartner H, Bonhoeffer P, De Groot NM, et al. ESC guidelines for the management of grown-up congenital heart disease (new version 2010). Eur Heart J 2010;31(23):2915–57.

25. Silversides CK, Kiess M, Beauchesne L, et al. Canadian Cardiovascular Society 2009 consensus conference on the management of adults with congenital heart disease: outflow tract obstruction, coarctation of the aorta, tetralogy of Fallot, Ebstein anomaly and Marfan's syndrome. Can J Cardiol 2010;26(3):e80–97.

26. Lee W, Yoo SJ, Roche SL, et al. Determinants and functional impact of restrictive physiology after repair of tetralogy of Fallot: new insights from magnetic resonance imaging. Int J Cardiol 2013; 167(4):1347–53.

27. Yoo BW, Kim JO, Kim YJ, et al. Impact of pressure load caused by right ventricular outflow tract obstruction on right ventricular volume overload in patients with repaired tetralogy of Fallot. J Thorac Cardiovasc Surg 2012;143(6):1299–304.

28. Norgard G, Gatzoulis MA, Josen M, et al. Does restrictive right ventricular physiology in the early postoperative period predict subsequent right ventricular restriction after repair of tetralogy of Fallot? Heart 1998;79(5):481–4.

29. Gatzoulis MA, Clark AL, Cullen S, et al. Right ventricular diastolic function 15 to 35 years after repair of tetralogy of Fallot. Restrictive physiology predicts superior exercise performance. Circulation 1995; 91(6):1775–81.

30. van den Berg J, Hop WC, Strengers JL, et al. Clinical condition at mid-to-late follow-up after transatrial-transpulmonary repair of tetralogy of Fallot. J Thorac Cardiovasc Surg 2007;133(2):470–7.

31. Lu JC, Cotts TB, Agarwal PP, et al. Relation of right ventricular dilation, age of repair, and restrictive right ventricular physiology with patient-reported quality of life in adolescents and adults with repaired tetralogy of fallot. Am J Cardiol 2010;106(12):1798–802.

32. Bonhoeffer P, Boudjemline Y, Saliba Z, et al. Percutaneous replacement of pulmonary valve in a right-ventricle to pulmonary-artery prosthetic conduit with valve dysfunction. Lancet 2000;356(9239): 1403–5.

33. Armstrong AK, Balzer DT, Cabalka AK, et al. One-year follow-up of the Melody transcatheter pulmonary valve multicenter post-approval study. JACC Cardiovasc Interv 2014;7(11):1254–62.

34. Butera G, Milanesi O, Spadoni I, et al. Melody transcatheter pulmonary valve implantation. Results from the registry of the Italian Society of Pediatric Cardiology. Catheter Cardiovasc Interv 2013;81(2):310–6.

35. McElhinney DB, Hellenbrand WE, Zahn EM, et al. Short- and medium-term outcomes after transcatheter pulmonary valve placement in the expanded multicenter US melody valve trial. Circulation 2010; 122(5):507–16.

36. Vezmar M, Chaturvedi R, Lee KJ, et al. Percutaneous pulmonary valve implantation in the young: 2-year follow-up. JACC Cardiovasc Interv 2010; 3(4):439–48.

37. Zahn EM, Hellenbrand WE, Lock JE, et al. Implantation of the melody transcatheter pulmonary valve in patients with a dysfunctional right ventricular outflow tract conduit: early results from the U.S. clinical trial. J Am Coll Cardiol 2009;54(18):1722–9.

38. Fraisse A, Aldebert P, Malekzadeh-Milani S, et al. Melody (R) transcatheter pulmonary valve implantation: results from a French registry. Arch Cardiovasc Dis 2014;107(11):607–14.

39. Patel M, Malekzadeh-Milani S, Ladouceur M, et al. Percutaneous pulmonary valve endocarditis: incidence, prevention and management. Arch Cardiovasc Dis 2014;107(11):615–24.

40. Malekzadeh-Milani S, Ladouceur M, Patel M, et al. Incidence and predictors of Melody(R) valve endocarditis: a prospective study. Arch Cardiovasc Dis 2015;108(2):97–106.

41. Van Dijck I, Budts W, Cools B, et al. Infective endocarditis of a transcatheter pulmonary valve in comparison with surgical implants. Heart 2015;101(10): 788–93.

42. Malekzadeh-Milani S, Ladouceur M, Cohen S, et al. Results of transcatheter pulmonary valvulation in native or patched right ventricular outflow tracts. Arch Cardiovasc Dis 2014;107(11):592–8.

43. Meadows JJ, Moore PM, Berman DP, et al. Use and performance of the melody transcatheter pulmonary valve in native and postsurgical, nonconduit right ventricular outflow tracts. Circ Cardiovasc Interv 2014;7(3):374–80.

44. Khairy P, Aboulhosn J, Gurvitz MZ, et al. Arrhythmia burden in adults with surgically repaired tetralogy of Fallot: a multi-institutional study. Circulation 2010; 122(9):868–75.

45. Gatzoulis MA, Balaji S, Webber SA, et al. Risk factors for arrhythmia and sudden cardiac death late after repair of tetralogy of Fallot: a multicentre study. Lancet 2000;356(9234):975–81.

46. Harrison DA, Siu SC, Hussain F, et al. Sustained atrial arrhythmias in adults late after repair of tetralogy of Fallot. Am J Cardiol 2001;87(5):584–8.

47. Roos-Hesselink J, Perlroth MG, McGhie J, et al. Atrial arrhythmias in adults after repair of tetralogy of Fallot. Correlations with clinical, exercise, and echocardiographic findings. Circulation 1995;91(8): 2214–9.

48. Cullen S, Celermajer DS, Franklin RC, et al. Prognostic significance of ventricular arrhythmia after repair of tetralogy of Fallot: a 12-year prospective study. J Am Coll Cardiol 1994;23(5):1151–5.

49. Diller GP, Kempny A, Liodakis E, et al. Left ventricular longitudinal function predicts life-threatening ventricular arrhythmia and death in adults with repaired tetralogy of Fallot. Circulation 2012;125(20):2440–6.

50. Ghai A, Silversides C, Harris L, et al. Left ventricular dysfunction is a risk factor for sudden cardiac death in adults late after repair of tetralogy of Fallot. J Am Coll Cardiol 2002;40(9):1675–80.

51. Khairy P, Dore A, Poirier N, et al. Risk stratification in surgically repaired tetralogy of Fallot. Expert Rev Cardiovasc Ther 2009;7(7):755–62.

52. Harrison DA, Harris L, Siu SC, et al. Sustained ventricular tachycardia in adult patients late after repair of tetralogy of Fallot. J Am Coll Cardiol 1997;30(5): 1368–73.

53. Czosek RJ, Anderson J, Khoury PR, et al. Utility of ambulatory monitoring in patients with congenital heart disease. Am J Cardiol 2013;111(5):723–30.

54. Khairy P, Landzberg MJ, Gatzoulis MA, et al. Value of programmed ventricular stimulation after tetralogy of Fallot repair: a multicenter study. Circulation 2004; 109(16):1994–2000.

55. Koyak Z, de Groot JR, Bouma BJ, et al. Symptomatic but not asymptomatic non-sustained ventricular tachycardia is associated with appropriate implantable cardioverter therapy in tetralogy of Fallot. Int J Cardiol 2013;167(4):1532–5.

56. Valente AM, Gauvreau K, Assenza GE, et al. Contemporary predictors of death and sustained ventricular tachycardia in patients with repaired tetralogy of Fallot enrolled in the INDICATOR cohort. Heart 2014;100(3):247–53.

57. Khairy P. Programmed ventricular stimulation for risk stratification in patients with tetralogy of Fallot: a Bayesian perspective. Nat Clin Pract Cardiovasc Med 2007;4(6):292–3.

58. Tan JL, Davlouros PA, McCarthy KP, et al. Intrinsic histological abnormalities of aortic root and ascending aorta in tetralogy of Fallot: evidence of causative mechanism for aortic dilatation and aortopathy. Circulation 2005;112(7):961–8.

59. Chong WY, Wong WH, Chiu CS, et al. Aortic root dilation and aortic elastic properties in children after repair of tetralogy of Fallot. Am J Cardiol 2006;97(6): 905–9.

60. Niwa K, Siu SC, Webb GD, et al. Progressive aortic root dilatation in adults late after repair of tetralogy of Fallot. Circulation 2002;106(11):1374–8.

61. Mongeon FP, Gurvitz MZ, Broberg CS, et al. Aortic root dilatation in adults with surgically repaired tetralogy of Fallot: a multicenter cross-sectional study. Circulation 2013;127(2):172–9.

62. Le Gloan L, Mongeon FP, Mercier LA, et al. Tetralogy of Fallot and aortic root disease. Expert Rev Cardiovasc Ther 2013;11(2):233–8.

63. Wijesekera VA, Kiess MC, Grewal J, et al. Aortic dissection in a patient with a dilated aortic root following tetralogy of Fallot repair. Int J Cardiol 2014;174(3):e33–4.

64. Nagy CD, Alejo DE, Corretti MC, et al. Tetralogy of Fallot and aortic root dilation: a long-term outlook. Pediatr Cardiol 2013;34(4):809–16.

65. Broberg CS, Aboulhosn J, Mongeon FP, et al. Prevalence of left ventricular systolic dysfunction in adults with repaired tetralogy of Fallot. Am J Cardiol 2011;107(8):1215–20.

66. Kempny A, Diller GP, Orwat S, et al. Right ventricular-left ventricular interaction in adults with tetralogy of Fallot: a combined cardiac magnetic resonance and echocardiographic speckle tracking study. Int J Cardiol 2012;154(3):259–64.

67. Norozi K, Wessel A, Alpers V, et al. Incidence and risk distribution of heart failure in adolescents and adults with congenital heart disease after cardiac surgery. Am J Cardiol 2006;97(8):1238–43.

68. Eindhoven JA, van den Bosch AE, Ruys TP, et al. N-terminal pro-B-type natriuretic peptide and its relationship with cardiac function in adults with congenital heart disease. J Am Coll Cardiol 2013; 62(13):1203–12.

69. Heng EL, Bolgor AP, Kempny A, et al. Neurohormonal activation and its relation to outcomes late after repair of tetralogy of Fallot. Heart 2015;101(6): 447–54.

70. Balci A, Drenthen W, Mulder BJ, et al. Pregnancy in women with corrected tetralogy of Fallot: occurrence and predictors of adverse events. Am Heart J 2011; 161(2):307–13.

71. Drenthen W, Pieper PG, Roos-Hesselink JW, et al. Outcome of pregnancy in women with congenital heart disease: a literature review. J Am Coll Cardiol 2007;49(24):2303–11.

72. Veldtman GR, Connolly HM, Grogan M, et al. Outcomes of pregnancy in women with tetralogy of Fallot. J Am Coll Cardiol 2004;44(1):174–80.

73. Khairy P, Ouyang DW, Fernandes SM, et al. Pregnancy outcomes in women with congenital heart disease. Circulation 2006;113(4):517–24.

74. Egidy Assenza G, Cassater D, Landzberg M, et al. The effects of pregnancy on right ventricular remodeling in women with repaired tetralogy of Fallot. Int J Cardiol 2013;168(3):1847–52.

Dextro-Transposition of the Great Arteries

Long-term Sequelae of Atrial and Arterial Switch

Christiane Haeffele, MD, MPH[a],*, George K. Lui, MD[a,b]

KEYWORDS

- Transposition of great arteries • Arterial switch • Atrial switch • Congenital heart disease

KEY POINTS

- Patients who have undergone the Mustard/Senning operation are at risk of heart failure, atrial arrhythmias, and sudden cardiac death that requires long-term follow-up.
- Compared with the Mustard/Senning operation, the long-term survival and event-free survival rates in the arterial switch operation (ASO) are superior, though these patients still require routine follow-up.
- Echocardiography is recommended in the long-term follow-up of both the atrial and arterial switch. For Mustard/Senning patients, evaluation of the systemic right ventricle and integrity of the baffle should be assessed. Coronary stenosis, neo-aortic regurgitation and branch pulmonary artery stenosis can be seen after ASO.
- Routine CT angiography or MRI is recommended in patients with D-TGA after atrial switch for patency of the baffles, baffle leak, and systemic right ventricular function.
- Chest pain or wall motion abnormalities should be evaluated promptly in the arterial switch patient, given the increased risk of coronary complications.

OVERVIEW

This article focuses on complete transposition of the great arteries, otherwise commonly referred to as dextro-transposition of the great arteries (D-TGA) and the 2 primary ways used to repair the lesion: the atrial switch procedure and the arterial switch operation (ASO).

TERMS

TGA is a congenital heart defect in which the aorta arises from the morphologic right ventricle (RV) and the pulmonary artery (PA) arises from the morphologic left ventricle.

In the term *D-TGA*, the *D* refers to either the ventricular loop or the spatial relationship of the aortic and pulmonary arteries. For this article, D-TGA represents situs solitus, atrioventricular (AV) concordance, and ventriculo-arterial discordance.

Atrial switch is the creation of an atrial baffle to direct venous flow to the contralateral AV valve and ventricle.

Senning operation is an atrial switch operation that creates a baffle out of autologous tissue.

[a] Division of Cardiovascular Medicine, Department of Medicine, Stanford University School of Medicine, 300 Pasteur Drive, Stanford, CA 94304, USA; [b] Division of Pediatric Cardiology, Department of Pediatrics, Stanford University School of Medicine, 725 Welch Road, Palo Alto, Stanford, CA 94304, USA
* Corresponding author. 300 Pasteur Avenue, Stanford, CA 94305.
E-mail address: haeffele@stanford.edu

Cardiol Clin 33 (2015) 543–558
http://dx.doi.org/10.1016/j.ccl.2015.07.012
0733-8651/15/$ – see front matter © 2015 Elsevier Inc. All rights reserved.

Mustard operation is an atrial switch operation that creates a baffle out of synthetic material.

ASO is surgery that restores normal physiologic relationships in D-TGA. The PA and aorta are transected above the sinuses and reimplanted to positions to restore normal blood flow. The coronary arteries are also detached and sewn onto the neo-aorta.

Complete Transposition of the Great Arteries

The most common form of TGA is a cyanotic heart lesion. The prevalence of TGA is between 20 and 30 per 100,000 live births.[1] It composes approximately between 5% and 7% of all congenital heart disease.[1]

In the most common form of transposition, also known as complete transposition or D-TGA, there is ventriculo-arterial discordance. Thus, the aorta arises from the morphologic RV and the PA arises from the morphologic left ventricle (LV), which creates 2 parallel circuits for blood flow. In one circuit, the deoxygenated blood returns via systemic venous return to the right atrium, travels to the RV, and then flows out to the body via the aorta. In the other circuit, the oxygenated blood returns from the lungs to the left atrium, flows into the LV, and then flows back to the lungs via the PA (**Fig. 1**A).

Because the blood runs in 2 parallel circuits, there must be a communication between the circuits to sustain life in the form of an atrial septal defect, ventricular septal defect (VSD), or patent ductus arteriosus. These communications allow mixing of oxygenated and deoxygenated blood.

If D-TGA is present with no other cardiac abnormalities, it is called *simple TGA*. If there are other anomalies present, that is, a VSD or LV outflow tract obstruction (LVOTO), this is often referred to as *complex TGA*. VSDs and LVOTO occur in approximately 50% and 25% of patients with D-TGA, respectively.[1]

Congenitally Corrected Transposition of the Great Arteries

There is another form of TGA: levo-TGA (L-TGA). Most patients with L-TGA also have ventricular inversion; thus, the commonly applied term for L-TGA is congenitally corrected TGA. In this defect, in addition to the transposed great arteries, there is ventricular inversion, with the LV receiving inflow from the right atrium and the RV receiving inflow from the left atrium. In this circuit, deoxygenated blood returns via the right atrium, goes into the morphologic LV, and then goes to the lungs through the PA. Once the blood is oxygenated in the lungs, it flows back into the left atrium through the pulmonary veins, into the morphologic RV, and then out to the aorta. Because there is also ventricular inversion, along

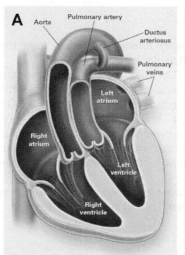 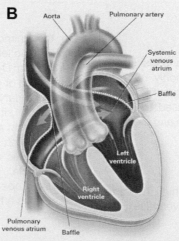 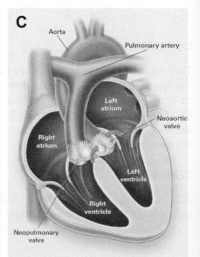

Fig. 1. (*A*) Diagram of typical TGA. The atria and ventricles are in their usual position, but the aorta arises anteriorly from the RV and the PA arises posteriorly from the LV. (*B*) Diagram of atrial-level repair for TGA. Both the Mustard and Senning repairs create a baffle within the atria that redirects the caval blood to the mitral valve and the pulmonary venous blood to the tricuspid valve. (*C*) Diagram of arterial repair for TGA. The PA and the aorta are excised from their respective positions and resewn into their correct anatomic positions. The coronary arteries are also excised and sewn onto the neo-aorta. (*From* Brickner ME, Hillis LD, Lange RA. Congenital heart disease in adults. Second of two parts. N Engl J Med 2000;342(13):338; with permission.)

with the transposed arteries, this anatomic double switch creates physiologically normal blood flow through the body. Thus, these patients are typically asymptomatic at birth and do not require early surgical intervention. Complications arise later in life, often in the form of heart failure, as the systemic RV is incapable of handling systemic-level pressure and volume loads over time.

The remainder of this article focuses exclusively on D-TGA and the long-term sequelae of the 2 surgical repairs used to correct the parallel circulations.

SURGICAL PALLIATION
Blalock-Hanlon

The earliest surgical palliation of D-TGA began with Drs Alfred Blalock and C. Rollins Hanlon who developed an atrial septectomy technique with Vivien Thomas in 1948.[2] The atrial septectomy allowed unrestricted mixing of blood at the atrial level; thus, cyanosis improved and infants survived longer.

Rashkind

The Blalock-Hanlon operation was later replaced with the Rashkind balloon septostomy in 1966.[3] In this procedure, a wire is advanced across the atrial septum in the catheterization laboratory. A balloon is inflated on the left atrial side and retracted into the right atrium, creating a hole in the septum to allow mixing of blood. Both procedures only palliate the child or infant, as patients remain cyanotic and high mortality is reported in infants after several weeks.[4]

Mustard/Senning Operation: the Atrial Switch

Dr Ake Senning, using flaps of autologous atrial tissue to make the atrial baffle, performed the first atrial switch operation in 1957.[4] Using this technique, Senning created a conduit that routes the deoxygenated blood from the superior vena cava (SVC) and inferior vena cava (IVC) into the mitral valve and LV. Pulmonary venous (oxygenated) blood then returned to the tricuspid valve, flowed into the morphologic RV, and then out the aorta to the body. Dr William Mustard, by contrast, excised the atrial septum and created a baffle out of prosthetic material in 1963 (see **Fig. 1**B). The net result of either operation is to restore a physiologically normal circulation, though with anatomic abnormalities in the form of venous redirection in the atria and with the morphologic RV as the systemic pump and the morphologic LV as the pulmonary pump.

Either atrial switch operation may be preceded by a Rashkind balloon septostomy or Blalock-Hanlon procedure.

Arterial Switch Operation

Unlike the atrial switch operation, the ASO restores both normal physiologic blood flow and the normal Ventriculo-arterial relationships of the heart. The aorta and PA are transected above the sinuses and attached to the correct ventricles. The PAs are translocated anterior to the aorta, which is known as the LeCompte maneuver. The coronary arteries are also detached and reimplanted on the neo-aorta (see **Fig. 1**C).

Before development of the ASO, early surgical attempts included a rudimentary form of the ASO and rerouting the pulmonary venous flow. Despite these palliative attempts, patients did not live for significant periods of time. Cardiopulmonary bypass was in its early stages, and the first attempts at the arterial switch were unable to successfully reimplant the coronary arteries. Dr Adib Jatene and colleagues[5] performed the first successful ASO in 1975.

Over time, the arterial switch has replaced the atrial switch as the preferred surgical intervention for D-TGA.[4] Although there are associated complications with each repair, the ASO has become the preferred intervention because of the restoration of normal cardiovascular anatomic and physiologic relationships (**Fig. 2**).

Data in the adult survivors of this operation are only now forthcoming, as the ASO became the predominant correction for D-TGA in the late 1980s once mortality rates decreased with improved surgical technique.[4]

Mustard/Senning Takedown with Arterial Switch

For some atrial switch patients in whom the RV is failing, a takedown of the Mustard/Senning operation with an arterial switch has been done. The procedure was first performed by Dr Roger Mee[6] in 1981 and may be considered in a highly selected group of Mustard/Senning patients. The goal of the operation is to restore the anatomic and physiologic relationships in hopes of mitigating the complications related to the systemic RV. Converting patients from a Mustard/Senning to an arterial switch is a multistep process in most patients that includes preparation of the morphologic LV for a new role of performing systemic work.

In most patients, LV training is done by placing a PA band to create an outflow obstruction to hypertrophy the LV and increase LV pressure. In rare

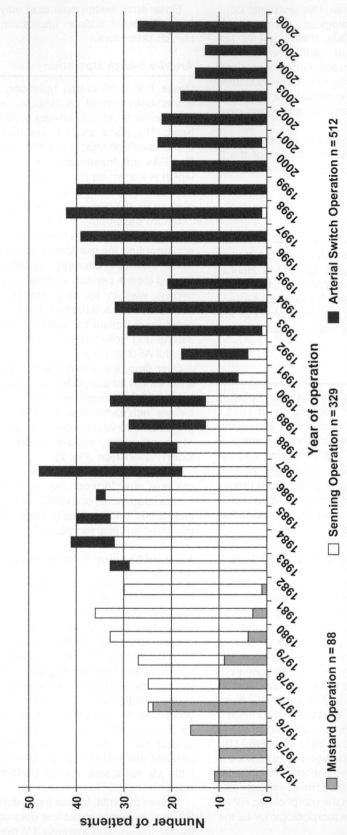

Fig. 2. Overall surgical trend from 1974 to 2006 for repair of TGA. The Mustard operation was the primary repair early on but was gradually replaced by the Senning procedure as surgical technique improved. The arterial switch had high mortality rates early on as the technique was introduced but, with experience, replaced the Senning as the operation of choice for D-TGA. Improvement in long-term survival after hospital discharge but not in freedom from reoperation after the change from atrial to arterial switch for transposition of the great arteries. J Thorac Cardiovasc Surg 2009;137(2):349; with permission.) (*From* Horer J, Schrieber C, Cleuziou J, et al.

patients, a naturally occurring outflow obstruction may already exist, obviating a surgical band. Before takedown of the atrial switch and ASO, there are multiple means of assessing the LV readiness to support the systemic circulation.[7] Successful ASO has been achieved in a select group of patients, but conditioning the LV remains a challenge.[7]

Pulmonary Artery Band

Use of the PA band has been used as a treatment of patients with D-TGA undergoing atrial switch by itself to help treat the failing systemic RV.[8,9] When the RV begins to fail, it dilates and the septum shifts toward the LV, increasing the amount of tricuspid regurgitation. By increasing LV pressure, the PA band moves the septum back to a more normal anatomic position and the tricuspid regurgitation is reduced (**Fig. 3**). Therefore, the PA band may improve RV function and tricuspid regurgitation and serve as a bridge to transplantation.[10]

LONG-TERM OUTCOMES
Survival

Atrial switch

After the Senning or Mustard procedure, the RV remains the systemic pump. Over time, studies have shown that the anatomy of this ventricle cannot sustain the demands of the systemic circulation and gradually fails.[11–14] Long-term complications include RV failure, atrial arrhythmias, and sudden cardiac death. In one series, Mustard patients had an 80% survival rate at the 20-year follow-up and 68% at 39 years.[11] Survival free of events, including heart transplantation, arrhythmias, reintervention, or heart failure, was only 19% at 39 years.

Some studies suggest Senning patients survive longer. In another series that compared Senning versus Mustard outcomes, Senning patients fared better at 15 years follow-up compared with their Mustard counterparts, with 94% and 77% survival rates, respectively.[12] However, the survival rate without complication or need for reintervention decreases significantly in adulthood. Most of these patients will require involved, long-term follow-up. In both groups, most late deaths were sudden.

Arterial switch

Emerging data from ASO indicate more favorable survival rates and decreased arrhythmia burden relative to the Mustard/Senning procedure. Initially, the ASO had a significant perioperative mortality rate between 5% and 20%.[15] Many of these poor outcomes were caused by complications associated with coronary transfer. With time and experience, the mortality rates of the ASO have decreased to less than 5%.[15–17] In one of the largest studies to date, 1200 patients with D-TGA were followed after ASO (**Table 1**). Survival at 10 and 15 years was 88%, and freedom from reintervention was 82% at 10 and 15 years. Reoperation was done in less than 10% of the patients, mostly for pulmonic stenosis[18] (**Table 2**).

Heart Failure

Atrial switch

RV failure and tricuspid regurgitation are both long-term complications in Mustard/Senning patients. The tricuspid regurgitation is often functional, resulting from progressive dilation of the RV,[9] which results in poor coaptation of the tricuspid valve leaflets. The mechanism of the RV

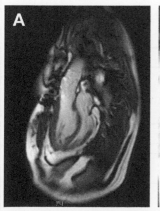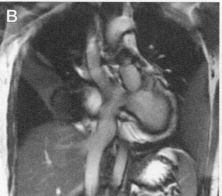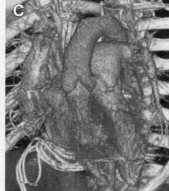

Fig. 3. MRI reconstructions of a patient with TGA with a Mustard repair following placement of a PA band. (*A*) Sagittal MRI view of PA band in a Mustard patient. (*B*) Coronal MRI view of PA band on Mustard patient; (*C*) Three-dimensional reconstruction of Mustard patient with a PA band.

Table 1
Monitoring of patients with D-TGA in the outpatient setting

	Baseline	Frequency
History and physical examination	√	Yearly[40]
EKG	√	Yearly[31,40]
Holter monitoring	√	Yearly (atrial switch patients)[31] Clinically indicated (arterial switch patients)[31]
Chest radiograph	√	Clinically indicated
Transthoracic echocardiogram	√	Yearly
MRI/CT[a]	√	Every 3–5 y (atrial switch patients)[40] Clinically indicated (arterial switch patients)[40]
Exercise testing[b]	√	Clinically indicated[31]
Cardiac catheterization		Clinically indicated[31,40]

[a] MRI contraindicated in patients with pacemakers. CT may be substituted to evaluate patients, though should be performed on limited basis because of radiation exposure.
[b] Consider cardiopulmonary exercise test for atrial switch patients and exercise or pharmacologic stress test for arterial switch patients.

failure is incompletely understood, but one study using late gadolinium enhancement with cardiac MRI showed evidence of myocardial fibrosis in the RV of patients with D-TGA. The fibrosis occurred more frequently in patients with documented syncope.[19] Myocardial perfusion studies and stress echocardiography have also demonstrated impaired ventricular function and perfusion defects during exercise suggestive of coronary insufficiency,[20,21] even in patients much less than 30 years of age.

Pulmonary hypertension occurs in approximately 5% to 7% of patients with D-TGA who underwent an atrial switch.[22,23] Late repair and elevated pulmonary pressures soon after surgical repair increase the risk for developing pulmonary vascular

disease.[22,23] Obstruction in the pulmonary venous pathway may cause pulmonary hypertension and should be evaluated as a possible cause.[9] Age of presentation tends to be decades after the initial repair,[23] but patients do seem to improve with use of pulmonary vasodilator therapy.[23]

Arrhythmia

Atrial switch
Rhythm issues in atrial switch patients range from sinus node dysfunction to atrial and ventricular tachyarrhythmias.[24–30]

Sinus node dysfunction becomes highly prevalent in the atrial switch population with time. In one series, only 40% of Mustard patients had a

Table 2
Summary of atrial versus arterial switch complications

Atrial Switch		Arterial Switch	
Complication	**Method of evaluation**	**Complication**	**Method of evaluation**
Baffle leak	TTE with saline contrast study, TEE[40]	**Coronary artery stenosis**	CT angiography, stress test (exercise or pharmacologic), catheterization[40]
Baffle stenosis	Cardiac MRI, catheterization, TTE[40]	**PA stenosis**	Cardiac MRI, CT angiography
RV failure	TTE, cardiac MRI[40]	**Neo-aortic root dilation**	TTE, cardiac MRI, CT angiography
Tricuspid regurgitation	TTE, cardiac MRI[40]	**Neo-aortic regurgitation**	TTE, cardiac MRI
Arrhythmias	Annual rhythm monitoring[31]	—	—

Abbreviations: TEE transesophageal echocardiography; TTE transthoracic echocardiography.

functional sinus node at the 20-year follow-up.[25] Senning patients have a slightly lower rate of sinus node dysfunction.[26] The high rates of sinus node dysfunction in the atrial switch population are presumed to be secondary to fibrosis from the surgical scars or damage to the sinus node artery during surgery.[24] Patients will often present in a junctional rhythm and are at increased risk of atrial arrhythmias. Approximately 10% of patients needed a pacemaker at the 20-year follow-up.[25]

Atrial flutter, also referred to as intra-atrial reentrant tachycardia, occurs frequently in this population with time. At the 20-year follow-up, nearly a third of patients have experienced an episode of atrial flutter.[25,26] The scar lines from the formation of the atrial baffle likely create the atrial flutter pathways.[26]

Sudden death, presumably from an arrhythmia, is the most frequent cause of late death in Mustard/Senning patients.[25,26] Occurrence of atrial flutter or atrial fibrillation is a predictor for sudden cardiac death.[27,28] Implantable cardioverter defibrillator (ICD) is indicated in atrial switch patients for secondary prevention when a reversible cause is not revealed.[31] However, indications for ICD placement in the case of primary prevention remain a challenge. In one study, there were 0.5% annual rates of appropriate shocks and 6.6% annual rates of inappropriate shocks.[30] One series documented a complication rate of almost 40%, indicating ICD placement in patients with D-TGA who have undergone an atrial switch must be done with caution.[30] Attempts to risk stratify which patients will benefit from ICD placement have been inconclusive. Patients with an older age at the time of repair, repairs done in the early surgical era for atrial switch, and onset of atrial arrhythmias all have increased risk for sudden death.[29]

Arterial switch
Late arrhythmias are unusual but can occur at a frequency of 2.4% to 9.6%.[32] Atrial arrhythmias often present in the setting of residual RV outflow tract obstruction or myocardial dysfunction. Sudden death has been reported in this population but generally isolated to the first few years after ASO and related to coronary obstruction with myocardial ischemia or infarction.[32]

ANATOMIC COMPLICATIONS
Atrial Switch

Baffle obstruction and leak is not uncommon. Small baffle leaks are best imaged by a saline contrast study performed during a transthoracic or transesophageal echocardiogram.[33] Much like a saline contrast study done for a patent foramen ovale, if agitated saline is injected into the venous system and seen within a few beats of the heart in the systemic RV, it indicates a baffle leak (**Fig. 4**). Small baffle leaks may lead to a cerebrovascular event via paradoxic embolus if tachyarrhythmias or a pacemaker/ICD lead is present.[9] Large shunts should be closed percutaneously or by surgery.[9]

Nonechocardiographic imaging (computed tomography [CT], MRI, catheterization) has a higher

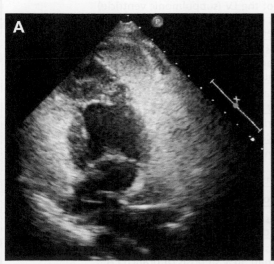
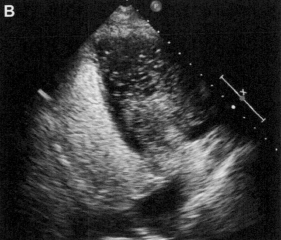

Fig. 4. Saline contrast study to evaluate for baffle leak in a Mustard/Senning patient. (*A*) Negative saline contrast study, apical 4-chamber view. Saline contrast injected into the subpulmonary LV. No bubbles visualized in the systemic RV. (*B*) Positive saline contrast study in a patient with TGA with dextrocardia, apical 4-chamber view. Saline contrast injected into the subpulmonary LV. Multiple bubbles visualized in the systemic RV.

sensitivity for detecting baffle obstruction than the conventional transthoracic echocardiogram (88% vs 16% by pulse-wave Doppler).[34,35] Obstruction of the SVC arm of the baffle is more common than IVC baffle obstruction.[9] Rates of baffle stenosis have been shown to be as high as 44%, which has implications for placement of a transvenous pacemaker, which many of these patients require later in life[34] (**Table 3**).

Arterial Switch

Coronary artery stenosis

Patients who undergo the arterial switch procedure are at risk for coronary artery complications, both in the immediate postoperative period and later in life. The pattern of coronary events in ASO survivors seems to be bimodal, as there is a resurgence of cardiac events in long-term survivors. In one series, 1198 patients were followed after discharge from their ASO. Coronary event-free initial survival was 93% at 59 months and 88% at 15 years.[33] In another series, of the patients that received catheterizations during follow-up, 8% had coronary lesions.[17]

Patients with single coronary patterns and intramural coronary arteries have the highest rates of mortality as seen in a meta-analysis.[36] Myocardial perfusion scans have also revealed perfusion defects.[37] It is not yet clear if these defects were acquired at the time of the original repair or indicate inadequate myocardial perfusion following coronary reimplantation with the ASO.

Although this population remains quite young to date, ASO patients may be at increased risk for coronary artery disease and peripheral vascular disease.[38] Proximal intimal thickening and abnormalities in coronary flow reserve have been seen in these patients following their surgical repair and reimplantation of the coronaries. Thus far, the population has not seemed to have significant cardiovascular events from these early changes; but how it will affect long-term outcomes remains to be seen. Some have recommended routine coronary angiography or CT to evaluate the coronary arteries, but current data do not support routine use.

Neo-aortic root dilation

The neo-aorta remains a site of vulnerability in arterial switch patients. The anastomosis site and new location of the aorta can be associated with either coarctation or dilation.[14] Reposition of the aorta during surgery may be complicated by compression either from the posterior displacement of the arch or from the nearby bronchus.[14] The neo-aortic root also seems to enlarge significantly in some patients over time (**Fig. 5**). In one

Table 3
Indications for intervention on complications

Complications of Atrial Switch	Indication for Intervention
Baffle leak	• Left to right shunt with Qp:Qs >1.5 • Dilation of the LV (subpulmonic ventricle) • Paradoxic embolus • Pacemaker/ICD (increased risk of paradoxic embolus)
Baffle stenosis	• Symptoms • Pacemaker/ICD implantation and stenosis prevents placement of pacemaker leads
Atrial flutter	• Catheter ablation if recurrent symptomatic or drug refractory
Severe tricuspid regurgitation	• Primary tricuspid valve disease • PA band can be considered as bridge to transplantation
Failing RV	• Heart transplant • PA band • Atrial switch takedown and ASO
Complications of Arterial Switch	**Indication for Intervention**
Coronary artery stenosis	• Symptoms • Evidence of ischemia by exercise testing or cardiac markers
PA stenosis	• Symptoms • Greater than 50% stenosis of branch PA • RV systolic pressure >50 mm Hg
Neo-aortic regurgitation	• Symptoms • Evidence of LV dysfunction or progressive LV dilation

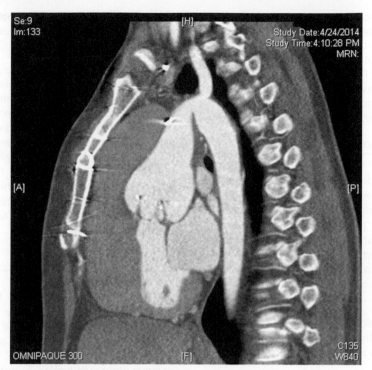

Fig. 5. MRI image of aortic root dilation in a patient with TGA following ASO.

series, more than half of the patients studied had aortic root enlargement more than 3 standard deviations greater than the expected normal value at 10 years.[39] Patients are also at risk of aortic regurgitation, though in a large longitudinal series of 1200 patients, only 10% of patients had significant aortic regurgitation. Of the patients with aortic dilation and valve regurgitation, only 1.1% required surgical intervention up to 15 years after repair.[17]

Pulmonary artery stenosis
Supravalvar pulmonary stenosis or branch pulmonary artery stenosis are frequent complications after ASO,[16] with reintervention needed in up to one-third of the patients in some series. Stenosis occurs at the level of the pulmonary trunk from scarring of the anastomotic site or prior history of PA banding. However, the traction from the Lecompte maneuver often results in more frequent stenosis at the bifurcation of the pulmonary trunk. These complications are often amenable to percutaneous balloon dilation and stent but sometimes require surgical palliation.

CLINICAL MANAGEMENT
For All Patients with Dextro-Transposition of the Great Arteries Patients

Per the 2008 American College of Cardiology (ACC) and American Heart Association's (AHA)

"Guidelines for the Management of Adults with Congenital Heart Disease,"[40] all repaired patients with D-TGA should be seen annually by a cardiologist with expertise in adult congenital heart disease.[40] Patients who are symptomatic should be seen more frequently.

Physical Examination

Atrial switch
The most common problems associated with an atrial switch repair are baffle complications and failure of the systemic RV. With a baffle stenosis, the superior limb is most commonly affected at 37% to 44%.[34] Patients with stenosis of the SVC baffle may present with head edema, flushing, and swelling in the arms but are often asymptomatic because of venous collaterals, such as the azygous vein. Inferior baffle stenosis may cause leg edema, hepatomegaly, and ascites. Failure of the systemic RV will present with heart failure symptoms, including exercise intolerance and/or pulmonary edema in acute situations. With auscultation, a murmur may indicate progressive tricuspid regurgitation or subpulmonary obstruction. A new fixed, split S2 may indicate pulmonary hypertension.[40]

Arterial switch
Symptoms should be elicited, with particular attention to exercise intolerance or chest pain. Exercise intolerance could indicate pulmonary

stenosis or coronary artery insufficiency, particularly if chest pain or pressure occurs with exertion. During auscultation, the clinician should evaluate for the presence of neo-aortic regurgitation or pulmonic stenosis. If PA stenosis is present in severe form, patients may have evidence of right-sided heart failure, including lower extremity edema and hepatomegaly.

Electrocardiogram

Atrial switch

Yearly electrocardiograms (EKGs) with the annual visit are recommended to monitor for the known progressive conduction disturbances seen in Mustard/Senning patients. Sinus node dysfunction is common, and patients will often present in a junctional rhythm. The EKG will typically show RV hypertrophy and right axis deviation, given that the RV is the systemic ventricle.

Arterial switch

Yearly EKGs should be performed in ASO patients. Changes suggestive of ischemia can sometimes be seen, either at rest or with exercise testing.[40]

Chest Radiograph

Atrial switch

Typical appearance of atrial switch patients will include the appearance of sternal wires. With progressive heart failure, the heart border may appear enlarged. Phrenic nerve injury was common in early Mustard repairs,[24] so right diaphragm elevation may be present. A pacemaker may be present, with leads present in the atrium and subpulmonic LV.

Arterial switch

Chest radiographs in ASO patients will have sternal wires but will otherwise be unremarkable.

Stress Testing

Atrial switch

Cardiopulmonary exercise test in atrial switch patients is reduced, though many patients will be asymptomatic. Mustard/Senning patients have reduced peak oxygen consumption (Vo_2) compared with age-matched cohorts. The proposed mechanism for the overall lower Vo_2 peaks in these patients is attributed to an inability to augment RV filling during exercise because of abnormal ventricular filling from the atrial baffle pathways and chronotropic incompetence.[41] Peak oxygen consumption (Vo_2) testing in Mustard/Senning patients revealed that a peak Vo_2 of 52.3% or less or a minute ventilation–carbon dioxide production relationship (VE/VCO$_2$ slope) slope of 35.4 or greater was predictive for a higher 4-year risk of death or emergency cardiac-related hospital admission.[13] Vo_2 testing may help risk stratify the patients at higher risk of death over the next 4 years.

Arterial switch

Exercise or pharmacologic stress testing may be used to assess for myocardial ischemia or infarction in patients after ASO. It is the preferred modality for physiologic assessment of obstructed coronary arteries. Stress testing can be performed with echocardiography, single-photon emission CT, PET, or cardiac MRI. Guidelines have recommended that all adults should have at least one evaluation of the coronary arteries after ASO.[40] However, the modality of choice among catheterization, MRI/CT angiography, and stress testing remains unknown.

Rhythm Monitors

Atrial switch

The Pediatric and Congenital Electrophysiology Society/Heart Rhythm Society 2014 consensus statement recommends annual rhythm monitors in asymptomatic patients after atrial switch repair to evaluate for the presence of atrial arrhythmias or sinus node dysfunction. Symptoms can be evaluated with clinically appropriate ambulatory monitors.

Arterial switch

Patients after ASO have not been demonstrated to have a significant arrhythmia risk unless there are residual hemodynamic abnormalities. Therefore, guidelines have not recommended routine surveillance. Cardiac monitoring may be useful in symptomatic patients.

Echocardiography

Atrial switch

Echocardiography allows for an assessment of systemic RV function, degree of tricuspid regurgitation, and integrity of the baffle (**Fig. 6**). Per the current ACC/AHA's guidelines, the study should be performed at a regional adult congenital heart disease center.[40] Obtaining saline contrast study during the transthoracic echocardiogram is useful to evaluate for baffle leak[40] (see **Fig. 4**). If unable to visualize the baffle or baffle leak adequately by transthoracic echocardiogram, transesophageal echocardiogram or MRI/CT can be useful. 3-dimensional echocardiography can also be used to better visualize the RV and systemic venous baffles, which is a complex structure and more difficult to see by conventional imaging (**Fig. 7**).

Arterial switch

Echocardiography is useful to evaluate for neo-aortic dilation, aortic regurgitation, supravalvar

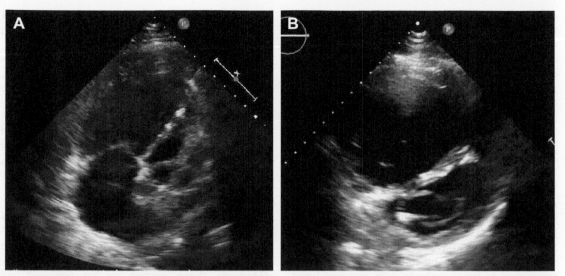

Fig. 6. Transthoracic echocardiogram. (*A*) Apical 4-chamber view, (*B*) short-axis view in a patient with TGA following Mustard repair. Note the enlarged systemic RV.

pulmonic stenosis, and branch pulmonary artery stenosis. Study should be done at a regional adult congenital heart disease center at least every 2 years.[40] In select patients, the PA anatomy may also be evaluated, although the PA and branches are often less well seen in the adult, as the PA is just below the sternum, which combined with scar tissue limits acoustic windows.

MRI/Computed Tomography

Atrial switch

MRI remains the best imaging modality to evaluate adult patients with D-TGA in which transthoracic windows may limit echocardiographic evaluation

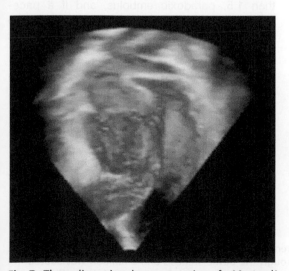

Fig. 7. Three-dimensional representation of a Mustard/ Senning patient.

of the prior repair. Biventricular function and detailed imaging of the baffle pathways are possible. Baffle leaks are not typically viewed well with MRI. CT may useful in either D-TGA patient population if patients cannot undergo MRI. Because many Mustard/Senning patients often have pacemakers or ICDs, they may require CT because of the inability to undergo MRI.

Arterial switch

Patients are prone to PA distortion, complications with the neo-aorta, and coronary artery stenosis. CT angiography provides superior spatial resolution to MRI for the evaluation of coronary arteries but is associated with radiation. MRI lacks the same resolution but adds functional information, including both ventricular and valvular function and flow. All ASO patients should have at least one evaluation of coronary artery patency.[40] The modality of choice remains a challenge.

MEDICAL MANAGEMENT
Atrial Switch

Optimal medical management for these patients, from both a heart failure and arrhythmia perspective, remains unclear. Studies on these patients for angiotensin-converting enzyme inhibitors do not indicate a favorable effect on survival, symptoms, or ventricular function, though studies have not necessarily had large enough numbers, high-risk patients, or long enough follow-up to know if there are groups of patients for whom there is benefit.[42] Beta blockers are also problematic, as Mustard and Senning patients are prone to sinus node dysfunction and AV block.[10,40] Nevertheless, despite the lack of data, the neurohormonal profiles of Mustard and Senning patients seem to be similar to that of patients with acquired heart disease. Current recommendations are to use conventional heart failure medications to treat patients with failing systemic RVs, as previous trials have not been powered sufficiently to determine efficacy.[43]

Arterial Switch

The ASO patient population is still quite young and to date has not required significant medical management. Should these patients manifest any valvular dysfunction or ventricular dysfunction, they should be managed with conventional therapies because they have normal anatomic relationships and would presumably have similar responses to those patients with acquired heart disease.

PREGNANCY
Atrial Switch

Patients with systemic RV are in the high-risk category for pregnancy and ideally should undergo a comprehensive evaluation at a center with expertise in adult congenital heart disease.[40] Women have increased risk for heart failure, arrhythmias, preeclampsia, and fetal complications when compared with a normal pregnancy.[44,45] In one series, 39 of the completed 49 pregnancies in 28 patients had complications, with arrhythmia being the most prevalent (22%).[46] Eleven of the 51 children were small for gestational age (22%). In another series, 16 women were followed for 28 completed pregnancies.[47] Six of the 16 women had a decline in their New York Heart Association functional class, and 2 did not return to their prepregnancy baseline following pregnancy. Four

women had a worsening of their systemic RV function, with 3 failing to recover function following delivery.[47]

If a woman has normal or mildly impaired systemic ventricular function and is asymptomatic, the maternal risk is likely acceptable to undergo pregnancy. Before delivery, she should have regular cardiology visits, a minimum of each trimester, with an echocardiogram to monitor the function of the RV. Vaginal delivery is generally favored if close obstetric and cardiology management is possible.[40]

Arterial Switch

Limited pregnancy data in the arterial switch population are available, as most of this population has only recently reached childbearing age. Generally, these women are low risk and can have vaginal deliveries.[44]

CATHETER-BASED INTERVENTION
Atrial Switch

Transcatheter intervention is the procedure of choice to alleviate baffle stenosis or baffle leaks if patients are symptomatic. Symptomatic baffle stenosis can be alleviated through the use of balloon dilation and stent placement in the baffle stenosis (**Fig. 8**). If a stenosis is not amenable to stenting, patients may require surgery.

Baffle leaks can also be addressed by transcatheter approach. Baffle leaks have been closed through the use of septal occluder devices. General indications for closure are as follows: presence of a left to right shunt, dilation of the subpulmonic ventricle, Qp:Qs greater than 1.5, paradoxic embolus, and if a pacemaker/ICD placement is desired. The presence of a pacemaker or ICD leads with a baffle leak

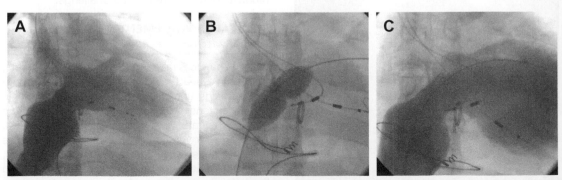

Fig. 8. (*A*) Injection into the inferior vena cava shows a stenosis in the inferior limb of baffle in a patient with TGA following an atrial switch. (*B*) A wire was advanced through the baffle stenosis and a balloon was dilated. (*C*) Following stent placement, injection into the inferior vena cava shows the inferior limb of the baffle stenosis to be improved.

present may increase the risk of a paradoxic embolus.

Arterial Switch

As mentioned, PA stenosis occurs in up to one-third of arterial switch patients and is a significant source of morbidity.[43] Neo-pulmonary valve stenosis after ASO is associated with growth failure of the valve annulus and is often associated with supravalvar pulmonary stenosis.[48] Peak incidence for reintervention occurs within the first year.[14] However, one large multicenter study showed that freedom from pulmonary stenosis was 95% at 1 year, 90% at 5 years, and 86% at 10 years, suggesting pulmonary stenosis may also develop long-term.[1] Catheter-based interventions, including ballooning and stenting, may relieve the obstruction.[49] Surgical patch augmentation of the branch PAs may be necessary in patients with anatomy not suitable for percutaneous intervention.

ELECTROPHYSIOLOGY
Atrial Switch

Many Mustard/Senning patients require pacemaker placement over time because of the high rate of sinus node dysfunction. Given the high rates of atrial tachyarrhythmias, patients also require a pacemaker to help facilitate medical treatment of the tachyarrhythmia. Placement of a transvenous pacemaker can prove challenging, as patients often will have stenosis of the SVC limb of their baffle. The atrial lead is placed in the systemic venous atrium. The ventricular lead is placed in the subpulmonic LV.[17] Patency of the baffle must be confirmed before placement.[17] If the patency of the SVC baffle is in question, epicardial pacing may be necessary.

Given the high rates of heart failure with the systemic RV, biventricular pacing has been explored in this population.[50] Limited data suggest that patients with D-TGA with a systemic RV may benefit from a biventricular pacing system. Of note, when considering biventricular pacing, the coronary sinus can drain to either side of the atrial baffle, into either the pulmonary venous atrium or the systemic venous atrium. Because the additional lead is usually placed in the coronary sinus, the anatomy of the coronary sinus must be identified before placing the lead. Alternatively, epicardial leads can be placed surgically for biventricular pacing if the coronary sinus anatomy is unfavorable.

Catheter ablation is generally indicated for patients with recurrent symptomatic or drug-refractory atrial arrhythmias. Mustard/Senning patients most commonly present with atrial flutter, which is specifically an intra-atrial reentrant tachycardia with a cavotricuspid isthmus-dependent reentry. As mentioned, the onset of atrial flutter is typically a poor prognostic sign in Mustard/Senning patients.

Traditional ablation procedures for Mustard/Senning patients are limited by the presence of the systemic venous baffles. Access to the common pulmonary venous atrium is difficult to reach from the systemic veins. Several institutions have performed transbaffle access during electrophysiology ablation procedures for atrial tachyarrhythmias.[51–53] This access has ranged from accessing the pulmonary venous atrium via a baffle leak or by direct baffle puncture. In patients who had transbaffle access and patients who had traditional ablation measures, there was a reduction in arrhythmia burden for both groups.[51] However, many of the patients with transbaffle access had a decline in their saturation level by 5% relative to their preprocedure baseline.[51] The coronary sinus must also be identified before ablation attempts to help with ablation. There is a high degree of success with electrophysiology ablation, but it can be complicated by complete heart block.[52,53] These procedures should be performed by electrophysiologists with congenital heart disease experience.

SURGICAL INTERVENTION
Atrial Switch

Surgical reintervention after an atrial switch procedure is rarely performed today with the advent of catheter-based interventions for baffle stenosis or leak. Other atrial switch complications include functional tricuspid regurgitation secondary to dilation of the systemic RV. Tricuspid valve repair or replacement may be considered in the setting of organic tricuspid valve disease or TR that may have resulted from a prior VSD closure. One series examined tricuspid valve repair and replacement in atrial switch patients and found a recurrence of TR in up to 40% of patients.[54] Other late surgical procedures include PA band and Mustard/Senning takedown and ASO. Finally, patients with systemic RV failure may ultimately require a ventricular assist device and/or transplantation.

Arterial Switch

Coronary stenosis following ASO is not uncommon. Both percutaneous coronary intervention and coronary artery bypass graft have been used to treat coronary stenoses.[55,56] In one series, of the late survivors, 5% had coronary lesions and 2% underwent coronary revascularization including stent placement and bypass.[56] Some patients may develop severe neo-aortic valve regurgitation, requiring surgical repair or replacement. Compared with the rates of pulmonic stenosis, the rates of significant neo-aortic regurgitation are significantly less. In one series, 9% of patients required a reoperation, mostly because of pulmonic stenosis. Although almost 10% of patients had grade II or greater aortic regurgitation at 15 years, only 1.1% of patients required an aortic valve intervention.[17]

SUMMARY

All patients with D-TGA should be followed by individuals with expertise in adult congenital heart disease. Regular imaging by echocardiography or advanced imaging, such as MRI/CT, is essential to evaluate the full anatomy and prior surgical repair in each patient. New symptoms or declining function on exercise tests should prompt a thorough investigation for underlying cause, particularly in patients with Mustard/Senning. Given that all patients with D-TGA are at risk for long-term sequelae from their original anatomy and subsequent repairs, thorough education should be provided and the need for long-term, regular medical care should be stressed.

REFERENCES

1. Gatzoulis MA, Webb GD, Daubeney PEF. Diagnosis and management of adult congenital heart disease. Edinburgh, Scotland: Churchill Livingstone; 2003.
2. Evans WN. The arterial switch operation before Jatene. Pediatr Cardiol 2009;30:119–24.
3. Rashkind WJ, Miller WW. Creation of an atrial septal defect without thoracotomy. JAMA 1966;196:173–5.
4. Konstantinov IE, Alexi-Meskishvili VV, Williams WG, et al. Atrial switch operation: past, present, and future. Ann Thorac Surg 2004;77(6):2250–8.
5. Jatene AD, Fontes VF, Paulista PP, et al. Successful anatomic correction of transposition of the great vessels. A preliminary report. Arq Bras Cardiol 1975;28(4):461–4.
6. Mee RB. Severe right ventricular failure after Mustard or Senning operation. Two stage repair: pulmonary artery banding and switch. J Thorac Cardiovasc Surg 1986;92:385–90.
7. Watanabe N, Mainwaring RD, Carrillo SA, et al. Left ventricular retraining and late arterial switch for d-transposition of the great arteries. Ann Thorac Surg 2015;99:1655–63.
8. Cools B, Brown SC, Louw J, et al. Pulmonary artery banding as 'open end' palliation of systemic right ventricles: an interim analysis. Eur J Cardiothorac Surg 2012;41(4):913–8.
9. Warnes CA. Transposition of the great arteries. Circulation 2006;114:2699–709.
10. Van Son JA, Reddy VM, Silverman NH, et al. Regression of tricuspid regurgitation after two-stage arterial switch operation for failing systemic ventricle after atrial inversion operation. J Thorac Cardiovasc Surg 1996;111:342–7.
11. Cuypers JA, Eindhoven JA, Slager MA, et al. The natural and unnatural history of the mustard procedure: long-term outcome up to 40 years. Eur Heart J 2014;35(25):1666–74.
12. Sarkar D, Bull C, Yates R, et al. Comparison of long-term outcomes of atrial repair of simple transposition with implications for a late arterial switch strategy. Circulation 1999;100:II-176–81.
13. Roos-Hesselink JW, Meijboom FJ, Spitaels SE, et al. Decline in ventricular function and clinical condition after mustard repair for transposition of the great arteries (a prospective study of 22-29 years). Eur Heart J 2004;25(14):1264–70.
14. Giardini AG. Ventilatory efficiency and aerobic capacity predict event-free survival in adults with atrial repair for complete transposition of the great arteries. J Am Coll Cardiol 2009;53(17):1548–55.
15. Mussatto K, Wernovsky G. Challenges facing the child, adolescent, and young adult after the arterial switch operation. Cardiol Young 2005;15(Suppl 1):111–21.
16. Khairy P, Clair M, Fernandes SM, et al. Cardiovascular outcomes after the arterial switch operation for d-transposition of the great arteries. Circulation 2013;127(3):331–9.
17. Tobler D, Williams WG, Jegatheeswaran A, et al. Cardiac outcomes in young adult survivors of the arterial switch operation for transposition of the great arteries. J Am Coll Cardiol 2010;56(1):58–64.
18. Losay J, Touchot A, Serraf A, et al. Late outcome after arterial switch operation for transposition of the great arteries. Circulation 2001;104:I-121–6.
19. Babu-Narayan SV, Goktekin O, Moon JC, et al. Late gadolinium enhancement cardiovascular magnetic resonance of the systemic right ventricle in adults with previous atrial redirection surgery for transposition of the great arteries. Circulation 2005;111(16):2091–8.
20. Lubiszewska B, Gosiewska E, Hoffman P, et al. Myocardial perfusion and function of the systemic right ventricle in patients after atrial switch procedure for complete transposition: long-term follow-up. J Am Coll Cardiol 2000;36(4):1365–70.
21. Li W, Hornung TS, Francis DP, et al. Relation of biventricular function quantified by stress echocardiography to cardiopulmonary exercise capacity in adults with mustard (atrial switch) procedure for transposition of the great arteries. Circulation 2004;110:1380–6.
22. Ebenroth ES, Hurwitz RA, Cordes TM. Late onset of pulmonary hypertension after successful mustard

surgery for d-transposition of the great arteries. Am J Cardiol 2000;85:127–30.

23. Yehya A, Lyle T, Pernetz MA, et al. Pulmonary arterial hypertension in patients with prior atrial switch procedure for d-transposition of great arteries (dTGA). Int J Cardiol 2010;143(3):271–5.

24. Oechslin EN, Harrison DA, Connelly MS, et al. Mode of death in adults with congenital heart disease. Am J Cardiol 2000;86:1111–6.

25. Gelatt M, Hamilton RM, McCrindle BW, et al. Arrhythmia and mortality after the mustard procedure: a 30-year single-center experience. J Am Coll Cardiol 1997;29(1):194–201.

26. Love BA, Mehta D, Fuster VF. Evaluation and management of the adult patient with transposition of the great arteries following atrial-level (Senning or Mustard) repair. Nat Clin Pract Cardiovasc Med 2008;5:454–67.

27. Kammeraad JAE, van Deurzen CH, Sreeram N, et al. Predictors of sudden cardiac death after mustard or Senning repair for transposition of the great arteries. J Am Coll Cardiol 2004;44(5):1095–102.

28. Chakrabarti S, Stuart AG. Terminal arrhythmia in a patient with Mustard's operation. Cardiol Young 2006;16:498–500.

29. Wheeler M, Grigg L, Zentner D. Can we predict sudden cardiac death in long-term survivors of atrial switch surgery for transposition of the great arteries? Congenit Heart Dis 2014;9(4):326–32.

30. Khairy P, Harris L, Landzberg MJ, et al. Sudden death and defibrillators in transposition of the great arteries with intra-atrial baffles: a multicenter study. Circ Arrhythm Electrophysiol 2008;1(4):250–7.

31. Khairy P, Van Hare GF, Balaji S, et al. PACES/HRS expert consensus on the recognition and management of arrhythmias in adults with CHD. Heart Rhythm 2014;11(10):e102–65.

32. Villafane J, Lantin-Hermoso MR, Bhatt AB, et al. D-transposition of the great arteries: the current era of the arterial switch operation. J Am Coll Cardiol 2014;64(5):498–511.

33. Kaulitz R, Stümper OF, Geuskens R, et al. Comparative values of the precordial and transesophageal approaches in the echocardiographic evaluation of atrial baffle function after an atrial correction procedure. Int J Cardiol 1990;28:299–307.

34. Bottega NA, Silversides CK, Oechslin EN, et al. Stenosis of the superior limp of the systemic venous baffle following a mustard procedure: an under-recognized problem. Int J Cardiol 2012; 154(1):32–7.

35. Legendre A, Losay J, Touchot-Koné A, et al. Coronary events after arterial switch operation for transposition of the great arteries. Circulation 2003; 108:II-186–90.

36. Pasquali S, Hasselblad V, Li JS, et al. Coronary artery pattern and outcome of arterial switch operation for transposition of the great arteries: a meta analysis. Circulation 2002;106(20):2575–80.

37. Vogel M, Smallhorn JF, Gilday D, et al. Assessment of myocardial perfusion in patients after the arterial switch operation. J Nucl Med 1991;32(2):237–41.

38. Lui GK, Fernandes S, McEhinney DB. Management of cardiovascular risk factors in adults with congenital heart disease. J Am Heart Assoc 2014;3: e001076.

39. Schwartz ML, Gauvreau K, del Nido P, et al. Long-term predictors of aortic root dilation and aortic regurgitation after arterial switch operation. Circulation 2004;110:II128–32.

40. Warnes CA, Williams RG, Bashore TM, et al. ACC/AHA 2008 guidelines for the management of adults with congenital heart disease: a report of the American College of Cardiology/American Heart Association Task Force on Practice Guidelines (Writing Committee to Develop Guidelines on the Management of Adults With Congenital Heart Disease). Circulation 2008;118(23):e714–833.

41. Derrick GP, Narang I, White PA, et al. Failure of stroke volume augmentation during exercise and dobutamine stress is unrelated to load-independent indexes of right ventricular performance after the mustard operation. Circulation 2000;102(19 Suppl 3):III154–9.

42. Hecter ST, Fredriksen PM, Liu P, et al. Angiotensin-converting enzyme inhibitors in adults after the mustard procedure. Am J Cardiol 2001;87:660–3.

43. Shaddy RE, Webb G. Applying heart failure guidelines to adult congenital heart disease patients. Expert Rev Cardiovasc Ther 2008;6(2):165–74.

44. Franklin WJ, Gandhi M. Congenital heart disease in pregnancy. Cardiol Clin 2012;30:383–94.

45. Hutter PA, Kreb DL, Mantel SF, et al. Twenty-five years' experience with the arterial switch operation. J Thorac Cardiovasc Surg 2002;124:790–7.

46. Drenthen W, Pieper PG, Ploeg M, et al. Risk of complications during pregnancy after Senning or mustard (atrial) repair of complete transposition of the great arteries. Eur Heart J 2005;26(23):2588–95.

47. Guedes A, Mercier LA, Leduc L, et al. Impact of pregnancy on the systemic right ventricle after a mustard operation for transposition of the great arteries. J Am Coll Cardiol 2004;44(2):433–7.

48. Nogi S, McCrindle BW, Boutin C, et al. Fate of the neopulmonary valve after the arterial switch operation in neonates. J Thorac Cardiovasc Surg 1998; 115:557–62.

49. Zeevi B, Keane JF, Perry SB, et al. Balloon dilation of postoperative right ventricular outflow obstructions. J Am Coll Cardiol 1989;14:401–8.

50. Dubin AM, Janousek J, Rhee E, et al. Resynchronization therapy in pediatric and congenital heart disease patients. J Am Coll Cardiol 2005;46(12): 2277–83.

51. Correa R, Sherwin ED, Kovach J, et al. Mechanism and ablation of arrhythmia following total cavopulmonary connection. Circ Arrhythm Electrophysiol 2015;8(2):318–25.

52. Kanter RJ, Papagiannis J, Carboni MP, et al. Radiofrequency catheter ablation of supraventricular tachycardia substrates after Mustard and Senning operations for d-transposition of the great arteries. J Am Coll Cardiol 2000;35:428–41.

53. Zrenner B, Dong J, Schreieck J, et al. Delineation of intra-atrial reentrant tachycardia circuits after mustard operation for transposition of the great arteries using biatrial electroanatomic mapping and entrainment mapping. J Cardiovasc Electrophysiol 2003;14:1302–10.

54. Scherptong RWC, Vliegen HW, Winter MM, et al. Tricuspid valve surgery in adults with a dysfunctional systemic right ventricle: repair or replace? Circulation 2009;119:1467–72.

55. El-Segaier M, Lundin A, Hochbergs B, et al. Late coronary complications after arterial switch operation and their treatment. Catheter Cardiovasc Interv 2010;76(7):1027–32.

56. Raisky O, Bergoend E, Agnoletti G, et al. Latecoroncoronary artery lesions after neonatal arterial switch operation: results of surgical coronary revascularization. Eur J Cardiothorac Surg 2007;31:894–8.

Fontan Repair of Single Ventricle Physiology
Consequences of a Unique Physiology and Possible Treatment Options

Anitha S. John, MD, PhD

KEYWORDS

- Single ventricle • Fontan • Hepatic dysfunction • Protein losing enteropathy • Heart failure

KEY POINTS

- Understand Fontan physiology.
- Identify Fontan related long-term complications.
- Design an individualized treatment plan.

INTRODUCTION

The Fontan operation is a unique strategy that attempts to create a circulation in series in a patient with single ventricle physiology.[1] Fontan physiology relies on nonpulsatile, passive flow of blood though the pulmonary circulation. Elevation of central venous pressure, elevated pulmonary vascular resistance (PVR), systolic and diastolic dysfunction, and chronic cyanosis can contribute to the phenotype of the "failing Fontan." As the causes of low cardiac output in a patient after the Fontan operation are multifold, treatment plans need to be individualized based on understanding the physiology and the patient's clinical picture. This review provides a summary of Fontan physiology, long-term complications, and potential treatment strategies.

SINGLE VENTRICLE EPIDEMIOLOGY, ANATOMY, AND PHYSIOLOGY

Functional single ventricle anatomy can also result from the inability to septate 2 well formed ventricular chambers.[2,3] These subtypes include, but are

not limited to, double inlet atrioventricular (AV) connections, valvular atresia or severe stenosis, and unbalanced AV septal defect. All are associated with a single ventricular cavity, but functional single ventricle anatomy can also result from the inability to septate 2 well-formed ventricular chambers. Given the heterogeneity of the anatomic subtypes, the prevalence of disease can be difficult to determine. Recent data from Marelli and colleagues[4] examining the population in Quebec in 2010 showed a prevalence ratio of univentricular heart to be 0.15 in 1000 in children and 0.05 in 1000 in adults. Hypoplastic left heart syndrome, the most common variant of univentricular heart, had a prevalence ratio of 0.09 in 1000 in children and 0.03 in 1000 in adults.[4]

The clinical presentation and physiology depend on the underlying heart defects; specifically, the presence of outflow tract obstruction, AV valve obstruction or regurgitation, and anomalous venous return determine the type of palliative procedure needed to stabilize the infant. In general, intracardiac mixing across an atrial septal defect and shunting of blood through a patent ductus arteriosus is needed for survival.

Financial Disclosure: The authors have no relevant financial disclosures.
Division of Cardiology, Children's National Medical Center, George Washington University, 111 Michigan Avenue Northwest, WW 3rd Floor, Washington, DC 20010, USA
E-mail address: anjohn@cnmc.org

cardiology.theclinics.com

Directionality of blood flow across the patent ductus arteriosus is determined by the degree and type of outflow tract obstruction. In the case of hypoplastic left heart syndrome, a patent atrial septum is needed for adequate delivery of oxygenated blood in addition to right-to-left flow across a patent ductus arteriosus to maintain systemic outflow. The goal of initial palliative surgery is to provide stable sources of both pulmonary and systemic blood flow with the eventual goal of separating deoxygenated venous return from oxygenated systemic output.

ANATOMIC AND PHYSIOLOGIC CONSIDERATIONS OF THE FONTAN OPERATION

First described in 1971 by Fontan and Baudet, the Fontan procedure attempts to circumvent the need for a subpulmonary ventricle by redirecting systemic venous return from the superior and inferior vena cava directly to the pulmonary arteries.[1] The classic Fontan operation involved a valved conduit from the right atrium to pulmonary artery, attempting to use the right atrium as a pump to the pulmonary arteries. This evolved to the classic Fontan, which involved a direct anastomosis of the right atrium to the pulmonary artery (**Fig. 1**A). Over time, the right atrium became severely dilated and modifications were proposed to improve hemodynamics and decrease the incidence of arrhythmias. In 1987, de Leval described creating an intraatrial tunnel using the right atrial posterior wall and an end-to-side anastomosis of the superior vena cava to the right pulmonary artery (see **Fig. 1**B).[5] This was followed by the development of an entirely extracardiac

conduit directing caval flow to the pulmonary arteries (see **Fig. 1**C).[6] In the newer modifications, a fenestration is often created in the Fontan baffle be creating a small opening between the Fontan pathway and the atrium, allowing for right to left shunting.[7] This shunting allows for augmentation of cardiac output in the early postoperative period, although this is in exchange for the cyanosis that results from the right-to-left shunt. Assessment can be performed as the patient ages to determine candidacy for fenestration closure.[8]

The Fontan operation produces a state of chronic low cardiac output.[9] The Fontan operation relies on nonpulsatile, passive flow of caval blood to the pulmonary arteries. Because there is not a subpulmonary ventricle, the circulation relies on low pulmonary pressures and low PVR. Forward flow through the pulmonary vasculature depends on a differential between the central venous pressure and left atrial pressure. The reasons for progression to the "failing Fontan" physiology are multifold and extend beyond systemic systolic ventricular dysfunction. Caval pressures and the nonpulsatile flow to the pulmonary vascular bed result in chronically elevated central venous pressure, which causes progressive hepatic dysfunction in addition to decreased cardiac output.[10] Increases in pulmonary pressures and PVR only compound these effects as does diastolic dysfunction. Elevation of ventricular end-diastolic pressure can not only cause impaired ventricular filling, but also impairs forward flow through the Fontan baffle and pulmonary arteries. Ventricular systolic dysfunction can occur, but frequently patients with Fontan failure have preserved ventricular systolic function.

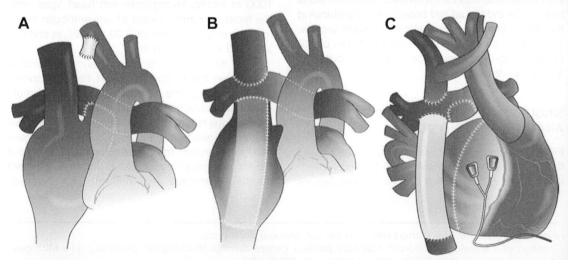

Fig. 1. Variations of the Fontan operation. (*A*) Modified classic right atrium to pulmonary artery Fontan. (*B*) Lateral tunnel Fontan. (*C*) Extracardiac conduit (with extracardiac pacemaker leads). (*From* Khairy P, Poirier N, Mercier L. Univentricular heart. Circulation 2007;115:804; with permission.)

A key component to the development of end-organ system manifestations and long-term cardiac failure is the inability to augment cardiac output during exercise.[11] With a normal biventricular circulation, cardiac output is augmented by 40–50% though increased pressures generated by the subpulmonary ventricle and a decrease in PVR.[12,13] Flow through Fontan baffle cannot generate similar pressures to augment cardiac output in response to exercise and, as such, the patient is even more dependent on the decrease in PVR to augment cardiac output during exercise. Given the physiology, the average peak oxygen consumption for patients after the Fontan operation ranges between 60% and 70% of predicted normative values.[11,14] Peak oxygen consumption decreases over time, with some studies showing a decrease of 2.6% per year.[15] Additionally, many patients after the Fontan operation have some degree of sinus node dysfunction and are unable to increase their heart rate appropriate for the level of exercise.[16] This further compounds the inability to increase cardiac output. Even in Fontan patients who have a "normal" cardiac index at rest, the inability to increase cardiac output with exercise contributes significantly to the long-term complications seen in this patient population.

LONG-TERM SURVIVAL AND MORTALITY

With advances in surgical, catheter, and medical therapies, patients with congenital heart disease are living well into adulthood, surpassing the number of children with congenital heart disease. From 2000 to 2010 in Quebec, Canada, the prevalence of congenital heart disease in the adult population increased by 57% compared with 11% in children with congenital heart disease.[4] This included the prevalence of severe congenital heart disease, which increased by 55% in the adult population but only by 19% in children with congenital heart disease.[4]

Following these trends, the survival rate of patients undergoing the Fontan operation has improved dramatically over time.[17,18] A recent single-center study shows that the perioperative mortality rate is less than 2%.[19] Freedom from death or transplantation has been reported to be 90% at 10 years, 83% at 20 years, and 70% at 25 years.[18] The most common causes of death in patients after the Fontan operation include cardiac failure, thromboemboli, or sudden death.[18] The incidence of sudden death has been shown to be 0.15% per year, with the presumed cause being arrhythmogenic events.[18] Most patients do well after the Fontan operation with the risk of heart failure and thromboembolic events increasing 10 and 15 years, respectively, after the Fontan completion.

CAUSES AND POTENTIAL TREATMENT STRATEGIES FOR DECREASED CARDIAC OUTPUT

The mainstay of treatment for the Fontan patient is to optimize and improve cardiac output. To determine the contributing mechanisms of decreased cardiac output, all patients should have a detailed evaluation aimed at identifying potential treatment strategies and potential end-organ system damage. A suggested evaluation is detailed in **Box 1**. In general, the treatment strategy needs to be tailored to each patient depending on the underlying mechanisms.

Arrhythmias

Atrial arrhythmias are extremely common in patients who have had the Fontan operation, occurring in up to 50% to 60% of patients with an atriopulmonary Fontan.[16,20] The incidence is reported to be lower in the newer modifications of the lateral tunnel Fontan and extracardiac Fontan, although there is likely a similar arrhythmia burden when comparing these newer modifications to each other.[21,22] Intraatrial reentrant tachycardia is the most common type of supraventricular tachycardia (SVT), accounting for 75% of SVT in these patients.[23] Focal atrial tachycardia can also occur, but at lower percentages. As the population ages, atrial fibrillation can also be seen.[24,25] Patients generally do not tolerate 1:1 conduction at rapid rates, and can quickly have clinical decompensation, especially those with elevated Fontan pressures and poor ventricular function. Atrial rates in tachycardia may be relatively slow owing to the altered anatomy and enlarged atrium; thus, rapid ventricular rates in a Fontan patient may be as low as 110 to 120 beats per minute and can be confused for sinus tachycardia. Given Fontan physiology, many patients will be symptomatic even at these heart rates. Direct current cardioversion should be used in cases of symptomatic rapid conduction, but radiofrequency ablation and medical therapy are often needed in addition.[24,26] Radiofrequency ablation can be helpful in reducing the occurrence of arrhythmia, but owing to new reentrant pathways emerging, the recurrence rate is 50% within 4 to 5 years.[27,28] Rate control can be an option in some patients, but most patients are dependent on AV synchrony to maintain cardiac output and can feel unwell without it. Coumadin anticoagulation needs to be initiated in patients with atrial arrhythmias, and careful assessment for thrombosis should be

Box 1
Suggested evaluation of patients with failing Fontan physiology

Detailed history and physical examination

 Onset of symptoms

 Arrhythmias symptoms

 Sleep apnea symptoms

 GI bleeding history

 Presence of ascites, edema, cyanosis

 Thyroid dysfunction

 Liver dysfunction

Cardiac catheterization ± cardiac MRI

 Obstruction in Fontan pathway

 Pressure in Fontan circuit

 Pulmonary vascular resistance

 Cardiac index

 Mixed venous saturation

 Ventricular end-diastolic pressures

 Presence of collateral vessels

Gastroenterology consultation

 Evaluation for hepatic dysfunction

 Rule out other etiologies of PLE

Echocardiogram

 Presence of fenestration

 Valve regurgitation

 Ventricular function

 Suggestion of Fontan obstruction

 Aortic coarctation

Electrophysiology assessment (ECG, 24-h Holter monitoring, exercise testing)

 Sinus node dysfunction

 Atrial arrhythmias

Laboratory assessment

 Complete blood count

 Basic metabolic profile with BUN/Cr

 Serum albumin and total protein

 Hepatic function testing

 Thyroid function testing

 Serum pregnancy testing

 Urine analysis for protein

 Stool alpha-1 antitrypsin level

Abbreviations: BUN, blood urea nitrogen; Cr, creatinine; ECG, electrocardiogram; GI, gastrointestinal; PLE, protein losing enteropathy.

performed. Fontan conversion of an atriopulmonary Fontan to an extracardiac conduit with atrial reduction surgery, MAZE procedure, and pacemaker insertion is also a potential strategy to treat refractory intraatrial reentrant tachycardia.[29] Careful selection of the ideal candidate needs to be performed because the procedure can carry a high mortality rate depending on the underlying risk factors. Older age and AV valve regurgitation have been shown to be predictors of perioperative death in patients undergoing Fontan conversion.[30]

Sinus node dysfunction is also commonly seen in patients after the Fontan operation, as injury to the sinus node can occur frequently during the surgery.[29] Epicardial pacemaker therapy is often needed, although there is the potential for successful placement of a transvenous atrial lead in atriopulmonary or lateral tunnel Fontan after careful consideration (necessitating anticoagulation). Ventricular arrhythmias can also occur in Fontan patients with poor ventricular function, likely accounting for the incidence of sudden death.[24]

Mechanical or Structural Lesions

Careful assessment for obstruction of the Fontan pathway, pulmonary arteries, and pulmonary veins should be performed by noninvasive imaging such as MRI or cardiac CT. Stenosis or narrowing can potentially be treated in the cardiac catheterization laboratory or operating room. In some cases of atriopulmonary Fontans, the pulmonary veins can be compressed mechanically from the giant right atrium.[31] Certain anatomic subtypes might also have components of outflow tract obstruction, such as subaortic obstruction in double inlet left ventricle with L-looping or coarctation of the aorta, which can be seen at sites neoaortic anastomosis, such as in the Norwood operation. Alleviating these obstructions can improve cardiac output. Patients with severe valve regurgitation may need valve replacement if symptomatic and showing signs of poor cardiac output.[32]

Cyanosis

There are several mechanical causes of cyanosis that need to be evaluated. Persistent fenestrations in the Fontan baffle can help to augment cardiac output but may result in cyanosis. Fenestration creation can be used in patients with protein losing enteropathy (PLE) as a mode of treatment, but in some patients worsening cyanosis can cause symptoms of fatigue and dyspnea.[33] Careful evaluation in the cardiac catheterization laboratory is needed to determine whether the hemodynamics are favorable for closure. Determining Fontan pressures, degree of right-to-left shunting, and measuring mixed venous saturations after test occluding the defect can guide whether the patient is dependent on the fenestration for cardiac output.[8] Venovenous collaterals are another source of chronic cyanosis, as are pulmonary arteriovenous malformations. Pulmonary arteriovenous malformations are seen commonly in patients who have an isolated Glenn shunt or who do not have inclusion of the hepatic veins into the Fontan circuit.[34] Surgical revision to include hepatic vein flow into the Fontan baffle can be performed to treat pulmonary arteriovenous malformations. Venovenous collaterals can be coiled, but Fontan pressures and patency should be assessed carefully as part of the evaluation.[35]

Elevated Pulmonary Vascular Resistance

A low PVR is critical to maintaining cardiac output in Fontan physiology. Increases in PVR leads to an increase in central venous pressure and decreased forward flow through the Fontan circuit. PVR increases with aging, but there are additional factors that contribute to abnormal pulmonary vasculature in the patient after the Fontan operation. Depending on the anatomic subtype, patients may have had unobstructed pulmonary blood flow or palliative shunts, which may have resulted in pulmonary overcirculation and increased PVR from a young age. After the Fontan, patients continue to have changes in the vascular bed with decreased capillary recruitment and medial hypertrophy.[36] This can result in altered nitric oxide synthesis and an increase in endothelin receptor expression.[37,38] Increased PVR has been associated with Fontan failure and was predictive of death in the population of patients with PLE.[39,40]

There are increasing data on using medical therapy to help target the pulmonary vasculature in Fontan patients. Sildenafil, a pulmonary vasodilator, decreases PVR and has been shown to improve some parameters of ventricular function and exercise capacity in patients after the Fontan operation.[41,42] More recently, endothelin receptor antagonists have also been shown to improve exercise capacity in adolescent and adult Fontan patients, targeting the increase in endothelin receptor expression.[43] Inhaled prostacyclins have also been shown to improve exercise capacity in patients after the Fontan operation.[44] Inhaled agents have the advantage of fewer systemic side effects, such as the systemic vasodilation that has been observed with sildenafil. Spironolactone has been shown to be effective in the treatment of PLE in Fontan patients.[45] Although the effects have been attributed to improved cardiac function and its diuretic properties, spironolactone has also

been shown to improve endothelial cell function and decrease inflammation.[46] Initial reports have been published suggest spironolactone in combination with endothelin-A receptor antagonists improve exercise capacity in patients with pulmonary arterial hypertension.[47]

Ventricular Dysfunction

Medical therapy for ventricular dysfunction in patients with single ventricle physiology is extrapolated from adult heart failure patients with a biventricular circulation. Angiotensin-converting enzyme inhibitors and β-blockers have been shown to have some benefit for systolic dysfunction of the single ventricle, but data are limited.[48,49] Carvedilol has been shown improve New York Heart Association class and ejection fraction in Fontan patients, but use of β-blockers may be limited by the degree of sinus node dysfunction.[50,51] Diuretic therapy with both loop diuretics and aldosterone antagonists can be used to treat fluid overload; additionally, aldosterone antagonists may have some positive effect on the pulmonary vascular bed.[47]

An additional modality to improve ventricular function is "cardiac resynchronization therapy" in a single ventricle, more accurately termed multisite pacing. There are no long-term data showing this improves ventricular function long-term, but there have been some improvements in cardiac function after surgery with multisite pacing.[52] The aim would be to "resynchronize" the dilated, dysfunctional single ventricle through multiple ventricular epicardial pacemaker leads.

Cardiopulmonary exercise and rehabilitation has been shown to be effective in the adult heart failure patient in improving physical capacity. Similarly, in adult congenital heart disease patients, those who exercise frequently had improved oxygen consumption as compared with sedentary adult congenital heart disease patients, including patients with a Fontan.[53] In the Fontan patient, both skeletal and respiratory muscle training aid in improved filling by helping with chest wall compliance and venous return. Physical exercise also helps with weight management and decreasing the risk of obesity-related complications such as obstructive sleep apnea, which can further hasten ventricular dysfunction and increase the risk of atrial arrhythmias.

PROTEIN LOSING ENTEROPATHY

PLE occurs in 5% to 15% of patients after the modified Fontan operation and, historically, has been a difficult complication to treat.[54,55] PLE is characterized by the enteric loss of proteins, such as albumin, immunoglobulins, and clotting factors. The protein loss that occurs leads to the clinical findings of peripheral edema, ascites, diarrhea, weight loss, and malabsorption. The exact mechanisms of this complication are poorly understood and the treatment strategies are varied.

Historically, patients with PLE after the Fontan operation have had a reported 50% mortality at 5 years after diagnosis.[54,55] Recent data from some centers show with treatment advances, survival has improved to 88% and 72% after diagnosis at 5 and 10 years, respectively.[40] Patients with PLE at greatest risk of mortality can be identified based on their hemodynamic parameters and laboratory assessment at initial diagnosis. Lower cardiac index, lower mixed venous saturation, New York Heart Association class greater than II, and higher serum creatinine were seen more commonly in patients who

died.[40] Additional factors seen more frequently in patients who died with PLE included Fontan pressures of greater than 15 mm Hg, decreased ventricular function, and elevated PVR. Low cardiac index has been thought to be one of the causal factors in the development of PLE after the Fontan operation, and it is not surprising that features that further decrease cardiac output were associated with increased mortality in this subgroup.[56] Similar to patients with failing Fontan physiology, the treatment strategy for PLE is individualized based on contributing factors and a comprehensive evaluation is recommended, similar to the failing Fontan population. A suggested treatment algorithm is presented in **Fig. 2**. Cardiac transplantation can be used as a potential treatment strategy in refractory cases. Recurrence rates of PLE after cardiac transplantation are low, and recent data suggest that the mortality rate is similar

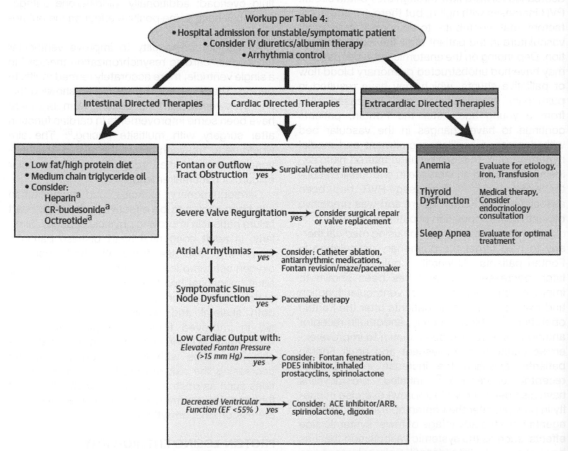

Fig. 2. Treatment algorithm for PLE therapies must be individualized for each patient given the number of possible contributing factors. ACE, angiotensin-converting enzyme; ARB, angiotensin receptor blocker; CR, controlled release; EF, ejection fraction; IV, intravenous; PDE5, phosphodiesterase 5. [a]Use with caution if hepatic dysfunction. (*From* John AS, Johnson JA, Khan M, et al. Clinical outcomes and improved survival in patients with protein-losing enteropathy after the Fontan operation. J Am Coll Cardiol 2014;64:59; with permission.)

among pediatric Fontan patients with and without PLE.[57]

EXTRACARDIAC ORGAN SYSTEM INTERACTION
Liver Disease

Liver disease has been increasingly recognized in the Fontan population, and is present in some degree in all adult Fontan patients. The etiology is likely multifold, with chronic venous congestion/increased central venous pressures, hypoxia, and decreased cardiac output all playing a role in development.[58] Owing to the nonpulsatile state, increased venous pressures leads to passive congestion, which then over time triggers injury and fibrosis.[59,60] Chronic hypoxia contributes further by stimulating genes that are part of the fibrosis pathway. Hepatic fibrosis can be either portal or sinusoidal, which is different from other causes of cardiac cirrhosis where the predominant feature is sinusoidal fibrosis.[61,62] In addition, the degree of portal fibrosis is more severe, perhaps owing to the contribution of a hypoxic state and poor cardiac output. The disease is heterogenous and can include nonuniform hepatic fibrosis, hypervascular nodules, cirrhosis, and rare cases of hepatocellular carcinoma.[59,63,64] Given the nonuniform area of disease, the small samples from liver biopsy may not represent the severity of disease accurately; in addition, biopsy carries inherent risks of bleeding and morbidity in this population. Screening has largely been accomplished with ultrasound or MRI. Recent studies have published techniques of MR elastography as a screening tool for liver disease in patients after the Fontan operation.[65] Elastography can quantitate the degree of fibrosis noninvasively, avoiding the risks of biopsies.

Most patients are asymptomatic, but those with advanced disease and cirrhosis can present with ascites and abdominal distension. Some patients have vague right upper quadrant pain that can be worsened with increased congestion and increased pulmonary pressures. Laboratory assessment may show mild elevation in indirect bilirubin and alkaline phosphatase in addition to decreased platelets.[66] There is no established screening or treatment protocol, although using therapies to maximize cardiac output, decrease pulmonary pressures and resistance, and optimize oxygen delivery are strategies that may delay the progression of disease. All patients should undergo evaluation for hepatitis B and C, especially those operated on before the initiation of routine screening for those diseases in donated blood.

Thromboembolic Complications

After the Fontan operation, patients have been reported to have numerous clotting abnormalities including deficiencies of protein C, protein S, and antithrombin III; in addition, increased platelet reactivity has also been observed.[67,68] Combined with decreased cardiac output, a nonpulsatile low flow state to the pulmonary circulation, atrial arrhythmias, and the presence of prosthetic material, the Fontan patient is at high risk for thrombus formation. Some studies have reported a rate of thrombus formation of up to 20% in patients after a Fontan procedure. This is not limited to the atriopulmonary type of Fontan. The incidence of thromboemboli after the extracardiac conduit is estimated to be 7.1% at 10 years after Fontan completion.[69–71] This can result in pulmonary emboli, acute and chronic; systemic emboli through patent fenestration or baffle leaks; and systemic thrombi in the atria, pulmonary artery stump, or rudimentary ventricle. Thromboemboli in the pulmonary vasculature can produce acute hemodynamic instability and chronically, resulting in increased Fontan pressures and increased PVR. Systemic sources of thrombi place the patient at risk for stroke and end-organ system damage. Prophylactic treatment guidelines recommend aspirin, heparin, or vitamin K antagonists, although the efficacy of each has not been well-established.

Pulmonary Complications

It is important to evaluate for pulmonary causes of elevated pulmonary pressures and sources of cyanosis. Pulmonary venous desaturation in the absence of venovenous collaterals should prompt a pulmonary evaluation for lung parenchymal disease. As mentioned, chronic thromboembolic disease can lead to pulmonary hypertension with increased PVR and decreased oxygenation. Pulmonary vasodilators and anticoagulation are 2 modes of treatment. Additionally, airway disease such as ciliary dysfunction has a high prevalence in patients with heterotaxy syndrome. These patients can present with impaired airway clearance and may require prolonged intubation after procedures, which can be harmful for a Fontan patient. Any single ventricle patient with heterotaxy should be evaluated for symptoms of ciliary dysfunction.[72]

Obstructive sleep apnea, very commonly seen in the general population, can also raise pulmonary pressures and increase PVR in the Fontan patient.[73,74] Sleep apnea also places the patient at higher risk for refractory atrial arrhythmias, and careful screening is recommended.[75] Although continuous positive airway pressure may seem harmful for the Fontan physiology, the increase in pressure during periodic obstruction causes greater alterations in Fontan filling and increase in Fontan pressure. Untreated sleep apnea can alter endothelial function, further compounding the vascular changes. Screening should be performed when clinically indicated.[73,74]

Finally, restrictive lung disease is very common in the adult congenital heart disease population.[76,77] Prior surgery, scoliosis, and obesity place the patient at higher risk. Many patients with the Fontan completion have had prior cardiac surgeries and chest wall mechanics may interfere with adequate filling of the Fontan pathway. Cardiopulmonary rehabilitation may be needed for respiratory muscle training to help with symptoms and increase forced vital capacity.[76,77]

MECHANICAL ASSIST DEVICES AND TRANSPLANTATION

Although survival has continued to improve in the Fontan population, cardiac transplantation is still reserved for the patient after all other medical and surgical therapies have failed. Survival has improved overall, although it is still significantly lower than the general population without congenital heart disease.[78,79] Patients who are transplanted owing to early Fontan failure have been observed to have worse outcomes than those patients who are transplanted with late Fontan failure. In addition, those patients who had failing Fontan physiology with preserved ventricular function and those on mechanical ventilator support also had higher mortality.[78,80] As part of the transplant workup, it is important to perform a multiorgan system evaluation to assess for liver, kidney, hematologic, and pulmonary dysfunction. In some cases, cardiac transplant needs to be performed in combination with another failing organ system. Cirrhosis and advanced liver disease are increasingly recognized and present additional challenges for transplantation. An additional challenge is that many Fontan patients also have high titers when tested with the panel of reactive antibodies owing to previous blood transfusions and procedures, which markedly increase the risk of organ rejection and make the wait for a suitable organ substantially longer.

The use of ventricular assist devices has gained increasing attention over the past few years. Devices have been used both as a subpulmonary pump to drive blood forward through the pulmonary circuit and also in the standard systemic ventricular position to pull blood through the Fontan circuit by lowering the left atrial pressure.[81,82] Placement of the device may depend on the underlying hemodynamics: systemic ventricular failure versus elevation of PVR. Further investigation of ideal device strategies and prototypes is needed, because ventricular assist device therapy has the potential to not only serve as a bridge to transplant, but as eventual destination therapy for this complex cohort of patients.

SUMMARY

The Fontan operation remains a unique operative strategy for a complex group of patients, creating a circulation in series with only one systemic ventricle. The unique physiology results in a chronic state of low cardiac output, which has long-term multiorgan system effects. Understanding the physiology is vital to guiding an individualized treatment plan for each patient. Although cardiac transplantation is still used as an option for patients who have failed medical and surgical therapies, the development of ventricular assist device strategies presents an exciting new treatment strategy for this patient population.

REFERENCES

1. Fontan F, Baudet E. Surgical repair of tricuspid atresia. Thorax 1971;26:240–8.
2. Anderson RH, Becker AE, Wilkinson JL. Proceedings: morphogenesis and nomenclature of univentricular hearts. Br Heart J 1975;37:781–2.
3. Vanpraagh R, Ongley PA, Swan HJ. Anatomic types of single or common ventricle in man. Morphologic and geometric aspects of 60 necropsied cases. Am J Cardiol 1964;13:367–86.
4. Marelli AJ, Ionescu-Ittu R, Mackie AS, et al. Lifetime prevalence of congenital heart disease in the general population from 2000 to 2010. Circulation 2014;130:749–56.
5. de Leval MR, Kilner P, Gewillig M, et al. Total cavopulmonary connection: a logical alternative to atriopulmonary connection for complex Fontan operations. Experimental studies and early clinical experience. J Thorac Cardiovasc Surg 1988;96:682–95.
6. Marcelletti C, Corno A, Giannico S, et al. Inferior vena cava-pulmonary artery extracardiac conduit. A new form of right heart bypass. J Thorac Cardiovasc Surg 1990;100:228–32.
7. Bridges ND, Mayer JE Jr, Lock JE, et al. Effect of baffle fenestration on outcome of the modified Fontan operation. Circulation 1992;86:1762–9.
8. Goff DA, Blume ED, Gauvreau K, et al. Clinical outcome of fenestrated Fontan patients after closure: the first 10 years. Circulation 2000;102:2094–9.

9. Rychik J. Forty years of the Fontan operation: a failed strategy. Semin Thorac Cardiovasc Surg 2010;13:96–100.

10. Piran S, Veldtman G, Siu S, et al. Heart failure and ventricular dysfunction in patients with single or systemic right ventricles. Circulation 2002;105: 1189–94.

11. Fernandes SM, McElhinney DB, Khairy P, et al. Serial cardiopulmonary exercise testing in patients with previous Fontan surgery. Pediatr Cardiol 2010;31:175–80.

12. Stickland MK, Welsh RC, Petersen SR, et al. Does fitness level modulate the cardiovascular hemodynamic response to exercise? J Appl Physiol (1985) 2006;100:1895–901.

13. Argiento P, Chesler N, Mule M, et al. Exercise stress echocardiography for the study of the pulmonary circulation. Eur Respir J 2010;35:1273–8.

14. Paridon SM, Mitchell PD, Colan SD, et al. A cross-sectional study of exercise performance during the first 2 decades of life after the Fontan operation. J Am Coll Cardiol 2008;52:99–107.

15. Giardini A, Hager A, Pace Napoleone C, et al. Natural history of exercise capacity after the Fontan operation: a longitudinal study. Ann Thorac Surg 2008; 85:818–21.

16. Collins KK. The spectrum of long-term electrophysiologic abnormalities in patients with univentricular hearts. Congenit Heart Dis 2009;4:310–7.

17. d'Udekem Y, Iyengar AJ, Cochrane AD, et al. The Fontan procedure: contemporary techniques have improved long-term outcomes. Circulation 2007; 116:I157–64.

18. Khairy P, Fernandes SM, Mayer JE Jr, et al. Long-term survival, modes of death, and predictors of mortality in patients with Fontan surgery. Circulation 2008;117:85–92.

19. Rogers LS, Glatz AC, Ravishankar C, et al. 18 years of the Fontan operation at a single institution: results from 771 consecutive patients. J Am Coll Cardiol 2012;60:1018–25.

20. Giannakoulas G, Dimopoulos K, Yuksel S, et al. Atrial tachyarrhythmias late after Fontan operation are related to increase in mortality and hospitalization. Int J Cardiol 2012;157:221–6.

21. Lee JR, Kwak J, Kim KC, et al. Comparison of lateral tunnel and extracardiac conduit Fontan procedure. Interact Cardiovasc Thorac Surg 2007;6:328–30.

22. Stamm C, Friehs I, Mayer JE Jr, et al. Long-term results of the lateral tunnel Fontan operation. J Thorac Cardiovasc Surg 2001;121:28–41.

23. Mondesert B, Marcotte F, Mongeon FP, et al. Fontan circulation: success or failure? Can J Cardiol 2013; 29:811–20.

24. Deal BJ. Late arrhythmias following Fontan surgery. World J Pediatr Congenit Heart Surg 2012;3:194–200.

25. Stephenson EA, Lu M, Berul CI, et al. Arrhythmias in a contemporary Fontan cohort: prevalence and clinical associations in a multicenter cross-sectional study. J Am Coll Cardiol 2010;56:890–6.

26. Deal BJ, Jacobs ML. Management of the failing Fontan circulation. Heart 2012;98:1098–104.

27. Akca F, Bauernfeind T, Witsenburg M, et al. Acute and long-term outcomes of catheter ablation using remote magnetic navigation in patients with congenital heart disease. Am J Cardiol 2012;110:409–14.

28. Yap SC, Harris L, Silversides CK, et al. Outcome of intra-atrial re-entrant tachycardia catheter ablation in adults with congenital heart disease: negative impact of age and complex atrial surgery. J Am Coll Cardiol 2010;56:1589–96.

29. Deal BJ, Mavroudis C, Backer CL. Arrhythmia management in the Fontan patient. Pediatr Cardiol 2007; 28:448–56.

30. Said SM, Burkhart HM, Schaff HV, et al. Fontan conversion: identifying the high-risk patient. Ann Thorac Surg 2014;97:2115–21 [discussion: 2121–2].

31. O'Donnell CP, Lock JE, Powell AJ, et al. Compression of pulmonary veins between the left atrium and the descending aorta. Am J Cardiol 2003;91: 248–51.

32. Menon SC, Dearani JA, Cetta F. Long-term outcome after atrioventricular valve surgery following modified Fontan operation. Cardiol Young 2011;21:83–8.

33. Vyas H, Driscoll DJ, Cabalka AK, et al. Results of transcatheter Fontan fenestration to treat protein losing enteropathy. Catheter Cardiovasc Interv 2007;69:584–9.

34. Kavarana MN, Jones JA, Stroud RE, et al. Pulmonary arteriovenous malformations after the superior cavopulmonary shunt: mechanisms and clinical implications. Expert Rev Cardiovasc Ther 2014;12:703–13.

35. Magee AG, McCrindle BW, Mawson J, et al. Systemic venous collateral development after the bidirectional cavopulmonary anastomosis. Prevalence and predictors. J Am Coll Cardiol 1998;32:502–8.

36. Presson RG Jr, Baumgartner WA Jr, Peterson AJ, et al. Pulmonary capillaries are recruited during pulsatile flow. J Appl Physiol (1985) 2002;92:1183–90.

37. Busse R, Fleming I. Pulsatile stretch and shear stress: physical stimuli determining the production of endothelium-derived relaxing factors. J Vasc Res 1998;35:73–84.

38. Ishida H, Kogaki S, Ichimori H, et al. Overexpression of endothelin-1 and endothelin receptors in the pulmonary arteries of failed Fontan patients. Int J Cardiol 2012;159:34–9.

39. Gentles TL, Mayer JE Jr, Gauvreau K, et al. Fontan operation in five hundred consecutive patients: factors influencing early and late outcome. J Thorac Cardiovasc Surg 1997;114:376–91.

40. John AS, Johnson JA, Khan M, et al. Clinical outcomes and improved survival in patients with protein-losing enteropathy after the Fontan operation. J Am Coll Cardiol 2014;64:54–62.

41. Goldberg DJ, French B, Szwast AL, et al. Impact of sildenafil on echocardiographic indices of myocardial performance after the Fontan operation. Pediatr Cardiol 2012;33:689–96.

42. Goldberg DJ, French B, McBride MG, et al. Impact of oral sildenafil on exercise performance in children and young adults after the Fontan operation: a randomized, double-blind, placebo-controlled, crossover trial. Circulation 2011;123:1185–93.

43. Hebert A, Mikkelsen UR, Thilen U, et al. Bosentan improves exercise capacity in adolescents and adults after Fontan operation: the TEMPO (Treatment With Endothelin Receptor Antagonist in Fontan Patients, a Randomized, Placebo-Controlled, Double-Blind Study Measuring Peak Oxygen Consumption) study. Circulation 2014;130:2021–30.

44. Rhodes J, Ubeda-Tikkanen A, Clair M, et al. Effect of inhaled iloprost on the exercise function of Fontan patients: a demonstration of concept. Int J Cardiol 2013;168:2435–40.

45. Ringel RE, Peddy SB. Effect of high-dose spironolactone on protein-losing enteropathy in patients with Fontan palliation of complex congenital heart disease. Am J Cardiol 2003;91:1031–2. A9.

46. Elinoff JM, Rame JE, Forfia PR, et al. A pilot study of the effect of spironolactone therapy on exercise capacity and endothelial dysfunction in pulmonary arterial hypertension: study protocol for a randomized controlled trial. Trials 2013;14:91.

47. Maron BA, Opotowsky AR, Landzberg MJ, et al. Plasma aldosterone levels are elevated in patients with pulmonary arterial hypertension in the absence of left ventricular heart failure: a pilot study. Eur J Heart Fail 2013;15:277–83.

48. Kouatli AA, Garcia JA, Zellers TM, et al. Enalapril does not enhance exercise capacity in patients after Fontan procedure. Circulation 1997;96:1507–12.

49. Shaddy RE, Boucek MM, Hsu DT, et al. Carvedilol for children and adolescents with heart failure: a randomized controlled trial. JAMA 2007;298: 1171–9.

50. Ishibashi N, Park IS, Takahashi Y, et al. Effectiveness of carvedilol for congestive heart failure that developed long after modified Fontan operation. Pediatr Cardiol 2006;27:473–5.

51. Ishibashi N, Park IS, Waragai T, et al. Effect of carvedilol on heart failure in patients with a functionally univentricular heart. Circ J 2011;75:1394–9.

52. Sojak V, Mazic U, Cesen M, et al. Cardiac resynchronization therapy for the failing Fontan patient. Ann Thorac Surg 2008;85:2136–8.

53. Ubeda Tikkanen A, Opotowsky AR, Bhatt AB, et al. Physical activity is associated with improved aerobic exercise capacity over time in adults with congenital heart disease. Int J Cardiol 2013;168: 4685–91.

54. Mertens L, Hagler DJ, Sauer U, et al. Protein-losing enteropathy after the Fontan operation: an international multicenter study. PLE study group. J Thorac Cardiovasc Surg 1998;115:1063–73.

55. Feldt RH, Driscoll DJ, Offord KP, et al. Protein-losing enteropathy after the Fontan operation. J Thorac Cardiovasc Surg 1996;112:672–80.

56. Rychik J, Gui-Yang S. Relation of mesenteric vascular resistance after Fontan operation and protein-losing enteropathy. Am J Cardiol 2002;90:672–4.

57. Schumacher KR, Gossett J, Guleserian K, et al. Fontan-associated protein-losing enteropathy and heart transplant: a Pediatric Heart Transplant Study analysis. J Heart Lung Transplant 2015;34(9): 1169–76.

58. Mori M, Aguirre AJ, Elder RW, et al. Beyond a broken heart: circulatory dysfunction in the failing Fontan. Pediatr Cardiol 2014;35:569–79.

59. Ghaferi AA, Hutchins GM. Progression of liver pathology in patients undergoing the Fontan procedure: chronic passive congestion, cardiac cirrhosis, hepatic adenoma, and hepatocellular carcinoma. J Thorac Cardiovasc Surg 2005;129:1348–52.

60. Kendall TJ, Stedman B, Hacking N, et al. Hepatic fibrosis and cirrhosis in the Fontan circulation: a detailed morphological study. J Clin Pathol 2008; 61:504–8.

61. Johnson JA, Cetta F, Graham RP, et al. Identifying predictors of hepatic disease in patients after the Fontan operation: a postmortem analysis. J Thorac Cardiovasc Surg 2013;146:140–5.

62. Schwartz MC, Sullivan L, Cohen MS, et al. Hepatic pathology may develop before the Fontan operation in children with functional single ventricle: an autopsy study. J Thorac Cardiovasc Surg 2012; 143:904–9.

63. Asrani SK, Warnes CA, Kamath PS. Hepatocellular carcinoma after the Fontan procedure. N Engl J Med 2013;368:1756–7.

64. Bryant T, Ahmad Z, Millward-Sadler H, et al. Arterialised hepatic nodules in the Fontan circulation: hepatico-cardiac interactions. Int J Cardiol 2011; 151(3):268–72.

65. Poterucha JT, Johnson JN, Qureshi MY, et al. Magnetic Resonance Elastography: a Novel Technique for the Detection of Hepatic Fibrosis and Hepatocellular Carcinoma After the Fontan Operation. Mayo Clin Proc 2015;90(7):882–94.

66. Schwartz MC, Sullivan LM, Glatz AC, et al. Portal and sinusoidal fibrosis are common on liver biopsy after Fontan surgery. Pediatr Cardiol 2013;34: 135–42.

67. Ravn HB, Hjortdal VE, Stenbog EV, et al. Increased platelet reactivity and significant changes in coagulation markers after cavopulmonary connection. Heart 2001;85:61–5.

68. Tomita H, Yamada O, Ohuchi H, et al. Coagulation profile, hepatic function, and hemodynamics following Fontan-type operations. Cardiol Young 2001;11:62–6.

69. Monagle P, Karl TR. Thromboembolic problems after the Fontan operation. Semin Thorac Cardiovasc Surg 2002;5:36–47.

70. Kim SJ, Kim WH, Lim HG, et al. Outcome of 200 patients after an extracardiac Fontan procedure. J Thorac Cardiovasc Surg 2008;136:108–16.

71. Marrone C, Galasso G, Piccolo R, et al. Antiplatelet versus anticoagulation therapy after extracardiac conduit Fontan: a systematic review and meta-analysis. Pediatr Cardiol 2011;32:32–9.

72. Nakhleh N, Francis R, Giese RA, et al. High prevalence of respiratory ciliary dysfunction in congenital heart disease patients with heterotaxy. Circulation 2012;125:2232–42.

73. Watson NF, Bushnell T, Jones TK, et al. A novel method for the evaluation and treatment of obstructive sleep apnea in four adults with complex congenital heart disease and Fontan repairs. Sleep Breath 2009;13:421–4.

74. Watson NF, Stout K. Management of obstructive sleep apnea in patients with congenital heart disease and Fontan procedures. Sleep Med 2007;8:537–8.

75. Gami AS, Pressman G, Caples SM, et al. Association of atrial fibrillation and obstructive sleep apnea. Circulation 2004;110:364–7.

76. Cohen SB, Ginde S, Bartz PJ, et al. Extracardiac complications in adults with congenital heart disease. Congenit Heart Dis 2013;8:370–80.

77. Ginde S, Bartz PJ, Hill GD, et al. Restrictive lung disease is an independent predictor of exercise intolerance in the adult with congenital heart disease. Congenit Heart Dis 2012;8:246–54.

78. Bernstein D, Naftel D, Chin C, et al. Outcome of listing for cardiac transplantation for failed Fontan: a multi-institutional study. Circulation 2006;114:273–80.

79. Kanter KR, Mahle WT, Vincent RN, et al. Heart transplantation in children with a Fontan procedure. Ann Thorac Surg 2011;91:823–9 [discussion: 829–30].

80. Kovach JR, Naftel DC, Pearce FB, et al. Comparison of risk factors and outcomes for pediatric patients listed for heart transplantation after bidirectional glenn and after Fontan: an analysis from the Pediatric Heart Transplant Study. J Heart Lung Transplant 2012;31:133–9.

81. Derk G, Laks H, Biniwale R, et al. Novel techniques of mechanical circulatory support for the right heart and Fontan circulation. Int J Cardiol 2014; 176:828–32.

82. Sinha P, Deutsch N, Ratnayaka K, et al. Effect of mechanical assistance of the systemic ventricle in single ventricle circulation with cavopulmonary connection. J Thorac Cardiovasc Surg 2014;147: 1271–5.

Arrhythmias in Adult Congenital Heart Disease
Diagnosis and Management

Saurabh Kumar, BSc(Med)/MBBS, PhD[a],
Usha B. Tedrow, MD, MSc[a], John K. Triedman, MD[b],*

KEYWORDS

- Adult congenital heart disease • Arrhythmia • Intra-atrial reentrant tachycardia • Atrial flutter
- Atrial fibrillation • Ventricular tachycardia • Catheter ablation

KEY POINTS

- An increasing number of children with congenital heart disease (CHD) now survive into adulthood, posing unique challenges in clinical care and health care utilization.
- Cardiac arrhythmias, due to underlying anatomic defects and methods of surgical repair, are a major source of morbidity and mortality in this population, and manifest both as bradyarrhythmias or tachyarrhythmias. Although specific associations exist between certain anatomic defects and arrhythmia subtypes, most patients suffer from intra-atrial reentrant tachycardias and sinus node dysfunction.
- Pharmacologic antiarrhythmic management is empiric and has limited efficacy; however, anticoagulant therapy is an important aspect of drug management, as thrombosis and thromboembolism are major issues faced by this population.
- Advances in catheter mapping, imaging, and ablation technology have significantly enhanced procedural efficacy, such that catheter ablation is the preferred option for management of many tachyarrhythmias in this population. In selected patients, surgical maze therapy also may be useful.
- Pacing, resynchronization, and defibrillation via device therapy pose particular challenges due to the anatomic defects and methods of surgical repair.
- Although sudden cardiac death is relatively rare in adult patients with CHD, certain high-risk subgroups exist from which patients may be selected for the primary prevention of sudden cardiac death with defibrillators.

INTRODUCTION

Advances in cardiopulmonary bypass, higher infant survival rates attributed to improvements in surgical techniques, and improved clinical care have culminated in a progressive increase in life expectancy of patients born with congenital heart disease (CHD).[1–4] The past decade has seen a dramatic shift in population demographics as

Disclosures: Dr S. Kumar is a recipient of the Neil Hamilton Fairley Overseas Fellowship cofunded by the National Health and Medical Research Council and the National Heart Foundation of Australia and the Bushell Overseas Traveling Fellowship by the Royal Australasian College of Physicians. Dr U.B. Tedrow receives consulting fees/honoraria from Boston Scientific Corp. and St. Jude Medical and research funding from Biosense Webster and St Jude Medical. Dr J.K. Triedman is a consultant for Biosense Webster. He is funded in part by NIH 1U10HL109816.
[a] Arrhythmia Service, Cardiovascular Division, Brigham and Women's Hospital, 75 Francis Street, Boston, MA 02115, USA; [b] Department of Cardiology, Children's Hospital, Boston, 300 Longwood Avenue, Boston, MA 02115, USA
* Corresponding author.
E-mail address: John.Triedman@cardio.chboston.org

cardiology.theclinics.com

survivors of childhood surgery reach adulthood, such that adults now outnumber children with CHD.[2,5] The expanding population of adults with CHD poses unique clinical challenges that combine the morbidity of the underlying congenital defect coupled with the effects of aging-associated illnesses, such as diabetes, hypertension, obesity, and coronary and renal disease.[6–9] Expert consensus statements have focused on improving care access and delivery to patients with adult CHD (ACHD) within regional centers of excellence comprising of a multidisciplinary team of cardiologists, cardiac surgeons, anesthesiologists, imaging specialists, interventional physicians, and electrophysiologists with expertise in ACHD.[2,10]

Cardiac arrhythmias are a common and onerous complication faced by this population. Both bradyarrhythmias and tachyarrhythmias result in symptoms, may be hemodynamically poorly tolerated, and potentially lead to mortality.[2,11,12] Arrhythmias are a leading cause for hospital admissions, morbidity, impaired quality of life, and mortality.[13–17]

Atrial arrhythmias are the most prevalent, with a lifetime risk of approximately 50% regardless of the severity of the CHD lesion, and they are often refractory to medical management.[18] Intra-atrial reentrant tachycardia (IART) localized to the right atrium is the most common form,[19–21] but the prevalence of atrial fibrillation (AF) is increasing.[2,22,23] Other forms of supraventricular tachycardias (SVT) can be mediated by presence of accessory pathways, atrioventricular (AV) nodal reentry, and focal atrial tachycardias. Ventricular arrhythmias are thought to be a leading cause of sudden cardiac death in certain subtypes of CHD, with estimates that the relative risk may be up to 100-fold higher than age-matched controls.[14,15] However, the absolute incidence of sudden death remains quite low in patients with CHD, approximately 0.1% per year in most major diagnostic categories.[2,15,24–28] Bradyarrhythmias can occur as a consequence of disorders of the sinus node, AV node, His-Purkinje system, or pathologic intra-atrial propagation due to the underlying anatomic defect and method of surgical repair. Their management may be complex due to limitations of anatomy and vascular access.

Prompt recognition and proper management of cardiac arrhythmias in ACHD requires the cardiologist to be cognizant of the underlying cardiac defect, postoperative anatomy, potential arrhythmia mechanism, and the strengths and limitations of varied treatment options. Although the anatomic classification of congenital heart defects is complex, most can be associated with 1 of 3 major categories contributing the highest burden of arrhythmia in patients with ACHD (**Fig. 1**).[6] Some important specific associations between anatomic and arrhythmia diagnosis also must be appreciated (eg, multiple accessory pathways and Ebstein anomaly, ventricular tachycardia and repaired tetralogy of Fallot [TOF], AV block and corrected transposition of the great arteries [I-TGA]). **Table 1** summarizes the risk of bradyarrhythmias and tachyarrhythmias in various forms of CHD.[2] This review provides a succinct overview of arrhythmia diagnosis and management in ACHD, including pharmacologic therapy, pacing, catheter ablation, and arrhythmia surgery, as well as prophylaxis of thromboembolism and sudden death risk stratification.

FORMS OF TACHYCARDIA IN ADULT CONGENITAL HEART DISEASE
Supraventricular Tachycardias Occurring in Patients with Congenital Heart Disease

Embryologic errors responsible for CHD may result in displacement of the AV node and His bundle away from the usual anatomic location, or lead to the development of accessory or duplicated AV connections.[11,29] Ebstein anomaly of the tricuspid valve can be associated with the presence of accessory pathway in approximately 20% of cases with nearly half having multiple accessory pathways.[30,31] Atrial enlargement over time can give rise to IART or AF with potential for rapid conduction over the abnormal pathway.[30,31] Similarly, patients with I-TGA not infrequently exhibit an Ebstein-like malformation with accessory pathways along their left-sided tricuspid valve.[32] Patients with single ventricle of the heterotaxy variety can have 2 separate AV nodes with a connecting fiber giving rise to multiple forms of supraventricular arrhythmias.[33]

Intra-atrial Reentry Tachycardia

Many patients with ACHD have arrhythmias that resemble atrial flutter, in that the arrhythmia substrate relies on the presence of an isthmus of atrial myocardium between the inferior vena cava and the right-sided AV valve. However, IARTs are often distinct from the "typical" form of atrial flutter that occurs in patients without CHD.[34] IARTs are highly organized and often associated with multiple, anatomically complex circuits.[35–39] These circuits are "channeled" into macro-reentrant loops by anatomic boundaries created by natural conduction barriers (such as valve annuli and caval ostia), surgical incisions, cannulation sites, prosthetic patches and baffles, and regions of atrial scarring caused by long exposure to adverse

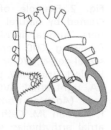

Mustard and Senning procedures

Patients born with transposition of the great vessels in the 1970s through the early 1990s were palliated by the construction of intra-atrial baffles using either synthetic material (the Mustard procedure) or by folding and augmentation of the atrial wall (the Senning procedure). Both redirect caval and pulmonary venous blood to correct cyanosis, utilising the right ventricle as the systemic ventricle. These operations have largely been abandoned in favour of the arterial switch procedure.

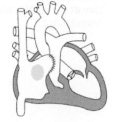

Fontan procedures

Many congenital heart defects have in common anatomical features that preclude surgical septation of the ventricles resulting in univentricular physiology. The common end point of staged surgical palliation is the Fontan procedure, which utilises the single ventricle as the systemic ventricle and sends blood directly from the systemic veins to the pulmonary arteries. Several approaches to this have been used; currently, an anastomosis between the superior vena cava and pulmonary artery is created, with an intercaval connection effected by tube graft or intra-atrial baffle.

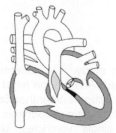

Repaired Tetralogy of Fallot (TOF)

The prevalence of TOF, its potential for survival through childhood without operation, and the early date at which reparative surgery became available have resulted in large group of patients with relatively homogenous clinical experience. Repair involves closure of the ventricular septal defect (VSD) and relief of right ventricular obstruction, often requiring both ventriculotomy and atriotomy.

Fig. 1. Congenital malformations associated with arrhythmias. (*From* Triedman JK. Arrhythmias in adults with congenital heart disease. Heart 2002;87:384; with permission.)

hemodynamic stresses and intermittent inflammatory effects of surgical intervention (**Fig. 2**).[7,12,24,35,40–43] The natural history of IART is characterized by gradual loss of normal sinus node function followed by increasingly frequent recurrences of tachycardia. Older age at operation and longer follow-up are prominent risk factors.[44,45] Ectopic atrial tachycardias are also

Table 1
Spectrum of bradyarrhythmias and tachyarrhythmias seen with selected CHD subtypes

CHD Type	IART	AF	WPW	VT/SCD	SA Node Dysfunction	Spontaneous AV Block	Acquired AV Block
VSD	+	—	—	+	—	—	+
ASD	++	+	—	—	—	—	—
TOF	+++	—	—	++	—	—	+
Aortic stenosis	—	+	—	++	—	—	+
d-TGA (Mustard or Senning)	+++	—	—	++	+++	—	—
CAVC	+	—	—	—	—	+	++
Fontan	+++	++	—	+	+++	—	—
l-TGA	+	—	+	+	—	++	+++
Ebstein's anomaly	++	—	+++	++	—	—	—

Abbreviations: AF, atrial fibrillation; ASD, atrial septal defect; AV, atrioventricular; IART, intra-atrial reentrant tachycardia; SA, sinoatrial; SCD, sudden cardiac death; TGA, transposition of the great arteries; TOF, tetralogy of Fallot; VSD, ventricular septal defect; VT, ventricular tachycardia.

Adapted from Walsh EP. Interventional electrophysiology in patients with congenital heart disease. Circulation 2007;115:3225.

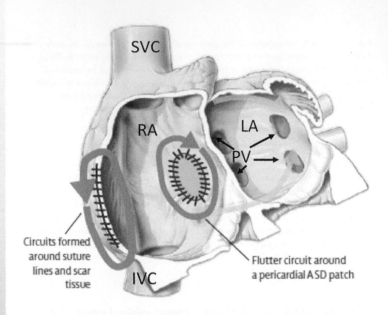

Fig. 2. Example of flutter circuit created by natural conduction barriers, surgical incisions or patches following CHD repair. ASD, atrial septal defect; IVC, inferior vena cava; LA, left atrium; PV, pulmonary veins; RA, right atrial; SVC, superior vena cava. (*Adapted from* Lee G, Sanders P, Kalman JM. Catheter ablation of atrial arrhythmias: state of the art. Lancet 2012;380:1512; with permission.)

SVC

RA

LA

PV —→

Circuits formed around suture lines and scar tissue

IVC

Flutter circuit around a pericardial A SD patch

seen, thought to be mediated by scarred tissues supporting micro-reentry.[46,47]

Patients with single ventricular physiology and Fontan circulation (particularly with right atrial to pulmonary artery connections), atrial baffles created by Mustard and Senning procedures for treatment of d-transposition of the great arteries (d-TGA), and repaired TOF are at greatest risk, but patients with simple atrial septal defect repair are also vulnerable years after repair.[2,7,11,23,48,49] Approximately 50% of patients with atriopulmonary Fontan repairs will develop IART within a decade of surgery and few patients with d-TGA will remain in sinus rhythm 10 years after Mustard or Senning repair.[44,50] Although ventricular arrhythmias are important in patients with TOF, IARTs are more prevalent and the main source of morbidity.[51]

IART has a stable cycle length and P-wave morphology. It tends to have slower atrial rates than typical atrial flutter (150–250 beats per minute). Atypical P waves are common, and multiple morphologies may be seen within one patient, suggesting "shift" from one circuit to another. In the presence of a healthy AV node, rapid conduction may cause symptomatic hemodynamic decompensation (**Fig. 3**).[18,20,52–54] Conversely, IART may masquerade as sinus rhythm when 2:1 or 3:1 conduction is present, thus the index of suspicion must be high. Hidden P waves may be uncovered by vagal maneuvers or diagnostic use of adenosine.[11]

Atrial Fibrillation

Prevalence of AF is increasing in the ACHD population, with a reported prevalence of 31% in one cardioversion study.[23] In patients with TOF, AF has surpassed IART as the most prevalent atrial arrhythmia in patients older than 55 years.[19] Aortic stenosis, mitral valve deformities, unrepaired (or unpalliated) single ventricles, unrepaired atrial septal defect (ASD), and to a lesser extent, Fontan surgery, are associated with development of AF.[22,23,55] Some concerning trends are that approximately 30% of patients who have previously undergone successful catheter ablation for IART develop AF at in follow-up and nearly 25% will develop AF many years after an ASD closure.[55,56] The mechanism of AF in the CHD population is likely linked to chronic hemodynamic stress and remodeling of the left atrium.

Ventricular Arrhythmias

Although ventricular ectopy and nonsustained ventricular tachycardia (VT) are common in ACHD populations, sustained monomorphic VT is quite rare.[2,57–60] The most common substrate for sustained VT is TOF. The prevalence of VT after TOF repair is estimated to be 3% to 14%,[25,26,51,61] and risk of sudden cardiac death (SCD) estimated to be 0.2% per year,[15,24–28] which may reach as high as 1% per year in adulthood by the fourth or fifth decade of life.[26,27] Greatest risk for ventricular arrhythmias is posed via 2 distinct mechanisms, which are not necessarily exclusive in a particular patient: (1) those who have undergone repair involving a ventriculotomy, and (2) those with long-standing hemodynamic overload causing ventricular dysfunction and/or hypertrophy independent of surgical incisions.[2,7,12,24,62–66]

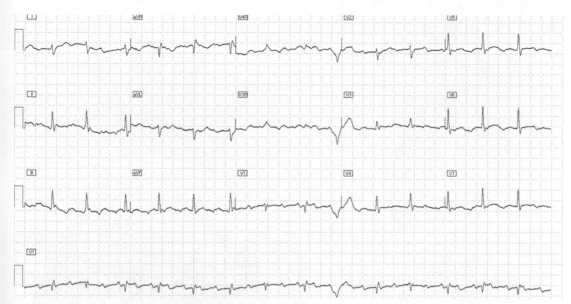

Fig. 3. Example of electrocardiogram of IART in a patient with adult CHD.

In patients with stable monomorphic VT, the arrhythmia substrate consists of 1 or more macro-reentrant circuits bounded by surgical incisions (often a ventriculotomy) and natural conduction barriers (eg, the septal defect or the edge of valve annulus). Mapping studies in patients with TOF have correlated VT circuits to the anatomic location of surgical scars that may be readily amenable to catheter ablation (**Fig. 4**).[57,67] In contrast, patients with ventricular dysfunction and a generalized myopathic process are more prone to disorganized polymorphic VT and/or ventricular fibrillation akin to that seen in the non-CHD adult population with dilated cardiomyopathy.[2,12,57,65]

Bradyarrhythmias

Bradyarrhythmias may be congenital or postoperative (**Table 2**).[2]

Sinus node dysfunction

Sinus node dysfunction (SND) is commonly associated with injury following cardiac surgery; patients with the Fontan, Glenn, Mustard, and Senning operations are at greatest risk.[6,21,44,50,68,69] Patients with ASD, TOF, arterial switch operation for TGA, and supracardiac total anomalous pulmonary venous return are also at risk.[2] Chronotropic incompetence limits exercise tolerance, aggravates AV valve regurgitation, and increases proclivity to IART and AF.[11,65] SND in patients with Fontan operation is associated with increased risk for plastic bronchitis and protein-losing enteropathy.[16,70]

Atrioventricular node dysfunction

The AV node may be congenitally abnormal in location and function, as in I-TGA or endocardial cushion defects.[71–73] In I-TGA, 3% to 5% will have complete AV block with another 20% developing by adulthood.[74,75] More commonly, however, trauma to the AV nodal tissue results in AV block (seen in 1%–3% of surgical cases).[76,77] Highest risk operations are those involving ventricular septal defect (VSD) closure, AV repair or replacement, and relief of left-heart outflow obstruction.[2]

MANAGEMENT OF ARRHYTHMIAS IN PATIENTS WITH CONGENITAL HEART DISEASE

Potentially curative therapies for tachyarrhythmias in patients with ACHD include catheter ablation and arrhythmia surgery. Other options for acute and chronic arrhythmia management include the use of antiarrhythmic drugs to restore and maintain sinus rhythm and/or control rate, device therapy to correct bradycardia and/or provide antitachycardia pacing, internal defibrillation (for ventricular arrhythmias), or external cardioversion.

Atrial Arrhythmias

SVTs dependent on AV nodal conduction and some focal atrial tachycardias may be terminated by vagal maneuvers, intravenous adenosine, or non-dihydropyridine calcium channel antagonists (ie, verapamil or diltiazem).

Acute termination of IARTs can be achieved by drug therapy, cardioversion, or by automatic or

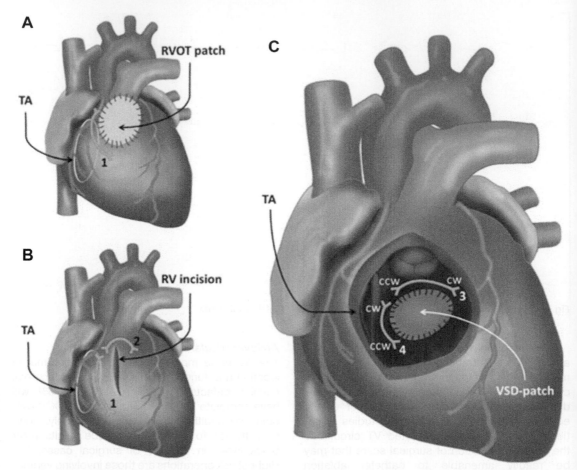

Fig. 4. Critical areas (also called an "isthmus") responsible for sustained monomorphic VT mapped in patients following TOF repair. Isthmus 1 is located between the tricuspid annulus (TA) and a RV incision/RV outflow tract (RVOT) patch (*A, B*). Isthmus 2 is located between an RV incision and pulmonary valve (PV; *B*). Isthmus 3, located between the PV and VSD patch. Isthmus 4 is located between the VSD patch and TA (*C*). Isthmus 3 and 4 are bordering on the septum. CW and CCW indicates counterclockwise and clockwise circuits. (*From* Kapel GF, Reichlin T, Wijnmaalen AP, et al. Left-sided ablation of ventricular tachycardia in adults with repaired tetralogy of Fallot: a case series. Circ Arrhythm Electrophysiol 2014;7:890; with permission.)

manual atrial overdrive pacing in paced patients.[78] Concerns for pharmacologic reversion include the risk of proarrhythmia with class IA (eg, quinidine, disopyramide) and IC drugs (eg, flecainide, propafenone) and severe conversion pauses in patients predisposed with underlying SND or AV nodal disease.[2] Ibutilide (class III antiarrhythmic drug) may be reasonable option for acute reversion being cognizant of the risk of torsades de pointes and severe bradycardia as potential severe side effects.[79,80] Antitachycardia pacing is generally effective for terminating atrial arrhythmias in approximately 50% of patients.[78,81,82] Disadvantages of atrial antitachycardia pacing include conversion to another form of atrial arrhythmia, degeneration into AF with rapid AV conduction, and worsened symptoms. Regardless, urgent cardioversion is indicated for atrial arrhythmias that

are not tolerated hemodynamically regardless of the arrhythmia duration or anticoagulation status. Anterior-posterior pad positioning may facilitate successful cardioversion in the face of marked atrial dilatation.[2]

Maintenance of AV synchrony with rhythm control may be hemodynamically useful in compromised physiologic states, such as univentricular hearts or systemic right ventricles. There is little literature informing pharmacologic arrhythmia prophylaxis in the ACHD population. Experience with chronic antiarrhythmic drug therapy using drugs such as sotalol, amiodarone and flecainide has been discouraging, resulting in a growing preference for nonpharmacological therapy.[11,45] Amiodarone is often used to maintain sinus rhythm in the presence of significant cardiac pathology.[2] Thyroid toxicity is heightened in patients with

Table 2
CHD substrates with high prevalence of congenital and postoperative SND and AV block

SND	AVB
Congenital	*Congenital*
Left atrial isomerism	Congenitally corrected TGA
Left-sided juxtaposition of atrial appendages	AV septal defect (endocardial cushion type)
—	L-looped single ventricles
Postoperative	*Postoperative*
Mustard baffle	Displaced AV conduction (congenitally corrected TGA, AV septal defect) undergoing cardiac surgery
Senning baffle	VSD
Hemi-Fontan or Fontan surgery; atriopulmonary and total cavopulmonary connections	MV surgery or multivalve surgery involved the TV
Glenn shunt	LV outflow tract surgery, subaortic stenosis
Sinus venosus ASD	—
Ebstein anomaly	—
Arterial switch for TGA	—
TOF	—

Abbreviations: ASD, atrial septal defect; AV, atrioventricular; LV, left ventricular; TGA, transposition of the great arteries; VSD, ventricular septal defect.

Adapted from Khairy P, Van Hare GF, Balaji S, et al. PACES/HRS expert consensus statement on the recognition and management of arrhythmias in adult congenital heart disease: developed in partnership between the Pediatric and Congenital Electrophysiology Society (PACES) and the Heart Rhythm Society (HRS). Endorsed by the governing bodies of PACES, HRS, the American College of Cardiology (ACC), the American Heart Association (AHA), the European Heart Rhythm Association (EHRA), the Canadian Heart Rhythm Society (CHRS), and the International Society for Adult Congenital Heart Disease (ISACHD). Can J Cardiol 2014;30:e1–63; with permission.

cyanotic heart disease, low body mass index, and univentricular hearts with Fontan palliation.[2] Dofetilide may be a reasonable alternative in the absence of metabolic, renal, and cardiac contraindications.[2] Current guidelines empirically suggest a variety of reasonable choices for prophylactic antiarrhythmic therapy of AF or IART in simple CHD, and use of amiodarone or dofetilide for rhythm control in more complex patients (**Fig. 5**).[83] Rate control with AV nodal blocking agents (eg, beta blocker, nondihydropyridine calcium channel blockers) may need to be used in many instances in which interventional options are not feasible or are unsuccessful.

Thromboprophylaxis in Atrial Arrhythmias

Prevention of thromboembolism is a major concern in patients with ACHD; the prevalence of thromboembolic complications is patients with ACHD is estimated to be 10-fold to 100-fold higher than in age-matched controls,[53] likely due to dilated chambers with sluggish flow, intracardiac prosthetic material, pacing/defibrillation leads, intracardiac shunts, and associated hypercoagulable states.[2,54] Pulmonary and systemic atrial thrombus has been observed in one series in 37% in patients undergoing transesophageal echo (TEE) before planned cardioversion,[84] although the observed rate of systemic thromboemboli observed at the time of cardioversion is low.[85] Recent studies have estimated the overall rate of stroke in patients with Fontan to be 2 to 3 per 1000 patient years with the rate of thrombosis (predominantly observed in the systemic venous circulation) estimated to be approximately 4 times that value.[86,87]

Fig. 6 summarizes the approach to thromboprophylaxis in the adult CHD population.[2] The presence of an atrial arrhythmia for ≥48 hours confers increased risk of thromboembolism; TEE is thus recommended to rule out intracardiac thrombus. Some severe CHD lesions (especially Fontan palliation), however are inherently associated with high thromboembolic risk, and one may consider a TEE regardless of arrhythmia duration (even if <48 hours)[88] or duration of therapeutic anticoagulation (even if ≥3 weeks).[84,89] It may be reasonable for such adults with simple nonvalvular forms of CHD to receive oral anticoagulation on

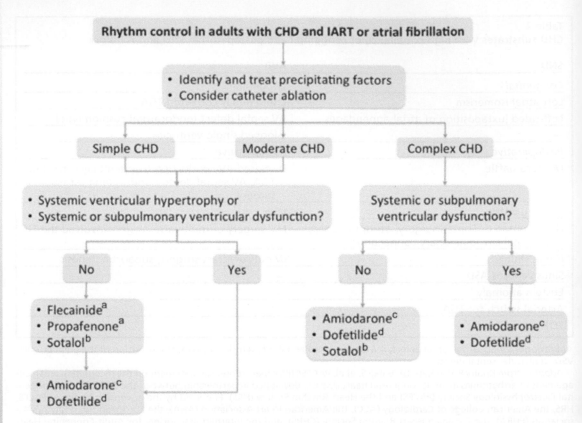

Fig. 5. Guideline recommendation for rhythm controls in adults with CHD and atrial arrhythmias. Drugs are listed in alphabetical order. [a] Class I antiarrhythmic agents are contraindicated in patients with coronary artery disease. [b] See text for cautionary note. [c] Amiodarone should be used with caution in patients with cyanotic heart disease, low body mass index, hepatic, pulmonary, or thyroid disease, and/or QT prolongation. [d] Dofetilide is subject to standard precautions and is contraindicated in patients with renal failure (creatinine clearance <20 mL/min), hypokalemia, or QT prolongation. (*From* Khairy P, Van Hare GF, Balaji S, et al. PACES/HRS expert consensus statement on the recognition and management of arrhythmias in adult congenital heart disease: developed in partnership between the Pediatric and Congenital Electrophysiology Society (PACES) and the Heart Rhythm Society (HRS). Endorsed by the governing bodies of PACES, HRS, the American College of Cardiology (ACC), the American Heart Association (AHA), the European Heart Rhythm Association (EHRA), the Canadian Heart Rhythm Society (CHRS), and the International Society for Adult Congenital Heart Disease (ISACHD). Can J Cardiol 2014;30:e15; with permission.)

the basis of established scores for stroke risk (congestive heart failure; Hypertension; Age (≥75 years, 2 points; 65–74 years, 1 point); diabetes; stroke, transient ischemic attack, or thromboembolism (2 points); vascular disease; sex category (female) [CHA$_2$DS$_2$-VASc]). In the absence of efficacy and safety data, novel oral anticoagulants (eg, dabigatran, apixaban) have not been recommended for use in patients with CHD, who may have a high prevalence of hepatic impairment and altered coagulation.[2]

Pharmacologic Management: Ventricular Arrhythmias

Hemodynamically poorly tolerated, ventricular arrhythmias require urgent cardioversion. For tolerated VT, pharmacologic reversion may be achieved with intravenous amiodarone, procainamide, or lidocaine.[2] Long-term drug therapy may be helpful in reducing shocks from the implantable cardioverter-defibrillator (ICD). Published literature on use of amiodarone, sotalol, or mexiletine for ventricular arrhythmias in ACHD is sparse.[90–92] Experience is drawn from non-CHD data where amiodarone in combination with a beta blocker is more efficacious than sotalol at preventing ICD shocks; use of class I drugs is not recommended in the presence of structural heart disease.[2,91]

Catheter Ablation

Supraventricular arrhythmias
Catheter ablation of supraventricular tachycardias can be acutely successful in 80% of patients[93,94]; lower acute success rates have been reported

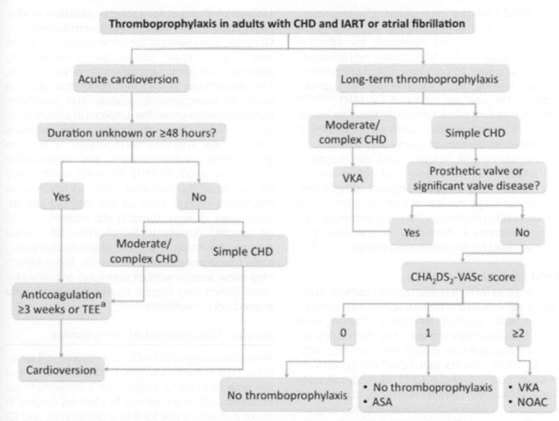

Fig. 6. Guideline recommendations for thromboprophylaxis in adults with CHD and atrial arrhythmias. ASA, aspirin; CHA$_2$DS$_2$-VASc, congestive heart failure; Hypertension; Age (≥75 years, 2 points; 65–74 years, 1 point); diabetes; stroke, transient ischemic attack, or thromboembolism (2 points); vascular disease; sex category (female); CHD, congenital heart disease; NOAC, newer oral anticoagulant; TEE, transesophageal echocardiography; VKA, vitamin K antagonist. [a] Patients with Fontan palliation are at particularly high risk of thromboembolic complications such that TEE may be prudent before cardioversion even if therapeutic anticoagulation is received for ≥3 weeks. (*From* Khairy P, Van Hare GF, Balaji S, et al. PACES/HRS expert consensus statement on the recognition and management of arrhythmias in adult congenital heart disease: developed in partnership between the Pediatric and Congenital Electrophysiology Society (PACES) and the Heart Rhythm Society (HRS). Endorsed by the governing bodies of PACES, HRS, the American College of Cardiology (ACC), the American Heart Association (AHA), the European Heart Rhythm Association (EHRA), the Canadian Heart Rhythm Society (CHRS), and the International Society for Adult Congenital Heart Disease (ISACHD). Can J Cardiol 2014;30:e17; with permission.)

with Ebstein anomaly with a higher risk for recurrences (27%–40%).[95,96] Referral is driven by drug-refractory and/or frequent symptoms. With the clinical success of the Cone procedure, many patients with Ebstein anomaly referral for preoperative intervention may be useful where not only accessory pathways can be mapped and ablated, but a high percentage of patients are found to have secondary arrhythmia substrates, such as atrial flutter or VT, which can ablated in the same session.[12,96] Should percutaneous ablation attempts fail, mapping can guide surgical ablation in the operating room as part of the Cone procedure or other repair.

Atrial arrhythmias

Advances in 3-dimensional mapping systems and image integration with computed tomography (CT), MRI, angiographic or fluoroscopic imaging, and/or intracardiac echo have made catheter ablation an early and preferred intervention for the management of IART.[97] Mapping systems allow for good reconstruction of distorted cardiac anatomy, allow visualization of scarred regions, caval ostia, prosthetic materials, and valve annuli. When combined with standard electrophysiological maneuvers, they enhance understanding of patient-specific arrhythmia mechanism (ie, reentrant or focal). Furthermore, imaging may detect myocardial changes from effective thermal abla-tion, reduce radiation exposure, and help guide catheter-tissue contact necessary for effective lesion formation.[12,65] When coupled with advance-ments in irrigated-tip catheters, which create more effective lesions, acute success rates of approxi-mately 81% can be achieved for IART.[2,98–102] IART recurrences occur frequently, however, espe-cially in older-style Fontan palliations (34%–54% of patients over 5 years of follow-up). Most recur-rences occur in the first year, and are thought to be related to progression of atrial myop-athy.[36,97,99,103,104] Despite recurrent arrhythmias, however, a large number of patients (40%–50%) remain in sinus rhythm and report improved symp-toms, reduction in frequency of episodes, and reduced need for long-term drug therapy.[100,105]

Atrial fibrillation

In contrast to IART, experience with catheter abla-tion for AF in ACHD is limited, with putative mech-anisms and ablation strategies inferred from experience in adults *without* CHD. One study re-ported a success rate of 42% with catheter abla-tion for AF in patients with ACHD compared with 55% in adults without CHD at approximately 1-year follow-up.[22] Given the paucity of published data on its mechanism, unclear ablation targets, and efficacy, specific recommendations for cath-eter ablation for AF have not yet been developed.

AV nodal ablation with permanent pacing may be also considered in patients with symptomatic atrial arrhythmia with poor rate control. Experience is limited to individual cases and small se-ries.[106,107] With potential adverse hemodynamic effects of pacing, potential difficulties in targeting the AV node for ablation, and limitations on place-ment of ventricular pacing leads (discussed later in this article), this option is rarely used except as a last resort.

Ventricular tachycardia

Experience with catheter ablation of sustained monomorphic VT is predominantly derived from repaired TOF where mapping studies have demonstrated key anatomic areas important for sustaining macro-reentrant VT circuits (see **Fig. 4**).[57,67] These areas are bounded by surgical incisions, patches, and prosthetic materials, such that linear ablation connecting these structures to adjacent anatomic structures, such as the valve annuli, yields good acute success rates.[57,58,60] Catheter ablation for VT provides useful adjunctive therapy to ICDs in patients with recurrent mono-morphic VT, VT storm, or multiple appropriate shocks that are not manageable by device reprog-ramming or drug therapy.

Unique challenges for catheter ablation in the adult congenital heart disease population

Given the complexity of the underlying CHD defect and surgical repair, knowledge of the existing anatomy and prior surgical repair is paramount. The procedure should be performed after a thorough hemodynamic workup and preproce-dural evaluation under the auspices of a multidisci-plinary ACHD team to optimize the patient's clinical state. This may be facilitated by invasive (right heart catheterization) and noninvasive testing (echo, CT, or MRI). Vascular access may be hampered by occluded veins, in which case alternative routes, such as the internal jugular, subclavian, or even transhepatic access, should be sought.[2] Access to the chamber of interest may require retrograde aortic or transbaffle punc-ture, hence assessment for baffle leaks (which may allow access without puncture) or baffle ste-nosis (which may require intervention before the procedure) is necessary.[2,108]

Surgical Management of Arrhythmias

Arrhythmia surgery in CHD is considered in 3 situa-tions: (1) in patients with preexisting arrhythmias at the time of planned surgery for a nonarrhythmia indication, (2) as an adjunct to planned surgery in those patients at risk for future arrhythmia, and (3) in patients with severe arrhythmia-related symp-toms or hemodynamic consequences where drugs and percutaneous catheter ablation have failed.

In patients with a prior history of arrhythmias who are scheduled to undergo open cardiac sur-gery for a nonarrhythmia indication, preoperative electrophysiological study may thus be useful to identify relevant arrhythmia substrate (eg, docu-mented accessory pathway, SVT, VT) that can be addressed at the time of surgery. Prophylactic arrhythmia surgery in the absence of documented arrhythmia is recommended only in moderate-high risk CHD lesions, such as in patients undergoing Fontan conversion or revision surgery or repair of Ebstein anomaly, repair of left-sided valvular heart disease. It is also prudent to consider left atrial appendage closure at the time of arrhythmia sur-gery to reduce thromboembolic risk.[2]

Device Therapy in Congenital Heart Disease

Indications for antibradycardia device therapy in adult CHD are similar to those for non-CHD patients for SND and AV nodal disease.[109,110] However, unique challenges exist in the adult CHD population with respect to leads placement. Intracardiac and venous anatomies are complex. Anatomic barriers and/or thromboembolic risk may prevent endocar-dial lead placement (especially in Fontan patients with single ventricle physiology and those with unrepaired intracardiac shunts), requiring surgical epicardial lead placement. Higher lead failure rates are observed.[12,65,111] Fontan patients, for example, lack a standard venous connection to their ventricle, and although transvenous atrial lead placement may be possible, it may also be at risk for thrombus. In patients with Mustard or Senning circulation, placement may be impeded by atrial baffle stenosis. Intracardiac shunts with right-to-left shunting need to be repaired before implantation to reduce the risk of systemic thromboembolism,[112,113] or alternatively, an epicardial implant has to be considered. Endocardial lead fixation to atrial muscle while avoiding patches, scars, and the left phrenic nerve may also prove challenging in patients with prior cardiac surgery.[12,65] Need for pacing may best be anticipated during surgeries for hemodynamic indication, thus providing epicardial for surgical lead fixation.[65]

Cardiac resynchronization therapy in CHD appears promising despite nonstandard indications and anatomic constraints on lead placement.[12,65,114] In contrast to patients without CHD, patients with CHD are much more likely to have right ventricle scarring and dysfunction and right bundle branch block. Improved in ventricular synchrony, improved New York Heart Association (NYHA) functional class status, and improved ejection fraction have been reported among patients with TOF and single ventricular physiology.[115–117] Limited access to a ventricular chamber (Fontan patients), abnormal coronary venous anatomy, or exclusion of the coronary sinus from the right heart by surgical patches are particular challenges[12]; many will require epicardial lead placement, which may be challenging in the context of prior cardiac surgeries. A hybrid approach consisting of transvenous lead insertion in the subpulmonary left ventricle (LV) and epicardial pacing of the systemic right ventricle may be needed in patients with Mustard or Senning baffles.[2] In addition to standard indications for cardiac resynchronization therapy (CRT) inferred from non-CHD implant guidelines,[118] patients with depressed systemic right ventricular ejection fraction ($\leq$35%), right ventricular dilation, ambulatory NYHA class II to IV symptoms, and complete right bundle branch block with a QRS complex of 150 ms or more may be suitable for CRT implantation.[2]

Risk Stratification for Sudden Cardiac Death and Implantable Cardiac Defibrillators

Approximately 20% to 25% of late total mortality in ACHD is attributed to SCD.[2,13–16,59,119] Overall, SCD risk is low (1% of patients per decade of follow-up) and largely concentrated in those with complicated hemodynamic lesions for whom the risk may approach 10% per decade of follow-up.[27,28] Although the mechanism originally was thought due to AV block (either by late-onset spontaneous AV block, device or lead failure[120]), it now appears that most SCDs are due to ventricular and atrial tachyarrhythmias, the latter causing hemodynamic instability from rapid AV conduction[20] and/or degeneration into a secondary ventricular arrhythmia.[52] Patients with TGA and systemic right ventricle (RV) after baffling operations, those with LV outflow obstruction, TOF, Eisenmenger syndrome, or those with single ventricular physiology appear to be at highest risk.[15,59,119] The presence of atrial arrhythmias and abnormal "systemic" ventricular function are also strongly associated with malignant arrhythmias.[20,24,52,121,122]

Specific risk factors have been examined in great detail in patients with TOF (**Table 3**)[24] and are used as a model for risk stratification in general. The presence of multiple risk factors may help guide ICD implantation for primary prevention of SCD, especially in patients with TOF.[26,123–130] Less well studied are patients with d- and l-TGA in whom the mechanism of malignant arrhythmia is attributed to a myopathic systemic RV.[52,119,121,131,132] In contrast to the TOF experience, programmed ventricular stimulation in transposition patients has not been shown to be predictive of SCD,[52] but longer follow-up, presence of syncope, atrial tachycardia, and depressed systemic RV function all appear to be risk factors (see **Table 3**).[24] SCD risk in Fontan palliation and single ventricular physiology is mitigated by a similar list of risk factors in addition to older Fontan techniques, such as the atrio-pulmonary connection.[21,23,133] Criteria for primary prevention ICDs are not refined in this population. In patients with LV outflow tract obstruction, LV hypertrophy and diastolic stiffness have been implicated in the mechanism of SCD predicated by risk factors along with elevated outflow tract gradients and ventricular dysfunction (see **Table 3**).[15,64,66]

Although the decision for a secondary prevention ICD implant is simple in survivors of cardiac arrest or spontaneous sustained ventricular arrhythmia, primary prevention criteria are less clear. Guidelines recommend primary prevention ICD implant in the setting of biventricular physiology and depressed systemic LV ejection fraction ($\leq$35%), NYHA class II or III symptoms. Furthermore ICD implantation should be considered in patients with single or systemic RV physiology, depressed ejection fraction ($\leq$35%), with or without presence of additional risk factors or elevated NYHA class, as well as patients with syncope of unknown etiology

Table 3
Risk factors for sudden cardiac death identified by prior studies in various high risk CHD substrates

	TOF	Atrial Switch for Transposition	Post Fontan	LV Outflow Tract Obstruction
Historical and clinical	Longer duration of follow-up Syncope, palpitations Older age at time of repair	Longer duration of follow-up Syncope, palpitations	Longer duration of follow-up Syncope, palpitations Older-type Fontan (atriopulmonary connection)	Longer duration of follow-up ≥2 episodes of syncope
Hemodynamic	Severe pulmonary regurgitation Severe RV enlargement ≥Moderate RV systolic dysfunction Extensive RV fibrosis ≥Moderate LV systolic dysfunction Elevated LV end-diastolic pressure	Depressed systemic RV function	Depressed single ventricular function	Outflow gradient >50 mm Hg High LV end-diastolic pressure Depressed LV systolic function Severe LV hypertrophy
Electrophysiological	Atrial tachycardia Nonsustained VT on Holter Inducible VT at EPS QRS duration ≥180 ms	Atrial tachycardia	Atrial tachycardia	Aortic regurgitation

Abbreviations: LV, left ventricular; RV, right ventricular; TOF, tetralogy of Fallot; VT, ventricular tachycardia.
Adapted from Walsh EP. Sudden death in adult congenital heart disease: risk stratification in 2014. Heart Rhythm 2014;11:1735–42; with permission.

with inducible ventricular arrhythmia at electrophysiology study or in those with moderate-severe CHD in whom there is a high clinical suspicion of ventricular arrhythmia.[2]

Appropriate ICD discharges among CHD recipients is similar to patients without CHD (7%–9% per year), but inappropriate discharges are reported in approximately 27% of patients and lead failures are more common than in patients without CHD.[134–136] Numerous configurations of coils and patches have been described for shock delivery when epicardial implantation is the only option.[137,138] However, epicardial implantation has the disadvantage of more invasive procedures, higher lead failure rates, and a possibility of developing restrictive "pericardial" physiology.[134,139] Subcutaneous array and coils originally designed for adjunctive use to lower the defibrillation threshold have been used as the sole defibrillation lead.[138,140] The novel subcutaneous ICD system also may be useful in those patients who do not require antibradycardia

pacing or antitachycardia pacing, as the system is capable of defibrillation only.[2]

SUMMARY

An increasing prevalence of children with CHD surviving into adulthood means that the adult cardiologist will be increasingly involved in the care of such patients. Cardiac arrhythmias are a major source of morbidity and mortality in adults with CHD. A multidisciplinary approach in a center specializing in the care of ACHD is most likely to have the expertise needed provide this care. Knowledge of the underlying anatomy, mechanism of arrhythmia, and potential management strategies is critical, as well as access and expertise in the use of advanced imaging and ablative technologies. Pharmacotherapy has key limitations in this cohort and there is a general preference for early catheter ablation, particularly for arrhythmias such as SVT, IART, and VT. Prevention of thromboembolism is paramount, as the moderate-complex ACHD population is at high risk. Pacing and defibrillation pose key challenges in terms of vascular, intracardiac, and epicardial access. Risk of SCD in the ACHD population is low overall, but certain high-risk groups exist in whom risk stratification for primary prevention of SCD need to be refined. Future challenges in management include refining the underlying mechanism and putative ablation targets for catheter ablation of AF, an arrhythmia rapidly rising in prevalence in this population.

REFERENCES

1. Khairy P, Ionescu-Ittu R, Mackie AS, et al. Changing mortality in congenital heart disease. J Am Coll Cardiol 2010;56:1149–57.

2. Khairy P, Van Hare GF, Balaji S, et al. PACES/HRS expert consensus statement on the recognition and management of arrhythmias in adult congenital heart disease: developed in partnership between the Pediatric and Congenital Electrophysiology Society (PACES) and the Heart Rhythm Society (HRS). Endorsed by the governing bodies of PACES, HRS, the American College of Cardiology (ACC), the American Heart Association (AHA), the European Heart Rhythm Association (EHRA), the Canadian Heart Rhythm Society (CHRS), and the International Society for Adult Congenital Heart Disease (ISACHD). Can J Cardiol 2014;30:e1–63.

3. Wren C, O'Sullivan JJ. Survival with congenital heart disease and need for follow up in adult life. Heart 2001;85:438–43.

4. van der Bom T, Zomer AC, Zwinderman AH, et al. The changing epidemiology of congenital heart disease. Nat Rev Cardiol 2011;8:50–60.

5. Marelli AJ, Mackie AS, Ionescu-Ittu R, et al. Congenital heart disease in the general population: changing prevalence and age distribution. Circulation 2007;115:163–72.

6. Mackie AS, Pilote L, Ionescu-Ittu R, et al. Health care resource utilization in adults with congenital heart disease. Am J Cardiol 2007;99:839–43.

7. Triedman JK. Arrhythmias in adults with congenital heart disease. Heart 2002;87:383–9.

8. Tutarel O, Kempny A, Alonso-Gonzalez R, et al. Congenital heart disease beyond the age of 60: emergence of a new population with high resource utilization, high morbidity, and high mortality. Eur Heart J 2014;35:725–32.

9. Moons P, Van Deyk K, Dedroog D, et al. Prevalence of cardiovascular risk factors in adults with congenital heart disease. Eur J Cardiovasc Prev Rehabil 2006;13:612–6.

10. Summary of recommendations–care of the adult with congenital heart disease. J Am Coll Cardiol 2001;37:1167–9.

11. Walsh EP, Cecchin F. Arrhythmias in adult patients with congenital heart disease. Circulation 2007; 115:534–45.

12. Sherwin ED, Triedman JK, Walsh EP. Update on interventional electrophysiology in congenital heart disease: evolving solutions for complex hearts. Circ Arrhythm Electrophysiol 2013;6:1032–40.

13. Nieminen HP, Jokinen EV, Sairanen HI. Causes of late deaths after pediatric cardiac surgery: a population-based study. J Am Coll Cardiol 2007; 50:1263–71.

14. Oechslin EN, Harrison DA, Connelly MS, et al. Mode of death in adults with congenital heart disease. Am J Cardiol 2000;86:1111–6.

15. Silka MJ, Hardy BG, Menashe VD, et al. A population-based prospective evaluation of risk of sudden cardiac death after operation for common congenital heart defects. J Am Coll Cardiol 1998;32:245–51.

16. Verheugt CL, Uiterwaal CS, van der Velde ET, et al. Mortality in adult congenital heart disease. Eur Heart J 2010;31:1220–9.

17. Kaemmerer H, Fratz S, Bauer U, et al. Emergency hospital admissions and three-year survival of adults with and without cardiovascular surgery for congenital cardiac disease. J Thorac Cardiovasc Surg 2003;126:1048–52.

18. Bouchardy J, Therrien J, Pilote L, et al. Atrial arrhythmias in adults with congenital heart disease. Circulation 2009;120:1679–86.

19. Khairy P, Aboulhosn J, Gurvitz MZ, et al. Arrhythmia burden in adults with surgically repaired tetralogy of Fallot: a multi-institutional study. Circulation 2010;122:868–75.

20. Khairy P, Fernandes SM, Mayer JE Jr, et al. Long-term survival, modes of death, and predictors of mortality in patients with Fontan surgery. Circulation 2008;117:85–92.

21. Ghai A, Harris L, Harrison DA, et al. Outcomes of late atrial tachyarrhythmias in adults after the Fontan operation. J Am Coll Cardiol 2001;37:585–92.

22. Philip F, Muhammad KI, Agarwal S, et al. Pulmonary vein isolation for the treatment of drug-refractory atrial fibrillation in adults with congenital heart disease. Congenit Heart Dis 2012;7:392–9.

23. Kirsh JA, Walsh EP, Triedman JK. Prevalence of and risk factors for atrial fibrillation and intra-atrial reentrant tachycardia among patients with congenital heart disease. Am J Cardiol 2002;90:338–40.

24. Walsh EP. Sudden death in adult congenital heart disease: risk stratification in 2014. Heart Rhythm 2014;11:1735–42.

25. Murphy JG, Gersh BJ, Mair DD, et al. Long-term outcome in patients undergoing surgical repair of tetralogy of Fallot. N Engl J Med 1993;329:593–9.

26. Gatzoulis MA, Balaji S, Webber SA, et al. Risk factors for arrhythmia and sudden cardiac death late

after repair of tetralogy of Fallot: a multicentre study. Lancet 2000;356:975–81.

27. Nollert G, Fischlein T, Bouterwek S, et al. Long-term survival in patients with repair of tetralogy of Fallot: 36-year follow-up of 490 survivors of the first year after surgical repair. J Am Coll Cardiol 1997;30: 1374–83.

28. Norgaard MA, Lauridsen P, Helvind M, et al. Twenty-to-thirty-seven-year follow-up after repair for Tetralogy of Fallot. Eur J Cardiothorac Surg 1999;16:125–30.

29. Anderson RH, Ho SY. The disposition of the conduction tissues in congenitally malformed hearts with reference to their embryological development. J Perinat Med 1991;19(Suppl 1):201–6.

30. Oh JK, Holmes DR Jr, Hayes DL, et al. Cardiac arrhythmias in patients with surgical repair of Ebstein's anomaly. J Am Coll Cardiol 1985;6:1351–7.

31. Smith WM, Gallagher JJ, Kerr CR, et al. The electrophysiologic basis and management of symptomatic recurrent tachycardia in patients with Ebstein's anomaly of the tricuspid valve. Am J Cardiol 1982;49:1223–34.

32. Saul JP, Walsh EP, Triedman JK. Mechanisms and therapy of complex arrhythmias in pediatric patients. J Cardiovasc Electrophysiol 1995;6: 1129–48.

33. Epstein MR, Saul JP, Weindling SN, et al. Atrioventricular reciprocating tachycardia involving twin atrioventricular nodes in patients with complex congenital heart disease. J Cardiovasc Electrophysiol 2001;12:671–9.

34. Kalman JM, Olgin JE, Saxon LA, et al. Activation and entrainment mapping defines the tricuspid annulus as the anterior barrier in typical atrial flutter. Circulation 1996;94:398–406.

35. Nakagawa H, Shah N, Matsudaira K, et al. Characterization of reentrant circuit in macroreentrant right atrial tachycardia after surgical repair of congenital heart disease: isolated channels between scars allow "focal" ablation. Circulation 2001;103:699–709.

36. de Groot NM, Lukac P, Blom NA, et al. Long-term outcome of ablative therapy of postoperative supraventricular tachycardias in patients with univentricular heart: a European multicenter study. Circ Arrhythm Electrophysiol 2009;2:242–8.

37. Love BA, Collins KK, Walsh EP, et al. Electroanatomic characterization of conduction barriers in sinus/atrially paced rhythm and association with intra-atrial reentrant tachycardia circuits following congenital heart disease surgery. J Cardiovasc Electrophysiol 2001;12:17–25.

38. Mandapati R, Walsh EP, Triedman JK. Pericaval and periannular intra-atrial reentrant tachycardias in patients with congenital heart disease. J Cardiovasc Electrophysiol 2003;14:119–25.

39. de Groot NM, Schalij MJ, Zeppenfeld K, et al. Voltage and activation mapping: how the recording technique affects the outcome of catheter ablation procedures in patients with congenital heart disease. Circulation 2003;108:2099–106.

40. Gandhi SK, Bromberg BI, Rodefeld MD, et al. Spontaneous atrial flutter in a chronic canine model of the modified Fontan operation. J Am Coll Cardiol 1997;30:1095–103.

41. Kalman JM, VanHare GF, Olgin JE, et al. Ablation of 'incisional' reentrant atrial tachycardia complicating surgery for congenital heart disease. Use of entrainment to define a critical isthmus of conduction. Circulation 1996;93:502–12.

42. Lee G, Sanders P, Kalman JM. Catheter ablation of atrial arrhythmias: state of the art. Lancet 2012;380: 1509–19.

43. Triedman JK, Jenkins KJ, Colan SD, et al. Intra-atrial reentrant tachycardia after palliation of congenital heart disease: characterization of multiple macroreentrant circuits using fluoroscopically based three-dimensional endocardial mapping. J Cardiovasc Electrophysiol 1997;8:259–70.

44. Fishberger SB, Wernovsky G, Gentles TL, et al. Factors that influence the development of atrial flutter after the Fontan operation. J Thorac Cardiovasc Surg 1997;113:80–6.

45. Garson A Jr, Bink-Boelkens M, Hesslein PS, et al. Atrial flutter in the young: a collaborative study of 380 cases. J Am Coll Cardiol 1985;6:871–8.

46. de Groot NM, Zeppenfeld K, Wijffels MC, et al. Ablation of focal atrial arrhythmia in patients with congenital heart defects after surgery: role of circumscribed areas with heterogeneous conduction. Heart Rhythm 2006;3:526–35.

47. De Groot NM, Blom N, Vd Wall EE, et al. Different mechanisms underlying consecutive, postoperative atrial tachyarrhythmias in a Fontan patient. Pacing Clin Electrophysiol 2009;32:e18–20.

48. Berger F, Vogel M, Kramer A, et al. Incidence of atrial flutter/fibrillation in adults with atrial septal defect before and after surgery. Ann Thorac Surg 1999;68:75–8.

49. Gatzoulis MA, Freeman MA, Siu SC, et al. Atrial arrhythmia after surgical closure of atrial septal defects in adults. N Engl J Med 1999;340:839–46.

50. Flinn CJ, Wolff GS, Dick M 2nd, et al. Cardiac rhythm after the Mustard operation for complete transposition of the great arteries. N Engl J Med 1984;310:1635–8.

51. Roos-Hesselink J, Perlroth MG, McGhie J, et al. Atrial arrhythmias in adults after repair of tetralogy of Fallot. Correlations with clinical, exercise, and echocardiographic findings. Circulation 1995;91: 2214–9.

52. Khairy P, Harris L, Landzberg MJ, et al. Sudden death and defibrillators in transposition of the great

arteries with intra-atrial baffles: a multicenter study. Circ Arrhythm Electrophysiol 2008;1:250–7.

53. Hoffmann A, Chockalingam P, Balint OH, et al. Cerebrovascular accidents in adult patients with congenital heart disease. Heart 2010;96:1223–6.

54. Khairy P. Thrombosis in congenital heart disease. Expert Rev Cardiovasc Ther 2013;11:1579–82.

55. Teh AW, Medi C, Lee G, et al. Long-term outcome following ablation of atrial flutter occurring late after atrial septal defect repair. Pacing Clin Electrophysiol 2011;34:431–5.

56. Katritsis DG. Transseptal puncture through atrial septal closure devices. Heart Rhythm 2011;8: 1676–7.

57. Zeppenfeld K, Schalij MJ, Bartelings MM, et al. Catheter ablation of ventricular tachycardia after repair of congenital heart disease: electroanatomic identification of the critical right ventricular isthmus. Circulation 2007;116:2241–52.

58. Gonska BD, Cao K, Raab J, et al. Radiofrequency catheter ablation of right ventricular tachycardia late after repair of congenital heart defects. Circulation 1996;94:1902–8.

59. Gallego P, Gonzalez AE, Sanchez-Recalde A, et al. Incidence and predictors of sudden cardiac arrest in adults with congenital heart defects repaired before adult life. Am J Cardiol 2012;110:109–17.

60. Morwood JG, Triedman JK, Berul CI, et al. Radiofrequency catheter ablation of ventricular tachycardia in children and young adults with congenital heart disease. Heart Rhythm 2004;1: 301–8.

61. Murphy JG, Gersh BJ, McGoon MD, et al. Long-term outcome after surgical repair of isolated atrial septal defect. Follow-up at 27 to 32 years. N Engl J Med 1990;323:1645–50.

62. Deanfield JE, McKenna WJ, Presbitero P, et al. Ventricular arrhythmia in unrepaired and repaired tetralogy of Fallot. Relation to age, timing of repair, and haemodynamic status. Br Heart J 1984;52:77–81.

63. Gatzoulis MA, Munk MD, Williams WG, et al. Definitive palliation with cavopulmonary or aortopulmonary shunts for adults with single ventricle physiology. Heart 2000;83:51–7.

64. Keane JF, Driscoll DJ, Gersony WM, et al. Second natural history study of congenital heart defects. Results of treatment of patients with aortic valvar stenosis. Circulation 1993;87:I16–27.

65. Walsh EP. Interventional electrophysiology in patients with congenital heart disease. Circulation 2007;115:3224–34.

66. Wolfe RR, Driscoll DJ, Gersony WM, et al. Arrhythmias in patients with valvar aortic stenosis, valvar pulmonary stenosis, and ventricular septal defect. Results of 24-hour ECG monitoring. Circulation 1993;87:I89–101.

67. Kapel GF, Reichlin T, Wijnmaalen AP, et al. Left-sided ablation of ventricular tachycardia in adults with repaired tetralogy of Fallot: a case series. Circ Arrhythm Electrophysiol 2014;7:889–97.

68. Edwards WD, Edwards JE. Pathology of the sinus node in d-transposition following the Mustard operation. J Thorac Cardiovasc Surg 1978;75:213–8.

69. Gillette PC, el-Said GM, Sivarajan N, et al. Electrophysiological abnormalities after Mustard's operation for transposition of the great arteries. Br Heart J 1974;36:186–91.

70. Escudero C, Khairy P, Sanatani S. Electrophysiologic considerations in congenital heart disease and their relationship to heart failure. Can J Cardiol 2013;29:821–9.

71. Anderson RH, Becker AE, Arnold R, et al. The conducting tissues in congenitally corrected transposition. Circulation 1974;50:911–23.

72. Papagiannis J, Avramidis D, Alexopoulos C, et al. Radiofrequency ablation of accessory pathways in children and congenital heart disease patients: impact of a nonfluoroscopic navigation system. Pacing Clin Electrophysiol 2011;34:1288–396.

73. Thiene G, Wenink AC, Frescura C, et al. Surgical anatomy and pathology of the conduction tissues in atrioventricular defects. J Thorac Cardiovasc Surg 1981;82:928–37.

74. Huhta JC, Maloney JD, Ritter DG, et al. Complete atrioventricular block in patients with atrioventricular discordance. Circulation 1983;67:1374–7.

75. Connelly MS, Liu PP, Williams WG, et al. Congenitally corrected transposition of the great arteries in the adult: functional status and complications. J Am Coll Cardiol 1996;27:1238–43.

76. Beauchesne LM, Warnes CA, Connolly HM, et al. Outcome of the unoperated adult who presents with congenitally corrected transposition of the great arteries. J Am Coll Cardiol 2002;40:285–90.

77. Graham TP Jr, Bernard YD, Mellen BG, et al. Long-term outcome in congenitally corrected transposition of the great arteries: a multi-institutional study. J Am Coll Cardiol 2000;36:255–61.

78. Stephenson EA, Casavant D, Tuzi J, et al. Efficacy of atrial antitachycardia pacing using the Medtronic AT500 pacemaker in patients with congenital heart disease. Am J Cardiol 2003;92:871–6.

79. Hoyer AW, Balaji S. The safety and efficacy of ibutilide in children and in patients with congenital heart disease. Pacing Clin Electrophysiol 2007; 30:1003–8.

80. Rao SO, Boramanand NK, Burton DA, et al. Atrial tachycardias in young adults and adolescents with congenital heart disease: conversion using single dose oral sotalol. Int J Cardiol 2009;136:253–7.

81. Balaji S, Johnson TB, Sade RM, et al. Management of atrial flutter after the Fontan procedure. J Am Coll Cardiol 1994;23:1209–15.

82. Rhodes LA, Walsh EP, Gamble WJ, et al. Benefits and potential risks of atrial antitachycardia pacing after repair of congenital heart disease. Pacing Clin Electrophysiol 1995;18:1005–16.

83. Anderson JL, Halperin JL, Albert NM, et al. Management of patients with atrial fibrillation (compilation of 2006 ACCF/AHA/ESC and 2011 ACCF/AHA/HRS recommendations): a report of the American College of Cardiology/American Heart Association Task Force on Practice Guidelines. J Am Coll Cardiol 2013;61:1935–44.

84. Feltes TF, Friedman RA. Transesophageal echocardiographic detection of atrial thrombi in patients with nonfibrillation atrial tachyarrhythmias and congenital heart disease. J Am Coll Cardiol 1994;24:1365–70.

85. Ammash NM, Phillips SD, Hodge DO, et al. Outcome of direct current cardioversion for atrial arrhythmias in adults with congenital heart disease. Int J Cardiol 2012;154:270–4.

86. Manlhiot C, Menjak IB, Brandão LR, et al. Risk, clinical features, and outcomes of thrombosis associated with pediatric cardiac surgery. Circulation 2011;124:1511–9.

87. McCrindle BW, Manlhiot C, Cochrane A, et al. Factors associated with thrombotic complications after the Fontan procedure: a secondary analysis of a multicenter, randomized trial of primary thromboprophylaxis for 2 years after the Fontan procedure. J Am Coll Cardiol 2013;61:346–53.

88. Idorn L, Jensen AS, Juul K, et al. Thromboembolic complications in Fontan patients: population-based prevalence and exploration of the etiology. Pediatr Cardiol 2013;34:262–72.

89. Fyfe DA, Kline CH, Sade RM, et al. Transesophageal echocardiography detects thrombus formation not identified by transthoracic echocardiography after the Fontan operation. J Am Coll Cardiol 1991;18:1733–7.

90. Moak JP, Smith RT, Garson A Jr. Mexiletine: an effective antiarrhythmic drug for treatment of ventricular arrhythmias in congenital heart disease. J Am Coll Cardiol 1987;10:824–9.

91. Deal BJ, Scagliotti D, Miller SM, et al. Electrophysiologic drug testing in symptomatic ventricular arrhythmias after repair of tetralogy of Fallot. Am J Cardiol 1987;59:1380–5.

92. Furushima H, Chinushi M, Sugiura H, et al. Ventricular tachycardia late after repair of congenital heart disease: efficacy of combination therapy with radiofrequency catheter ablation and class III antiarrhythmic agents and long-term outcome. J Electrocardiol 2006;39:219–24.

93. Chetaille P, Walsh EP, Triedman JK. Outcomes of radiofrequency catheter ablation of atrioventricular reciprocating tachycardia in patients with congenital heart disease. Heart Rhythm 2004;1:168–73.

94. Zachariah JP, Walsh EP, Triedman JK, et al. Multiple accessory pathways in the young: the impact of structural heart disease. Am Heart J 2013;165:87–92.

95. Reich JD, Auld D, Hulse E, et al. The pediatric radiofrequency ablation Registry's experience with Ebstein's anomaly. Pediatric Electrophysiology Society. J Cardiovasc Electrophysiol 1998;9:1370–7.

96. Roten L, Lukac P, DE Groot N, et al. Catheter ablation of arrhythmias in Ebstein's anomaly: a multicenter study. J Cardiovasc Electrophysiol 2011;22:1391–6.

97. Triedman JK, Bergau DM, Saul JP, et al. Efficacy of radiofrequency ablation for control of intraatrial reentrant tachycardia in patients with congenital heart disease. J Am Coll Cardiol 1997;30:1032–8.

98. Yap SC, Harris L, Silversides CK, et al. Outcome of intra-atrial re-entrant tachycardia catheter ablation in adults with congenital heart disease: negative impact of age and complex atrial surgery. J Am Coll Cardiol 2010;56:1589–96.

99. de Groot NM, Atary JZ, Blom NA, et al. Long-term outcome after ablative therapy of postoperative atrial tachyarrhythmia in patients with congenital heart disease and characteristics of atrial tachyarrhythmia recurrences. Circ Arrhythm Electrophysiol 2010;3:148–54.

100. Triedman JK, Alexander ME, Love BA, et al. Influence of patient factors and ablative technologies on outcomes of radiofrequency ablation of intra-atrial reentrant tachycardia in patients with congenital heart disease. J Am Coll Cardiol 2002;39:1827–35.

101. Seiler J, Schmid DK, Irtel TA, et al. Dual-loop circuits in postoperative atrial macro re-entrant tachycardias. Heart 2007;93:325–30.

102. Tanner H, Lukac P, Schwick N, et al. Irrigated-tip catheter ablation of intraatrial reentrant tachycardia in patients late after surgery of congenital heart disease. Heart Rhythm 2004;1:268–75.

103. de Groot NM, Lukac P, Schalij MJ, et al. Long-term outcome of ablative therapy of post-operative atrial tachyarrhythmias in patients with tetralogy of Fallot: a European multi-centre study. Europace 2012;14:522–7.

104. Kannankeril PJ, Anderson ME, Rottman JN, et al. Frequency of late recurrence of intra-atrial reentry tachycardia after radiofrequency catheter ablation in patients with congenital heart disease. Am J Cardiol 2003;92:879–81.

105. Correa R, Sherwin ED, Kovach J, et al. Mechanism and ablation of arrhythmia following total cavopulmonary connection. Circ Arrhythm Electrophysiol 2015;8:318–25.

106. Bae EJ, Ban JE, Lee JA, et al. Pediatric radiofrequency catheter ablation: results of initial 100 consecutive cases including congenital heart anomalies. J Korean Med Sci 2005;20:740–6.

107. Friedman RA, Will JC, Fenrich AL, et al. Atrioventricular junction ablation and pacemaker therapy in patients with drug-resistant atrial tachyarrhythmias after the Fontan operation. J Cardiovasc Electrophysiol 2005;16:24–9.

108. Correa R, Walsh EP, Alexander ME, et al. Transbaffle mapping and ablation for atrial tachycardias after Mustard, Senning, or Fontan operations. J Am Heart Assoc 2013;2:e000325.

109. Epstein AE, DiMarco JP, Ellenbogen KA, et al. ACC/AHA/HRS 2008 guidelines for device-based therapy of cardiac rhythm abnormalities: a report of the American College of Cardiology/American Heart Association Task Force on Practice Guidelines (writing committee to revise the ACC/AHA/NASPE 2002 guideline update for implantation of cardiac Pacemakers and Antiarrhythmia devices) developed in collaboration with the American Association for Thoracic Surgery and Society of Thoracic Surgeons. J Am Coll Cardiol 2008;51:e1–62.

110. Gregoratos G, Abrams J, Epstein AE, et al. ACC/AHA/NASPE 2002 guideline update for implantation of cardiac pacemakers and antiarrhythmia devices–summary article: a report of the American College of Cardiology/American Heart Association Task Force on Practice Guidelines (ACC/AHA/NASPE Committee to update the 1998 pacemaker guidelines). J Am Coll Cardiol 2002;40:1703–19.

111. Cecchin F, Atallah J, Walsh EP, et al. Lead extraction in pediatric and congenital heart disease patients. Circ Arrhythm Electrophysiol 2010;3:437–44.

112. Knauth AL, Lock JE, Perry SB, et al. Transcatheter device closure of congenital and postoperative residual ventricular septal defects. Circulation 2004;110:501–7.

113. Khairy P, Landzberg MJ, Gatzoulis MA, et al. Transvenous pacing leads and systemic thromboemboli in patients with intracardiac shunts: a multicenter study. Circulation 2006;113:2391–7.

114. van Geldorp IE, Bordachar P, Lumens J, et al. Acute hemodynamic benefits of biventricular and single-site systemic ventricular pacing in patients with a systemic right ventricle. Heart Rhythm 2013;10:676–82.

115. Thambo JB, De Guillebon M, Xhaet O, et al. Biventricular pacing in patients with Tetralogy of Fallot: non-invasive epicardial mapping and clinical impact. Int J Cardiol 2013;163:170–4.

116. Cecchin F, Frangini PA, Brown DW, et al. Cardiac resynchronization therapy (and multisite pacing) in pediatrics and congenital heart disease: five years experience in a single institution. J Cardiovasc Electrophysiol 2009;20:58–65.

117. Janousek J, Gebauer RA, Abdul-Khaliq H, et al. Cardiac resynchronisation therapy in paediatric and congenital heart disease: differential effects in various anatomical and functional substrates. Heart 2009;95:1165–71.

118. Tracy CM, Epstein AE, Darbar D, et al. 2012 ACCF/AHA/HRS focused update of the 2008 guidelines for device-based therapy of cardiac rhythm abnormalities: a report of the American College of Cardiology Foundation/American Heart Association Task Force on Practice Guidelines and the Heart Rhythm Society. [corrected]. Circulation 2012;126:1784–800.

119. Koyak Z, Harris L, de Groot JR, et al. Sudden cardiac death in adult congenital heart disease. Circulation 2012;126:1944–54.

120. Perry JC. Sudden cardiac death and malignant arrhythmias: the scope of the problem in adult congenital heart patients. Pediatr Cardiol 2012;33:484–90.

121. Kammeraad JA, van Deurzen CH, Sreeram N, et al. Predictors of sudden cardiac death after Mustard or Senning repair for transposition of the great arteries. J Am Coll Cardiol 2004;44:1095–102.

122. Janousek J, Paul T, Luhmer I, et al. Atrial baffle procedures for complete transposition of the great arteries: natural course of sinus node dysfunction and risk factors for dysrhythmias and sudden death. Z Kardiol 1994;83:933–8.

123. Kavey RE, Thomas FD, Byrum CJ, et al. Ventricular arrhythmias and biventricular dysfunction after repair of tetralogy of Fallot. J Am Coll Cardiol 1984;4:126–31.

124. Gatzoulis MA, Till JA, Somerville J, et al. Mechanoelectrical interaction in tetralogy of Fallot. QRS prolongation relates to right ventricular size and predicts malignant ventricular arrhythmias and sudden death. Circulation 1995;92:231–7.

125. Valente AM, Gauvreau K, Assenza GE, et al. Contemporary predictors of death and sustained ventricular tachycardia in patients with repaired tetralogy of Fallot enrolled in the INDICATOR cohort. Heart 2014;100:247–53.

126. Park SJ, On YK, Kim JS, et al. Relation of fragmented QRS complex to right ventricular fibrosis detected by late gadolinium enhancement cardiac magnetic resonance in adults with repaired tetralogy of Fallot. Am J Cardiol 2012;109:110–5.

127. Kempny A, Diller GP, Orwat S, et al. Right ventricular-left ventricular interaction in adults with tetralogy of Fallot: a combined cardiac magnetic resonance and echocardiographic speckle tracking study. Int J Cardiol 2012;154:259–64.

128. Ghai A, Silversides C, Harris L, et al. Left ventricular dysfunction is a risk factor for sudden cardiac death in adults late after repair of tetralogy of Fallot. J Am Coll Cardiol 2002;40:1675–80.

129. Khairy P, Landzberg MJ, Gatzoulis MA, et al. Value of programmed ventricular stimulation after tetralogy of Fallot repair: a multicenter study. Circulation 2004;109:1994–2000.

130. Alexander ME, Walsh EP, Saul JP, et al. Value of programmed ventricular stimulation in patients with congenital heart disease. J Cardiovasc Electrophysiol 1999;10:1033–44.

131. Schwerzmann M, Salehian O, Harris L, et al. Ventricular arrhythmias and sudden death in adults after a Mustard operation for transposition of the great arteries. Eur Heart J 2009;30:1873–9.

132. Gatzoulis MA, Walters J, McLaughlin PR, et al. Late arrhythmia in adults with the Mustard procedure for transposition of great arteries: a surrogate marker for right ventricular dysfunction? Heart 2000;84: 409–15.

133. Cecchin F, Johnsrude CL, Perry JC, et al. Effect of age and surgical technique on symptomatic arrhythmias after the Fontan procedure. Am J Cardiol 1995;76:386–91.

134. Atallah J, Erickson CC, Cecchin F, et al. Multi-institutional study of implantable defibrillator lead performance in children and young adults: results of the Pediatric Lead Extractability and Survival Evaluation (PLEASE) study. Circulation 2013;127:2393–402.

135. Khanna AD, Warnes CA, Phillips SD, et al. Single-center experience with implantable cardioverter-defibrillators in adults with complex congenital heart disease. Am J Cardiol 2011; 108:729–34.

136. Czosek RJ, Bonney WJ, Cassedy A, et al. Impact of cardiac devices on the quality of life in pediatric patients. Circ Arrhythm Electrophysiol 2012;5: 1064–72.

137. Cannon BC, Friedman RA, Fenrich AL, et al. Innovative techniques for placement of implantable cardioverter-defibrillator leads in patients with limited venous access to the heart. Pacing Clin Electrophysiol 2006;29:181–7.

138. Stephenson EA, Batra AS, Knilans TK, et al. A multicenter experience with novel implantable cardioverter defibrillator configurations in the pediatric and congenital heart disease population. J Cardiovasc Electrophysiol 2006;17:41–6.

139. Radbill AE, Triedman JK, Berul CI, et al. System survival of nontransvenous implantable cardioverter-defibrillators compared to transvenous implantable cardioverter-defibrillators in pediatric and congenital heart disease patients. Heart Rhythm 2010;7:193–8.

140. Nery PB, Green MS, Khairy P, et al. Implantable cardioverter-defibrillator insertion in congenital heart disease without transvenous access to the heart. Can J Cardiol 2013;29(254):e1–3.

Heart Failure in Adult Congenital Heart Disease
Nonpharmacologic Treatment Strategies

Lisa LeMond, MD[a], Tuan Mai, MD[a], Craig S. Broberg, MD[a], Ashok Muralidaran, MD[b], Luke J. Burchill, MBBS, PhD[a],*

KEYWORDS

- Adult congenital heart disease • Heart failure • Biomarkers • Arrhythmia • Cardiac surgery
- Structural intervention

KEY POINTS

- Heart failure (HF) accounts for one-quarter of deaths in the adult congenital heart disease (ACHD) population; there has been an 80% increase in ACHD admissions involving HF.
- ACHD patients have lifelong adaptations to physiologic derangements related to their disease. Typical features of HF may not be present in this population.
- Whereas a diagnosis of acquired HF leads to standardized medical therapy, treating HF in ACHD relies on nonpharmacologic strategies, namely, transcatheter interventions and arrhythmias along with cardiac surgery.
- In addition to invasive treatment strategies, adjuvant palliative measures are important for reducing suffering associated with the condition.

UNDERSTANDING HEART FAILURE IN ADULT CONGENITAL HEART DISEASE

Heart failure (HF) accounts for one-quarter of deaths in the adult congenital heart disease (ACHD) population.[1] In parallel with a dramatic increase in the number of hospitalizations for ACHD, there has been an 80% increase in the number of ACHD admissions involving HF during the last decade.[2] HF in ACHD patients is both multifactorial and lesion specific.[3] Those at greatest risk for developing HF are patients with a systemic right ventricle (RV; d-transposition of the great arteries postatrial switch and congenitally corrected transposition of the great arteries), residual valvular dysfunction (ie, pulmonary

regurgitation after tetralogy of Fallot repair, congenital aortic stenosis), patients with a single ventricle circulation with or without Fontan palliation and patients with atrial or ventricular level shunt complicated by pulmonary hypertension. The observation that "repaired" ACHD patients also present with late-onset HF is a reminder that intrinsic myocardial structural and functional abnormalities predispose to HF even after the removal of the original anatomic or hemodynamic substrate.[4]

ACHD patients have had lifelong adaptations to physiologic derangements related to their underlying cardiac pathology. Thus, typical features of HF may not be present in this population. Chronic exercise intolerance is well-recognized, but is

Conflict of Interest: The authors have no conflict of interest to declare.

Disclosures: The authors have no grant or other funding disclosures.

[a] Adult Congenital Heart Disease Program, Knight Cardiovascular Institute, Oregon Health & Science University, Portland, OR 97239, USA; [b] Pediatric Cardiac Surgery, Doernbecher Children's Hospital, Oregon Health & Science University, Portland, OR 97239, USA

* Corresponding author. UHN 62, Knight Cardiovascular Institute, 3181 S.W. Sam Jackson Park Road, Portland, OR 97239.

E-mail address: burchilu@ohsu.edu

frequently underestimated. Cardiopulmonary exercise testing confirms universal reductions in peak oxygen uptake and circulatory dysfunction across the spectrum of congenital heart disease complexity.[5]

Whereas a diagnosis of acquired HF leads to standardized medical therapy for improvement of symptoms and prognosis, HF management in ACHD frequently rests on nonpharmacologic strategies. Clinicians caring for ACHD patients consider a wide array of factors that conspire to cause HF in this context. This article reviews emerging perspectives on nonpharmacologic treatment strategies for ACHD-related HF, including transcatheter interventions for structural heart disease, invasive electrophysiology strategies, and cardiac surgery. Whereas heart transplantation is beyond the scope of this review, the importance of palliative care in patients with end-stage disease is discussed.

INVASIVE HEMODYNAMIC EVALUATION AND TRANSCATHETER INTERVENTIONS IN ADULT CONGENITAL HEART DISEASE–RELATED HEART FAILURE

Invasive hemodynamic evaluation plays a crucial role in the evaluation and treatment of patients with ACHD. Accurate assessment of HF patients' hemodynamic state by physical examination often underestimates severity,[6] particularly in younger ACHD patients who may not demonstrate classic physical findings of increased ventricular filling pressures, such as peripheral and pulmonary edema, until late in the course of their HF trajectory. The initial assessment of ACHD patients presenting with newly diagnosed HF begins with noninvasive investigations including electrocardiographs, laboratory tests, echocardiography, and imaging (chest x-ray, MRI, CT) directed by the history and physical examination. Depending on the results of these initial investigations, invasive hemodynamic assessment may be considered (**Fig. 1**).

In addition to facilitating tailored (diuretic and other) therapy, cardiac catheterization identifies residual lesions that may be contributing to HF pathophysiology. Residual cardiac lesions suitable for catheter-based interventions include[1] pressure and/or volume overload lesions,[2] intracardiac and extracardiac shunting and,[3] lesion-specific interventions for unique ACHD subgroups, namely d-transposition of the great arteries after atrial switch (Senning or Mustard) and those with failing Fontan physiology.

Mustard/Senning patients are at increased risk of HF owing to systemic ventricular dysfunction,

systemic atrioventricular (AV) valve regurgitation, atrial arrhythmias, and pulmonary hypertension. Baffle complications are common with leaks reported in up to 25%[7] and varying degrees of baffle stenosis (superior vena cava > inferior vena cava) in 5% to 15% of patients.[8,9] Baffle leaks and stenoses often coexist. Depending on shunt volume and direction, baffle leaks may lead to ventricular volume overload (left-to-right shunt), systemic arterial desaturation, and systemic embolization (right-to-left shunt). When significant, systemic venous baffle stenosis can increase systemic venous pressure and impede venous return leading to reduced cardiac output. However, superior vena cava baffle stenosis is often asymptomatic owing to venous collaterals and azygous flow reversal developing as an alternative route for venous return to the heart. Inferior vena cava baffle stenosis or obstruction is less well-tolerated and may lead to hepatic venous congestion, hepatomegaly, and ascites. Pulmonary venous baffle obstruction leading to increased pulmonary venous pressure is a potentially reversible cause of pulmonary edema and hypertension that should be considered in Mustard/Senning patients presenting with these conditions.

Transthoracic echocardiography with saline contrast injection is helpful for confirming the presence of a baffle leak, although additional imaging with MRI and/or transesophageal echocardiography is usually needed to localize the leak. Cardiac catheterization remains the gold standard for evaluating hemodynamic status and should be undertaken in Mustard/Senning patients presenting with HF. Owing to high perioperative mortality for surgical baffle reintervention,[10] transcatheter procedures are now widely preferred as a lower risk alternative. For some patients, relief of baffle leaks and/or stenosis can translate to significant improvements in functional class and hemodynamics.[11] Percutaneous interventions include balloon angioplasty for baffle stenosis with or without stent placement. Baffle leaks can also be treated with deployment of a covered stent.

Adults with failing Fontan physiology typically demonstrate evidence of chronic systemic venous hypertension, low cardiac output, and ventricular diastolic dysfunction.[12] These changes progress over time and contribute to additional manifestations of HF, including atrial arrhythmia, hepatic venous and splanchnic congestion, ascites, protein-losing enteropathy (PLE), and plastic bronchitis. Other contributors that should be sought in patients presenting with failing Fontan physiology include pulmonary venous obstruction secondary to right atrial dilation, ventricular outflow tract obstruction, AV valve regurgitation, and residual

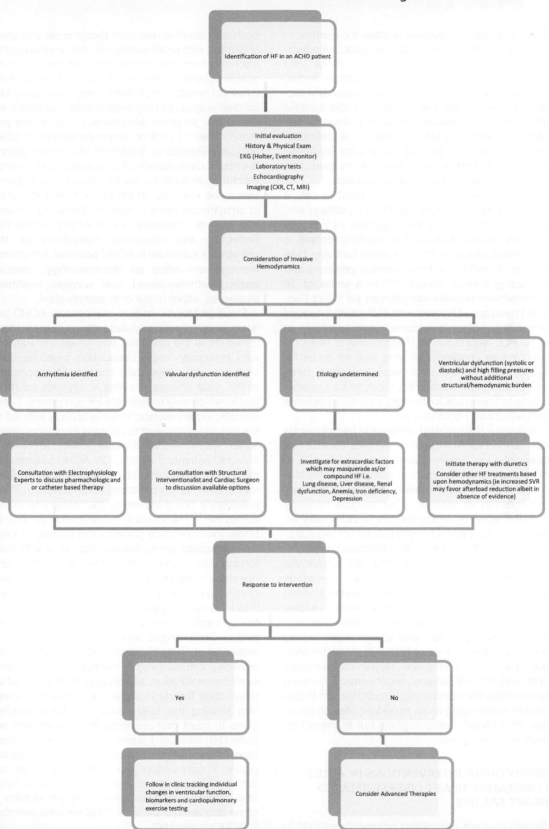

Fig. 1. The initial assessment of adult congenital heart disease (ACHD) patients presenting with newly diagnosed heart failure (HF). CXR, chest x-ray; EKG, electrocardiograph; SVR, systemic vascular resistance.

aortic coarctation. Surgery is often the best technical solution for these cardiac residua, but operative risk is not low, particularly in those with extracardiac disease, including hypoalbuminemia, cachexia, liver, and renal and pulmonary dysfunction. Transcatheter interventions in this context offer lower risk options including balloon angioplasty of pulmonary artery stenosis, coil embolization of collateral vessels to reduce systemic desaturation and/or ventricular volume load, and redilation/restenting of aortic coarctation.

Transcatheter puncture and creation of a communication between the Fontan pathway and common atrium has been suggested as a bridge to heart transplantation. The theoretic benefit is that decompression of the Fontan pathway may help by lowering systemic venous pressure and increasing cardiac output.[13,14] In a series of 16 transcatheter fenestration creation for failing Fontans (mean age, 18 years) with PLE, postprocedural fenestration closure occurred spontaneously in 63%. PLE recurred in all.[15] High rates of fenestration closure coupled with long wait list times for ACHD patients listed for heart transplant mean that fenestration creation is unlikely to be a reliable bridge to transplant for the vast majority of patients with advanced Fontan failure.

Arguably, the greatest advance in percutaneous intervention for ACHD within the past decade has been Melody valve implantation in the RV to pulmonary artery conduits or pulmonary valve bioprostheses in adults with residual pulmonary regurgitation or stenosis after surgical tetralogy of Fallot repair or others with RV to pulmonary artery conduits. Failure to treat pulmonary regurgitation in the long term is associated with HF secondary to both right and left ventricular dysfunction, which may manifest as venous congestion, ventricular arrhythmia, and/or sudden cardiac death. Melody valve implantation is widely accepted as an alternative to operative intervention and is associated with excellent procedural outcomes. Primary valve failure is rare after Melody valve implant. However, reintervention occurs in almost 20% of patients, most commonly owing to recurrent RV outflow tract obstruction.[16] Endocarditis is emerging as an important late complication after Melody valve implant, but its impact on mortality is not clear.

ARRHYTHMIA INTERVENTIONS IN ADULT CONGENITAL HEART DISEASE-RELATED HEART FAILURE

Arrhythmias are associated commonly with HF in ACHD patients, both as a cause and consequence of impaired hemodynamics. Tachyarrhythmias such as intraatrial reentrant tachycardia and atrial fibrillation with rapid ventricular response are common and frequently trigger HF. Conversely, acute exacerbations of HF in which progressive fluid overload leads to increased filling pressures, low cardiac output, and hypoxemia may precipitate arrhythmias. Whether arrhythmia or HF is the primary driver of clinical decompensation is often unclear. Regardless, treatment of both conditions is critical. Optimization of fluid status and ventricular function is necessary for antiarrhythmic therapies to be effective. At the same time, elimination of arrhythmias helps to reverse the hemodynamic and clinical manifestations of ACHD-related HF. Reflecting the increasing complexity of the arrhythmia substrate in ACHD patients, arrhythmia management relies on pharmacologic, device-based, catheter-based, and surgical treatment strategies, either alone or in combination.

Sinus and/or AV node dysfunction in ACHD patients is common, particularly after surgery in close proximity to the sinoatrial and AV nodes. Patients with inherently fragile conduction systems, such as those with congenitally corrected transposition of the great arteries, are also at high risk for heart block, which may exacerbate HF symptoms. Chronotropic incompetence, which is broadly defined as the inability of the heart to increase its rate commensurate with increased physical activity, is common in ACHD patients.[17] Among 727 ACHD patients undergoing cardiopulmonary exercise testing, 62% met criteria for chronotropic incompetence,[18] this prevalence being similar to that observed in acquired HF.[19] The increase in prevalence of chronotropic incompetence parallels the decline in peak oxygen uptake across the spectrum of ACHD, reinforcing the notion that preserved heart rate response is one of the strongest contributors to aerobic exercise ability. The lesson for ACHD clinicians is to look beyond peak oxygen uptake when undertaking cardiopulmonary exercise tests in HF patients. Chronotropic incompetence and related measures such as heart rate reserve and recovery provide additional insights into patients' symptoms, exercise intolerance, and prognosis. In terms of interventions for chronotropic incompetence, exercise training has been used to achieve modest gains in heart rate response in patients with acquired HF, although the precise mechanisms underlying these changes are unclear.[20] Rate adaptive pacing in conjunction with cardiac resynchronization has been associated with increased heart rate, exercise time, and peak oxygen uptake in some acquired HF patients,[21] but remains untested in ACHD-related HF.

The lifetime incidence of atrial arrhythmias in ACHD patients increases with age and is associated with a 2- to 3-fold increased risk of congestive HF.[22] Of the atrial arrhythmias occurring in ACHD patients, intraatrial reentrant tachycardia is the most common.[22,23] Intraatrial reentrant tachycardia is caused by a macro reentrant loop caused by areas of fibrosis from suture lines or patches combined with normal conduction barriers (valve or caval orifices and crista terminalis).[24] It usually has an atrial rate of 150 to 250 bpm, which may enable 1:1 conduction leading to hemodynamic compromise and cardiac arrest.[25] Initial success rate for intraatrial reentrant tachycardia ablation in CHD patients is greater than 80%, but recurrence can be up to 40% within 2 years of ablation for Fontan patients.[24,26]

Atrial fibrillation is frequently associated with ventricular dysfunction and decompensated HF. Standard therapeutic decisions apply in ACHD patients including rate versus rhythm control (with most needing rhythm control), the need for anticoagulation based on stroke risk (recognizing the limited applicability of $CHADS_2VASC$ and other risk scores in this population), and potential bleeding risk in those with kidney and liver disease. When antiarrhythmic drugs fail or are tolerated poorly, catheter-based ablation is often considered although various technical challenges need to be overcome in ACHD patients, including poor vascular access, significant atrial enlargement, and navigating catheters through baffles and conduits. A study evaluating the initial procedural success of pulmonary vein isolation in mostly simple forms of CHD (atrial septal defects) versus noncongenital structural heart disease reported early success in almost half undergoing the procedure with no difference between congenital and noncongenital patients (congenital heart disease, 42% vs noncongenital, 53%; $P = .46$). Four years after pulmonary vein isolation, one-third of congenital patients remained free of atrial fibrillation.[27] Atrial arrhythmia recurrence is significantly higher in ACHD patients with greater defect complexity, occurring in 50% within 6 months of ablation.[28] Repeat ablation is an important consideration in ACHD-related HF, particularly in those where a vicious cycle exists between arrhythmia and decompensated HF. Emerging technologies may improve future ablation outcomes for ACHD patients. Robotic, magnetic-guided catheter ablation system can be directed at less accessible areas and ablate complex circuits across baffles and conduits with immediate success rate of greater than 85% in a small number of CHD patients.[29]

Ventricular arrhythmias are a leading cause of sudden cardiac death in ACHD.[30] ACHD patients are predisposed to ventricular tachycardia owing to the presence of surgical scars from ventriculotomy and/or patch forming macroreentry conduction pathways, as well as chronic volume and pressure overload conditions. Sudden cardiac arrest owing to ventricular arrhythmia may be the first manifestation of HF in ACHD patients. As for ACHD patients presenting with atrial arrhythmias, a thorough hemodynamic assessment is indicated to rule out HF or other cardiac residua amenable to intervention. Although implantable cardioverter defibrillator implantation is clearly indicated in cases of aborted sudden cardiac arrest, consideration should also be given to ACHD patients recurrent unexplained syncope with ventricular dysfunction or inducible ventricular arrhythmias on an electrophysiology study (class IIa indications, level of evidence B).[31] Treatments shown to decrease future ventricular tachycardia burden, including antiarrhythmics and catheter-based ventricular tachycardia ablation, should also be discussed at the time of implantable cardioverter defibrillator implantation.[32]

Cardiac resynchronization therapy (CRT) is recommended in adults with acquired HF with ejection fraction of less than 35% and a QRS duration of greater than 120 ms secondary to left bundle branch block.[33] Improvements in New York Heart Association (NYHA) class, exercise tolerance, and ejection fraction have also been observed with CRT in ACHD populations, indicating that this therapy should be considered in those presenting with HF, particularly when other pacemaker indications exist. The benefits of CRT seem to be greatest for patients with ACHD with biventricular anatomy and a decreased left ventricular ejection fraction.[34] Presence of a systemic left ventricle is an independent predictor of a greater improvement in ventricular function and remodeling after CRT.[35] Standard CRT criteria apply to a small fraction (5%) of patients with a systemic RV. Improvements in NYHA class, RV ejection fraction, and peak oxygen uptake have, however, been reported leading the 2014 CRT guidelines on ACHD from the Heart Rhythm Society to give a class IIb recommendation for consideration of CRT in patients with a systemic RV.[36] Whether CRT is useful for patients with single ventricle circulation is unclear, with mixed results to date.[37,38]

OPERATIVE INTERVENTIONS IN ADULT CONGENITAL HEART DISEASE–RELATED HEART FAILURE

Prudence dictates that only patients with potentially reversible HF should undergo major "corrective" heart surgery. The challenge for clinicians is how to quantify the potential for reversibility given the multifactorial nature of HF in ACHD. Among adults with congenitally corrected transposition of the great arteries it can be difficult to determine whether tricuspid (systemic AV) valve regurgitation is the primary cause or a secondary complication of systemic RV dysfunction. Even after successful pulmonary valve replacement, patients with tetralogy of Fallot seldom demonstrate improvements in RV ejection fraction,[39] despite improved remodeling and decreased RV volumes. Fontan conversion improves hemodynamics and arrhythmia burden, although a subgroup of patients (5%) proceed to heart transplantation, indicating that conversion does not address the fundamental limitations of single ventricle circulation. Early operative intervention before the onset of significant ventricular dysfunction and clinical HF has been recommended for various ACHD subgroups. However, the risks of future reoperation along with the impact of complications not addressed or even compounded by surgical intervention, such as arrhythmia and conduction disturbance, need to be considered.

Assessing risk of mortality in ACHD patients undergoing cardiac surgery is highly individualized with little research upon which to make evidence-based recommendations. Greater mortality has been observed in ACHD patients with an increased brain natriuretic peptide (BNP; >100 pg/mL); however, low sensitivity (53%) and positive predictive value (35%) for mortality after cardiac surgery means that BNP cannot be reliably used for surgical selection.[40] Variation in BNP within and between ACHD lesions[41,42] further undermines the predictive value of BNP before and after cardiac surgery. By accounting for defect and operative complexity surgical risk scoring systems, such as Aristotle, Society of Thoracic Surgery-European Association for Cardio-Thoracic Surgery (STAT), and Risk Adjustment for Congenital Heart Surgery (RACHS-1), may be more helpful for assessing operative risk in ACHD patients.[43] Even though these scoring systems were derived and validated in pediatric congenital heart disease populations their predictive ability seems to translate to ACHD patients. The incremental predictive value of the presence or absence of HF to these scores has not been assessed.

The 2008 American College of Cardiology (ACC)/American Heart Association (AHA) guidelines on management of adults with congenital heart disease provide the following indications for operative intervention in repaired tetralogy of Fallot patients: a peak right ventricular outflow tract gradient on echocardiography of greater than 50 mm Hg, a right-to-left ventricular pressure

ratio of greater than 0.7, residual ventricular septal defects with a pulmonary to systemic flow (Qp:Qs) of higher than 1.5, and severe pulmonary regurgitation with associated RV dilation/dysfunction and associated moderate to severe tricuspid regurgitation (TR).[44] Causes of significant TR in this population are unclear, although progressive RV and tricuspid annular dilation secondary to pulmonary regurgitation are most likely. Whether to proceed with concomitant tricuspid valve repair at the time of PVR remains controversial.[45,46]

Systemic RV failure is a major cause of morbidity among adults with congenitally corrected transposition of the great arteries and is the cause of death in more than 50% of patients.[47] Systemic RV failure and severe systemic TR often coexist, even in the absence of other associated lesions such as an Ebstein-like malformation of the tricuspid valve. Discerning whether TR is the cause or consequence of RV dilation and dysfunction remains a challenge.[48] Progressive RV dysfunction and HF after tricuspid valve surgery has led some centers to recommend early tricuspid valve intervention in select patients before the onset of significant RV dilation.

Older children and adults presenting with Ebstein anomaly have better outcomes compared with fetal and neonatal presentations of this disease.[49] The ACC/AHA guidelines recommend surgery for Ebstein anomaly for symptoms of deteriorating exercise capacity, cyanosis, paradoxic embolism, progressive cardiomegaly on chest x-ray, progressive RV dilation, and RV dysfunction.[44] Concomitant arrhythmia surgery is indicated if atrial or ventricular arrhythmias are not amenable to catheter treatments or have been unsuccessfully managed. A wide array of operative approaches has been used, including valve replacement, valve repair, and palliative shunts.[50] Tricuspid valve repair and replacement have each been associated with good long-term outcomes, although significant ventricular systolic dysfunction before surgery should alert clinicians to increased operative mortality risk. Additional factors associated with higher mortality at the time of surgery include cyanosis, right ventricular outflow tract obstruction, hypoplastic pulmonary arteries, cyanosis, and mitral regurgitation.[51] For patients with advanced Ebstein's malformation and severe RV dilation/dysfunction, the construction of a bidirectional cavopulmonary shunt either as a planned or as a rescue procedure has been advocated in association with tricuspid valve repair to unload the RV with encouraging early results.[52]

Recommendations for surgery in adults with a prior Fontan procedure include but are not limited to repair or replacement of a significantly regurgitant AV valve, significant subaortic obstruction, Fontan pathway obstruction, and recurrent atrial fibrillation or flutter requiring a Fontan conversion (revision of an atriopulmonary connection to a lateral tunnel or an extracardiac conduit).[44] Defining HF in this population is difficult; in some respects, all Fontan patients have evidence of HF with low cardiac output, elevated systemic venous pressures and end-organ dysfunction. In those with older style (atriopulmonary) Fontan connections, declining functional status, worsening NYHA class, and arrhythmias refractory to medical therapy should prompt consideration for conversion. A landmark paper from Mavroudis and colleagues[53] describing their outcomes for patients undergoing Fontan conversion with concomitant arrhythmia surgery set the benchmark for clinical outcomes. The authors reported a 0.9% early mortality, 5.4% transplantation rate, and arrhythmia recurrence rate of 7.8%, the latter improving with their modifications to the Maze procedure over time. PLE, moderate to severe AV valve regurgitation, and the presence of a right or ambiguous ventricle were among the preoperative risk factors for death and need for transplantation. Other centers have reported higher mortality rates of up to 10%.[54] A 2015 publication has questioned the traditional indications for the conversion procedure, citing a high (86%) 8-year transplant-free survival among patients undergoing "early conversion."[55] Early Fontan conversion improved NYHA class and reduced arrhythmia burden, although these findings need to be confirmed prospectively before this approach can be recommended as standard of care.

PALLIATIVE CARE IN ADULT CONGENITAL HEART DISEASE–RELATED HEART FAILURE

HF, when not caused by a reversible underlying process, is a highly morbid condition and is associated with both physical and psychological suffering. This may be particularly true for patients with HF and ACHD, where patients may suffer from both conventional HF symptoms such as dyspnea, fatigue, pain, and depression in addition to lesion-specific symptoms. Failing Fontan patients may develop PLE, symptoms of hepatic congestion, plastic bronchitis, or other systemic complaints. Although the mainstay of therapy for ACHD-related HF consists of therapies directed to the underlying cause, it is important to consider adjuvant palliative measures to reduce the suffering associated with the condition. There is an apparent disconnect between symptom burden and symptom relief in ACHD-related HF.

In one study of ACHD patients at the end of life, only 19% had been referred to palliative care services.[56]

A strong correlation has been demonstrated between HF in acquired heart disease and depression, with at least 21% of all HF patients experiencing depression. In a study of 280 moderate and severe complexity ACHD patients, 22% of those interviewed met criteria for at least mild depression and 12% met criteria for moderate to severe depression.[57] This study went on to note that 30% of all patients who met diagnostic criteria for at least one mood disorder had never previously had mental health treatment. The sum of this evidence suggests a high likelihood of undertreatment of depression in this population.

In addition to symptom relief, palliative care providers contribute expertise to end-of-life discussions and advanced care planning. End-of-life discussions are complex and extend beyond defining code status. Learning between ACHD and palliative care providers is often reciprocal. ACHD providers develop new skills and knowledge in providing symptom relief to HF patients. Palliative care providers encounter a younger patient group who often regard themselves as survivors who have "beaten the odds" to defy death in the past. Managing expectations in this setting requires close interdisciplinary collaboration and clear goals regarding the direction of care. Continuing involvement of the ACHD team in patients with end-stage HF is important for maintaining clinical continuity along with the patients trust that providers are not abandoning them owing to medical futility, but rather helping them to navigate the next phase of their ACHD history. Studies of end of life have demonstrated that fewer than 1% of these patients reported having discussions with their providers regarding end-of-life issues. Fewer than 10% of patients who died in the hospital had documented end-of-life discussions before their deaths. Early initiation of end-of-life discussions, before diagnosis with life-threatening complications, was favored by 62% of patients but only 38% of providers.[56] In caring for patients with HF, ACHD clinicians clearly have an opportunity to improve how we care and communicate with those presenting with end-stage disease.

SUMMARY

HF is a leading cause of morbidity and mortality in ACHD patients. A variety of factors influence each patient's HF trajectory including anatomy, age, reoperations, ventricular and valvular function, residual pressure and volume overload, arrhythmias, chronotropic incompetence, and associated mood disorders. Consideration of nonpharmacologic strategies for treating ACHD-related HF and its complications is important when caring for this growing patient population. This approach relies heavily on collaboration between ACHD cardiologists, advanced HF specialists, structural interventional cardiologists, electrophysiologists, and congenital heart surgeons. Although much of the focus is on identifying anatomic, hemodynamic, and electrophysiologic targets for intervention, clinicians should also take time to consider the patients experience including the emergence of anxiety and depression. For patients with end-stage cardiac disease, palliative care involvement is important for end-of-life discussions, advanced care planning, and helping patients *and providers* make the transition from cardiac interventions to symptom-based treatment.

REFERENCES

1. Zomer AC, Vaartjes I, Uiterwaal CS, et al. Circumstances of death in adult congenital heart disease. Int J Cardiol 2012;154(2):168–72.
2. Opotowsky AR, Siddiqi OK, Webb GD. Trends in hospitalizations for adults with congenital heart disease in the U.S. J Am Coll Cardiol 2009;54(5):460–7.
3. Dinardo JA. Heart failure associated with adult congenital heart disease. Semin Cardiothorac Vasc Anesth 2013;17(1):44–54.
4. Broberg CS, Burchill LJ. Myocardial factor revisited: the importance of myocardial fibrosis in adults with congenital heart disease. Int J Cardiol 2015;189: 204–10.
5. Kempny A, Dimopoulos K, Uebing A, et al. Reference values for exercise limitations among adults with congenital heart disease. Relation to activities of daily life–single centre experience and review of published data. Eur Heart J 2012;33(11):1386–96.
6. Stevenson LW, Perloff JK. The limited reliability of physical signs for estimating hemodynamics in chronic heart failure. JAMA 1989;261(6):884–8.
7. Park SC, Neches WH, Mathews RA, et al. Hemodynamic function after the Mustard operation for transposition of the great arteries. Am J Cardiol 1983; 51(9):1514–9.
8. Castaneda AR, Trusler GA, Paul MH, et al. The early results of treatment of simple transposition in the current era. J Thorac Cardiovasc Surg 1988;95(1): 14–28.
9. Moons P, Gewillig M, Sluysmans T, et al. Long term outcome up to 30 years after the Mustard or Senning operation: a nationwide multicentre study in Belgium. Heart 2004;90(3):307–13.
10. Khairy P, Landzberg MJ, Lambert J, et al. Long-term outcomes after the atrial switch for surgical correction

11. of transposition: a meta-analysis comparing the Mustard and Senning procedures. Cardiol Young 2004;14(3):284–92.
11. Hill KD, Fleming G, Curt Fudge J, et al. Percutaneous interventions in high-risk patients following Mustard repair of transposition of the great arteries. Catheter Cardiovasc Interv 2012;80(6):905–14.
12. Ohuchi H, Ikado H, Noritake K, et al. Impact of central venous pressure on cardiorenal interactions in adult patients with congenital heart disease after biventricular repair. Congenit Heart Dis 2013;8(2): 103–10.
13. Bridges ND, Lock JE, Castaneda AR. Baffle fenestration with subsequent transcatheter closure. Modification of the Fontan operation for patients at increased risk. Circulation 1990;82(5):1681–9.
14. Laks H, Pearl JM, Haas GS, et al. Partial Fontan: advantages of an adjustable interatrial communication. Ann Thorac Surg 1991;52(5):1084–94 [discussion: 1094–5].
15. Vyas H, Driscoll DJ, Cabalka AK, et al. Results of transcatheter Fontan fenestration to treat protein losing enteropathy. Catheter Cardiovasc Interv 2007;69(4):584–9.
16. Cheatham JP, Hellenbrand WE, Zahn EM, et al. Clinical and hemodynamic outcomes up to 7 years after transcatheter pulmonary valve replacement in the US melody valve investigational device exemption trial. Circulation 2015;131(22):1960–70.
17. Brubaker PH, Kitzman DW. Chronotropic incompetence: causes, consequences, and management. Circulation 2011;123(9):1010–20.
18. Diller GP, Dimopoulos K, Okonko D, et al. Heart rate response during exercise predicts survival in adults with congenital heart disease. J Am Coll Cardiol 2006;48(6):1250–6.
19. Roche F, Pichot V, Da Costa A, et al. Chronotropic incompetence response to exercise in congestive heart failure, relationship with the cardiac autonomic status. Clin Physiol 2001;21(3):335–42.
20. van Tol BA, Huijsmans RJ, Kroon DW, et al. Effects of exercise training on cardiac performance, exercise capacity and quality of life in patients with heart failure: a meta-analysis. Eur J Heart Fail 2006;8(8): 841–50.
21. Tse HF, Siu CW, Lee KL, et al. The incremental benefit of rate-adaptive pacing on exercise performance during cardiac resynchronization therapy. J Am Coll Cardiol 2005;46(12):2292–7.
22. Bouchardy J, Therrien J, Pilote L, et al. Atrial arrhythmias in adults with congenital heart disease. Circulation 2009;120(17):1679–86.
23. Walsh EP, Cecchin F. Arrhythmias in adult patients with congenital heart disease. Circulation 2007; 115(4):534–45.
24. Triedman JK, Alexander ME, Berul CI, et al. Electroanatomic mapping of entrained and exit zones in

patients with repaired congenital heart disease and intra-atrial reentrant tachycardia. Circulation 2001; 103(16):2060–5.

25. Khairy P, Harris L, Landzberg MJ, et al. Sudden death and defibrillators in transposition of the great arteries with intra-atrial baffles: a multicenter study. Circ Arrhythm Electrophysiol 2008;1(4):250–7.

26. Triedman JK, Bergau DM, Saul JP, et al. Efficacy of radiofrequency ablation for control of intraatrial reentrant tachycardia in patients with congenital heart disease. J Am Coll Cardiol 1997;30(4): 1032–8.

27. Philip F, Muhammad KI, Agarwal S, et al. Pulmonary vein isolation for the treatment of drug-refractory atrial fibrillation in adults with congenital heart disease. Congenit Heart Dis 2012;7(4):392–9.

28. Shuplock J, Barker G, Radbill A, et al. Recurrence of atrial arrhythmias following ablation in adults with congenital heart disease: new substrate formation or late procedural failure? Circulation 2014;130: A11683.

29. Ernst S, Babu-Narayan SV, Keegan J, et al. Remote-controlled magnetic navigation and ablation with 3D image integration as an alternative approach in patients with intra-atrial baffle anatomy. Circ Arrhythmia Electrophysiol 2012;5(1):131–9.

30. Silka MJ, Hardy BG, Menashe VD, et al. A population-based prospective evaluation of risk of sudden cardiac death after operation for common congenital heart defects. J Am Coll Cardiol 1998; 32(1):245–51.

31. Russo AM, Stainback RF, Bailey SR, et al. ACCF/HRS/ AHA/ASE/HFSA/SCAI/SCCT/SCMR 2013 appropriate use criteria for implantable cardioverter-defibrillators and cardiac resynchronization therapy: a report of the American College of Cardiology Foundation appropriate use criteria task force, Heart Rhythm Society, American Heart Association, American Society of Echocardiography, Heart Failure Society of America, Society for Cardiovascular Angiography and Interventions, Society of Cardiovascular Computed Tomography, and Society for Cardiovascular Magnetic Resonance. Heart Rhythm 2013;10(4):e11–58.

32. Motonaga KS, Khairy P, Dubin AM. Electrophysiologic therapeutics in heart failure in adult congenital heart disease. Heart Fail Clin 2014;10(1):69–89.

33. Cleland JG, Daubert JC, Erdmann E, et al. The effect of cardiac resynchronization on morbidity and mortality in heart failure. N Engl J Med 2005;352(15): 1539–49.

34. Thambo JB, De Guillebon M, Xhaet O, et al. Biventricular pacing in patients with Tetralogy of Fallot: non-invasive epicardial mapping and clinical impact. Int J Cardiol 2013;163(2):170–4.

35. Janousek J, Gebauer RA, Abdul-Khaliq H, et al. Cardiac resynchronisation therapy in paediatric and congenital heart disease: differential effects in various anatomical and functional substrates. Heart 2009; 95(14):1165–71.

36. Khairy P, Van Hare GF, Balaji S, et al. PACES/HRS expert consensus statement on the recognition and management of arrhythmias in adult congenital heart disease: developed in partnership between the Pediatric and Congenital Electrophysiology Society (PACES) and the Heart Rhythm Society (HRS). Endorsed by the governing bodies of PACES, HRS, the American College of Cardiology (ACC), the American Heart Association (AHA), the European Heart Rhythm Association (EHRA), the Canadian Heart Rhythm Society (CHRS), and the International Society for Adult Congenital Heart Disease (ISACHD). Heart Rhythm 2014;11(10):e102–65.

37. Cecchin F, Frangini PA, Brown DW, et al. Cardiac resynchronization therapy (and multisite pacing) in pediatrics and congenital heart disease: five years experience in a single institution. J Cardiovasc Electrophysiol 2009;20(1):58–65.

38. Dubin AM, Janousek J, Rhee E, et al. Resynchronization therapy in pediatric and congenital heart disease patients: an international multicenter study. J Am Coll Cardiol 2005;46(12):2277–83.

39. Hazekamp MG, Kurvers MM, Schoof PH, et al. Pulmonary valve insertion late after repair of Fallot's tetralogy. Eur J Cardiothorac Surg 2001; 19(5):667–70.

40. Kurokawa SY, Kenji T, Shihoko D, et al. Clinical features and risk assessment for cardiac surgery in adult congenital heart disease: three years at a single Japanese center. Egypt J Anaesth 2014;30(2): 203–10.

41. Atz AM, Zak V, Breitbart RE, et al. Factors associated with serum brain natriuretic peptide levels after the Fontan procedure. Congenit Heart Dis 2011; 6(4):313–21.

42. Niedner MF, Foley JL, Riffenburgh RH, et al. B-type natriuretic peptide: perioperative patterns in congenital heart disease. Congenit Heart Dis 2010; 5(3):243–55.

43. Kogon B, Oster M. Assessing surgical risk for adults with congenital heart disease: are pediatric scoring systems appropriate? J Thorac Cardiovasc Surg 2014;147(2):666–71.

44. Warnes CA, Williams RG, Bashore TM, et al. ACC/ AHA 2008 Guidelines for the Management of Adults with Congenital Heart Disease: a report of the American College of Cardiology/American Heart Association Task Force on Practice Guidelines (writing committee to develop guidelines on the management of adults with congenital heart disease). Circulation 2008;118(23):e714–833.

45. Cramer JW, Ginde S, Hill GD, et al. Tricuspid repair at pulmonary valve replacement does not alter outcomes in tetralogy of Fallot. Ann Thorac Surg 2015;99(3):899–904.

46. Kogon B, Mori M, Alsoufi B, et al. Leaving moderate tricuspid valve regurgitation alone at the time of pulmonary valve replacement: a worthwhile approach. Ann Thorac Surg 2015;99(6):2117–23.

47. Connelly MS, Liu PP, Williams WG, et al. Congenitally corrected transposition of the great arteries in the adult: functional status and complications. J Am Coll Cardiol 1996;27(5):1238–43.

48. Graham TP Jr, Bernard YD, Mellen BG, et al. Long-term outcome in congenitally corrected transposition of the great arteries: a multi-institutional study. J Am Coll Cardiol 2000;36(1):255–61.

49. Celermajer DS, Bull C, Till JA, et al. Ebstein's anomaly: presentation and outcome from fetus to adult. J Am Coll Cardiol 1994;23(1):170–6.

50. Sarris GE, Giannopoulos NM, Tsoutsinos AJ, et al. Results of surgery for Ebstein anomaly: a multicenter study from the European Congenital Heart Surgeons Association. J Thorac Cardiovasc Surg 2006;132(1):50–7.

51. Brown ML, Dearani JA, Danielson GK, et al. The outcomes of operations for 539 patients with Ebstein anomaly. J Thorac Cardiovasc Surg 2008;135(5):1120–36, 1136.e1–7.

52. Raju V, Dearani JA, Burkhart HM, et al. Right ventricular unloading for heart failure related to Ebstein malformation. Ann Thorac Surg 2014;98(1):167–73 [discussion: 173–4].

53. Mavroudis C, Deal BJ, Backer CL, et al. J. Maxwell Chamberlain memorial paper for congenital heart surgery. 111 Fontan conversions with arrhythmia surgery: surgical lessons and outcomes. Ann Thorac Surg 2007;84(5):1457–65 [discussion: 1465–6].

54. Hiramatsu T, Iwata Y, Matsumura G, et al. Impact of Fontan conversion with arrhythmia surgery and pacemaker therapy. Eur J Cardiothorac Surg 2011;40(4):1007–10.

55. Poh CL, Cochrane A, Galati JC, et al. Ten-year outcomes of Fontan conversion in Australia and New Zealand demonstrate the superiority of a strategy of early conversion. Eur J Cardiothorac Surg 2015. [Epub ahead of print].

56. Tobler D, Greutmann M, Colman JM, et al. End-of-life care in hospitalized adults with complex congenital heart disease: care delayed, care denied. Palliat Med 2012;26(1):72–9.

57. Kovacs AH, Saidi AS, Kuhl EA, et al. Depression and anxiety in adult congenital heart disease: predictors and prevalence. Int J Cardiol 2009;137(2):158–64.

Pulmonary Hypertension in Congenital Heart Disease
Beyond Eisenmenger Syndrome

Eric V. Krieger, MD[a],*, Peter J. Leary, MD, MS[b],
Alexander R. Opotowsky, MD, MPH[c]

KEYWORDS

- Adult congenital heart disease • Pulmonary hypertension
- Pulmonary arterial hypertension disease management
- Humans vasodilator agents/diagnostic use/therapeutic use

KEY POINTS

- Pulmonary hypertension is present in approximately 5% of patients with adult congenital heart disease. These patients have worse functional status and increased mortality.
- There are various causes of pulmonary hypertension in patients with congenital heart disease. These causes include increased pulmonary blood flow, pulmonary vascular remodeling, and pulmonary venous hypertension. There is considerable overlap in patients with congenital heart disease.
- Effective treatment is not possible unless the underlying physiology of pulmonary hypertension is defined and requires a multidisciplinary approach from imagers, experts in congenital heart disease, and experts in pulmonary hypertension.
- Care for adults with congenital heart disease with pulmonary hypertension should be at specialized centers with experience in congenital heart disease.

INTRODUCTION AND DEMOGRAPHICS

Approximately 3% to 10% of adults with congenital heart disease (ACHD) will develop pulmonary hypertension (PH).[1–3] The causes of PH in congenital heart disease (CHD) are diverse. For example, patients with septal defects may have pulmonary arterial hypertension (PAH) with vascular remodeling and increased pulmonary vascular resistance (PVR), whereas patients with left-sided lesions may have PH due to pulmonary venous hypertension. In addition to different causes of PH associated with different defects, individual patients

Disclosures: Dr E.V. Krieger has received research grant funding from Actelion Pharmaceuticals US Inc. Dr P.J. Leary has nothing to disclose. Dr A.R. Opotowsky has received research grant funding from Actelion Pharmaceuticals US Inc and Merck & Co., Inc. Dr A.R. Opotowsky is supported by the Dunlevie Family Fund.
a Seattle Adult Congenital Heart Service, Division of Cardiology, Department of Medicine, University of Washington School of Medicine, 1959 Northeast Pacific Street, Seattle, WA 98195, USA; b Pulmonary Vascular Disease Program, Division of Pulmonary and Critical Care Medicine, Department of Medicine, University of Washington School of Medicine, 1959 Northeast Pacific Street, Seattle, WA 98195, USA; c Boston Adult Congenital Heart and Pulmonary Hypertension Service, Department of Cardiology, Boston Children's Hospital and Brigham and Women's Hospital, 300 Longwood Avenue, Boston, MA 02115, USA
* Corresponding author. Seattle Adult Congenital Heart Service, Division of Cardiology, Department of Medicine, University of Washington School of Medicine, 1959 NE Pacific Street, Seattle, WA 98195.
E-mail address: ekrieger@u.washington.edu

Cardiol Clin 33 (2015) 599–609
http://dx.doi.org/10.1016/j.ccl.2015.07.003
0733-8651/15/$ – see front matter © 2015 Elsevier Inc. All rights reserved.

may also have several different processes contributing to elevated pulmonary pressures. Because patients can have more than one congenital defect and because CHD is often associated with other congenital and acquired diseases, pathologic processes can overlap, leading to ambiguous phenotypes of PH.

Although the trend toward earlier repair has likely decreased the proportion of ACHD patients with PH, the absolute number of ACHD patients with PH is increasing because more patients with CHD survive to adulthood. The increased prevalence of PH is particularly true for patients with previously fatal and complex forms of CHD. These patients with complex CHD are at elevated risk to develop PH later in life.[4,5]

All patients with ACHD are at risk for developing PH; however, PH is most common in women, older patients, and those with shunt defects. For patients with ACHD, PH is associated with a more than 2-fold increase in mortality, increased hospital admissions, and 3-fold higher costs.[2] Observational administrative data also suggest that ACHD patients with PH have worse functional capacity and higher health care utilization compared with ACHD patients without PH.[2,4,6,7]

Classification and Mechanisms of Pulmonary Hypertension in Congenital Heart Disease

The World Health Organization (WHO) classification is used clinically to identify groups that may share similar pathophysiology and response to treatment.[8,9] This schema describes 5 distinct groups: (1) PAH, defined as PH due to elevated PVR with normal pulmonary venous pressure; (2) PH secondary to left heart disease; (3) PH secondary to lung diseases or hypoxia; (4) chronic thromboembolic PH; and (5) PH with unclear or multifactorial mechanisms.[9] Until 2013, PH-CHD was solely included in WHO group 1/PAH. There are 4 clinical phenotypes of PH-CHD associated with PAH that occur in patients with a congenital systemic-to-pulmonary shunt.[8] These WHO group 1/PAH forms of ACHD-PH include Eisenmenger syndrome; PAH associated with a systemic-to-pulmonary shunt; PAH associated with a small cardiac defect; and PAH after corrective surgery.

The most recent PH classification scheme acknowledges that PH in ACHD may also be related to increased PVR with pulmonary venous hypertension (WHO group 2PH). ACHD-PH with pulmonary venous hypertension related to left heart inflow/outflow obstruction or congenital cardiomyopathy is identified as causes of WHO group 2 PH in ACHD.[9] CHD lesions usually predispose to either WHO group I or WHO group II PH, although there are also less common scenarios wherein CHD is associated with other types of PH (examples include group III, kyphoscoliosis; group IV, in situ thrombosis or thromboembolism in Eisenmenger syndrome or the Fontan circulation; group V, extrinsic compression of the pulmonary arteries).

Although a particular ACHD lesion or repair is often associated with a specific cause of PH, these associations must be placed in the overall clinical context. Relationships between CHD anatomy and the resultant type of PH are complex, and prediction solely based on the underlying lesion is unreliable. For example, a moderate-sized patent ductus arteriosus (PDA) may lead to PH from left heart failure or PAH due to pulmonary vascular remodeling. Patients with CHD may also develop PH due to causes unrelated to the underlying heart defect, such as sleep apnea, human immunodeficiency virus, autoimmune disease, toxins, or drugs. Because of these areas of uncertainty, ACHD patients with PH should undergo a comprehensive evaluation to define physiology and assess for alternative causes of PH.

One must define the underlying hemodynamics to understand PH pathophysiology in ACHD. Elevated mean pulmonary artery pressure has 3 possible causes: high pulmonary resistance (associated with reduced arterial compliance), high pulmonary venous pressure, or high pulmonary blood flow (**Fig. 1**).[10] Overlap among these 3 causes is more common in ACHD-PH than in non-ACHD-PH (**Fig. 2**). For example, a patient with a large left-to-right shunt may have high pulmonary blood flow, pulmonary venous hypertension, and elevated PVR. Chronic pulmonary venous hypertension (eg, from mitral stenosis) is often accompanied by increased PVR and low vascular compliance.[11-13] This mixture of pathologic abnormality can also obscure relevant physiology as in the case of an ASD, which can mask the presence of important left heart diastolic dysfunction.[14] These factors make it challenging to characterize phenotypes of ACHD into the existing WHO classification and make it difficult to predict whether an intervention will provide benefit or cause harm over the long term. Despite the difficulty and uncertainty, a comprehensive and nuanced understanding is critical to making informed clinical decisions.

CLINICAL EVALUATION
Physical Examination and Bedside Tests Including 6-minute Walk Testing

The physical examination provides insight regarding the presence, severity, and consequences of PH in

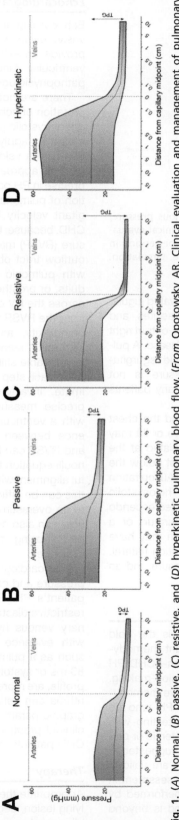

Fig. 1. (A) Normal, (B) passive, (C) resistive, and (D) hyperkinetic pulmonary blood flow. (*From* Opotowsky AR. Clinical evaluation and management of pulmonary hypertension in the adult with congenital heart disease. Circulation 2015;131:201; with permission.)

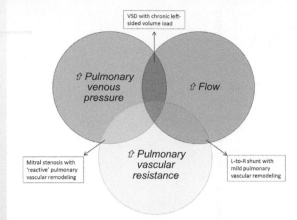

Fig. 2. Overlap among pulmonary venous pressure, flow, and PVR. (*From* Opotowsky AR. Clinical evaluation and management of pulmonary hypertension in the adult with congenital heart disease. Circulation. 2015;131:202; with permission.)

patients with CHD. Hepatomegaly, elevated jugular venous pressure, peripheral edema, ascites, and cool extremities are consistent with low-output right heart failure and suggest advanced disease. A pulsatile liver suggests substantial tricuspid regurgitation. Elevated jugular venous pressure is not specific for PAH and is present in many patients with PH due to left heart disease.

The right ventricle is directly behind the chest wall and a right ventricular (RV) heave or lift may be palpable with RV dilation, appreciated at the inferior left lower sternal border or just below the xiphoid process during inspiration. Auscultation may demonstrate a loud P2, a holosystolic tricuspid regurgitation murmur, a decrescendo diastolic pulmonary regurgitation murmur, or a right-sided S3. Tricuspid regurgitation may have a character similar to mitral regurgitation (lateral, high pitched) with very high RV pressure and an enlarged RV.

Invasive Hemodynamics

Invasive hemodynamic assessment is the gold standard for understanding relevant hemodynamic phenotypes in ACHD and non-ACHD-PH alike and is pivotal in treatment decision-making. A standardized approach to invasive hemodynamic assessment in patients with PH who do not have ACHD (including dynamic testing with intravascular volume, exercise, or systemic or pulmonary vasodilators) has been suggested.[15] Although some of these suggestions are valid in ACHD-PH, invasive hemodynamic assessment in ACHD is complex, should only be performed by those with specialized expertise, and is beyond the scope of this review.

Echocardiography

Echocardiography remains a key tool in the noninvasive evaluation of PH. An echocardiogram can provide an estimate of pulmonary pressure and ventricular function and suggest clues about pathophysiology.

There are notable potential pitfalls in the interpretation of echocardiograms in CHD. Pulmonary artery systolic pressure (PASP) is commonly estimated by applying the simplified Bernoulli equation to the velocity of the tricuspid regurgitation jet. This approach is only moderately reliable and precise in PH patients without ACHD.[16] Extrapolation of pulmonary pressures from tricuspid regurgitant velocity is further limited in patients with CHD because the right ventricular systolic pressure (RVSP) may differ from the PASP due to RV outflow tract obstruction; this is seen in patients with pulmonic stenosis, pulmonary artery conduits, or prosthetic pulmonic valves. The gradient across the RV outflow tract should be subtracted from the RVSP to estimate the PASP. With higher complexity, as in cases of long segment or sequential stenoses, echo-derived gradients are less reliable still with sequential measurement error at each step and should be considered approximate. Invasive hemodynamics are required if precise measurement is needed.[17] In patients with a ventricular septal defect (VSD), the difference between left ventricular systolic pressure and RVSP can be estimated by applying the Bernoulli equation the velocity of the VSD jet.[18] Careful alignment with the Doppler beam is critical, and this can be difficult in a membranous VSD leading to an overestimation of RVSP. Membranous VSD flow can also contaminate tricuspid regurgitation, predisposing to overestimation of pulmonary pressures.

Echocardiography may suggest an elevated pressure and can also help clarify the cause of a patient's PH. Patients with left atrial dilation or restrictive diastolic filling are likely to have pulmonary venous hypertension. Conversely, patients with evidence of pulmonary vascular disease, such as a pulmonary acceleration time less than 80 ms or systolic notching of the RV outflow tract profile, are more likely to have PAH.[19] Simple algorithms can estimate PVR based on echocardiographic parameters but are not widely applied in clinical practice and have not been validated in CHD patients.[20,21]

Therapy

Appropriate therapy for PH-CHD varies by underlying lesion, degree of pulmonary vascular remodeling, and associated pathophysiology.

Patent Left-to-Right Shunts with Normal Pulmonary Vascular Resistance and High Flow

Defect closure is the treatment of choice for patent left-to-right shunts with normal pulmonary vascular resistance and high flow. Long-term prognosis is good, especially if performed early in life.[22,23] This approach may not be fully curative, and evidence of residual subclinical RV dysfunction and pulmonary vascular disease can be exposed with exercise, even in patients with early repair and normal testing at rest.[24–28] Nevertheless, closure ameliorates most long-term sequelae in most patients with favorable hemodynamics in both young and old patients alike. Some caution should be used in elderly patients, particularly those with diastolic dysfunction, because closure of an atrial septal defect (ASD) can increase left heart filling and unmask diastolic heart failure.[29] Test occlusion of the ASD with simultaneous measurement of left atrial pressure can predict patients who may develop pulmonary congestion after closure. Fenestrated ASD occlusion devices have been used for patients at high risk.[30]

Atrial Septal Defect with Elevated Pulmonary Vascular Resistance

Most adults with an ASD do not develop pulmonary vascular remodeling and PAH regardless of the size of the defect or the magnitude or duration of shunt; however, 5% to 10% of patients with unrepaired ASD do develop PAH.[31] This amount is in contrast to patients with posttricuspid shunts (VSD, aortopulmonary windows, or PDA), who invariably develop irreversible PAH and Eisenmenger syndrome unless repaired in early childhood.[9]

A small subset of adults with a pre-tricuspid shunt has an elevated PVR consistent with PAH. Patients with sinus venosus defects seem more likely to develop PAH than patients with secundum ASDs despite similar magnitude of shunt.[32] Some studies suggest that PAH is more common in female patients with ASD. Size of the defect and age at repair have been inconsistently linked to the development of PAH.[33–35] If the PVR is severely elevated, closure of the pre-tricuspid shunt is contraindicated.

Decision-making in patients with ASD and mild to moderately elevated PVR is challenging; the best approach to management remains unclear. Acute right heart failure is uncommon, and most symptomatic patients improve directly after closure. Some patients, however, develop progressive, irreversible pulmonary vascular disease despite closure, and the absence of a "pop-off valve" can worsen pressure-volume overload of the right ventricle in these patients.

It would be ideal to identify those patients with mild or moderate elevations in PVR who will ultimately progress to severe PAH because these patients would be poor candidates for closure. Unfortunately, there is no definitive way to identify prospectively which patients are at highest risk for progressive worsening of PVR and PAH. Patients who develop progressive PAH after ASD or VSD closure tend to have higher baseline PVR (>5 WU) and pulmonary:systemic vascular resistance (R_p:R_s >0.33).[36] However, these criteria are not specific and many patients with elevated PVR and R_p:R_s do not develop PAH. In those who do not develop progressive PAH, closure has distinct advantages in terms of symptoms and functional capacity. There have been many reports using pulmonary vasodilators to bridge borderline patients to eventual repair and improvement, but no randomized data.[37–39] One algorithm to determine when to close an ASD, when to bridge with pulmonary vasodilators, and when not to close has been proposed (**Fig. 3**).

Recommendations tend to base the decision to close a shunt largely on a single resting catheterization.[9,40,41] This narrow perspective does not reflect the reality of clinical practice and ignores additional sources of information, which are likely to hone clinical decision-making and more reliably identify the best treatment strategy. Additional data, including exercise hemodynamics, response to acute pulmonary vasodilator challenge, response to balloon occlusion of the defect during catheterization, cardiopulmonary exercise testing, response to medical therapy, and changes in these variables with time, should provide a more holistic and accurate appraisal of underlying pulmonary vascular disease.[24–26,42,43] That said, even meticulous, comprehensive, dynamic assessment is an imperfect predictor of long-term outcome, and more reliable predictors are needed.[36]

Elevated Pulmonary Vascular Resistance (Pulmonary Arterial Hypertension) After Shunt Closure or in the Context of a Small Shunt

Management of patients with elevated PVR consistent with PAH with small shunt or after shunt closure is more straightforward and is considered, within the limitations of contemporary understanding, to have the same pathophysiology as other forms of WHO group 1 PAH (such as idiopathic PAH). As such, these patients should be managed accordingly by clinicians and centers with

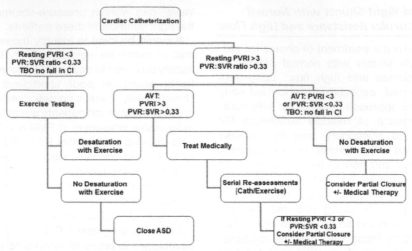

Fig. 3. One algorithm for treatment of an ASD in patients with ASD and PH. Specified cut points are arbitrary given limited available data, and there is marked heterogeneity between expert clinicians. Nonetheless, this algorithm highlights the important role of an iterative process in determining which patients are most likely to benefit from ASD closure. ASD-PH clinical management algorithm: individualized case approach. AVT, acute vasodilator testing; PVR:SVR ratio, ratio of pulmonary vascular resistance to systemic vascular resistance; PVRI, pulmonary vascular resistance indexed to body surface area; TBO, temporary balloon occlusion. (*From* Rosenzweig EB, Barst RJ. Congenital heart disease and pulmonary hypertension: pharmacology and feasibility of late surgery. Prog Cardiovasc Dis 2012;55:132; with permission.)

appropriate expertise. Some PAH medications may have advantageous medium- and long-term pulmonary vascular remodeling effects and improve right heart adaptation. These benefits are largely speculative, and no definitive drug exists that alters the natural history of pulmonary vasculopathy.[44] For those with a small shunt, the defect should not be closed because of the potential benefit of having a "relief valve" in the event of progressive right heart failure.

Other Mechanical and Structural Intervention

Clinicians have long understood the benefit of a "relief valve" by observing patients with Eisenmenger syndrome or non-Eisenmenger PAH associated with CHD.[45,46] One small study hinted that patients with non-ACHD PAH and a patent foramen ovale (n = 4) may have longer survival relative to those without patency (n = 30).[47] A small shunt allows continuous or intermittent right-to-left flow. Although this results in cyanosis, it also mitigates pressure-volume overload of the right ventricle, allows the right ventricle to remain in a position of mechanical advantage, and preserves cardiac output.

Several approaches have been explored to create an equivalent situation in patients who do not have any residual shunt (or who never had such a shunt). Percutaneous atrial septostomy has been performed in patients with end-stage PAH and in resource-limited countries. Early

reports of atrial septostomy in unselected PAH patients suggested very high periprocedural mortality often related to uncontrolled right-to-left shunting and cyanosis; however, avoidance of patients with high right atrial pressures (right atrial pressure <20 mm Hg or <15 mm Hg) has led to lower rates of periprocedural mortality and improvement in overall survival.[48,49]

Recent series have also reported on results of surgical and catheter creation of a Potts shunt (communication between left pulmonary artery and descending aorta).[50–52] These procedures seem feasible, although are associated with acute risk. Historical support for a Potts shunt is suggested by the observation that patients with Eisenmenger syndrome and PDA are less breathless than those with ASD or VSD, which may be related to relatively less hypoxemia in the head and neck vessels, which are rich in chemoreceptors.[53] In addition to this potential advantage over an atrial level shunt, the size of shunt can be precisely tailored with the Potts approach; therefore, uncontrolled cyanosis is not a significant concern (**Fig. 4**). In patients with very small shunts or after shunt closure, both atrial septostomy and Potts shunt are options.

Mechanical support and lung or heart-lung transplant are alternatives for some patients with refractory right heart failure despite medical therapy.[54,55] ACHD with or without prior intervention may be associated with additional and

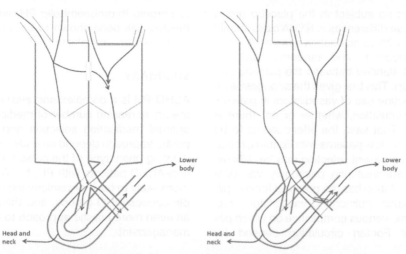

Fig. 4. (*left*) An atrial septostomy allows right-to-left shunting at the atrial level, supplementing cardiac output at the expense of hypoxemia to the entire systemic circulation. (*right*) A Potts shunt provides a conduit from the left pulmonary artery to the descending aorta. This allows right-to-left shunting at the arterial level below the takeoff of the head and neck vessels. As with atrial septostomy, systemic cardiac output is augmented; in contrast, however, the blood perfusing the head and neck is fully oxygenated. This, along with the capability to precisely define shunt size, provides advantages compared with an uncontrolled atrial level shunt.

patient-specific risks for such advanced interventions, and care should be limited to referral centers with extensive experience operating on these patients.

PULMONARY HYPERTENSION IN SPECIAL POPULATIONS
Pulmonary Vascular Disease in Patients with Fontan Circulation

More than other forms of CHD, the Fontan circulation demands a low PVR. Because there is no subpulmonary ventricle in the Fontan circulation, chronically elevated central venous pressures drive blood through the lungs. If the transpulmonary gradient increases in the Fontan circulation, then central venous pressure must increase as well. Once the limited capacity to elevate central venous pressure is surpassed, cardiac output and ventricular preload will decrease. The inability to augment cardiac output further leads to impaired ventricular filling and diminished preload reserve[56] and contributes to these patients' poor exercise capacity.[57,58] Therefore, treatments aimed at lowering pulmonary resistance are conceptually appealing.

Although very few patients with Fontan circulation meet the definition of PH (mean pulmonary artery pressure >25 mm Hg),[9] it has been speculated that nonpulsatile pulmonary blood flow leads to decreased expression of intrinsic pulmonary vasodilators.[59] Despite low absolute values for pulmonary pressure, PVR may be elevated in this

population, improvements in PVR even within the range of normal may be beneficial, and PVR may be modified by pulmonary vasodilators.[60]

There have been several studies testing pulmonary vasodilators in patients with Fontan circulation. Early studies showed that phosphodiesterase type 5 (PDE5) inhibitors were well tolerated and acutely led to small improvements in Fontan pressures, PVR, and maximal oxygen uptake during exercise.[61,62] One notable exception was a randomized trial of sildenafil in children and young adults, which did not meet the primary endpoint of improving maximal oxygen uptake but did demonstrate improvement in a secondary endpoint of ventilatory efficiency.[63] Van De Bruaene and colleagues[64] performed invasive hemodynamic studies showing that sildenafil improves cardiac index by approximately 20%, an effect that was even more pronounced during exercise. Sildenafil was well tolerated and did not worsen shunting.

The largest prospective study of pulmonary vasodilators in Fontan patients is the TEMPO study. This double-blind randomized trial compared bosentan, a nonselective endothelin receptor antagonist, to placebo in a relatively young and healthy group of Fontan patients. Subjects did not need to have elevated PVR to be eligible for the trial. Those receiving bosentan had a small (+5%) improvement in peak oxygen consumption and exercise duration compared with the placebo group. Importantly, in this double-blind trial, one-third of patients receiving bosentan improved by one New York Heart Association (NYHA) functional class, whereas no subject in the placebo group improved. These differences in NYHA class should be interpreted with some caution because it was a secondary endpoint, and randomization was somewhat unbalanced between the placebo and bosentan group. This trial gives the strongest support yet for routine use of vasodilators in patients with Fontan circulation, whether or not there is elevated PVR. That said, the effect seems to be modest, and very few patients with Fontan circulation have PH, so patient selection may be difficult. Furthermore, administering pulmonary vasodilators in this population has the potential for complications, because pulmonary vasodilators can impact systemic venous compliance on which patients with a Fontan circulation depend for preload.[65,66]

Segmental Pulmonary Hypertension

Some forms of CHD are characterized by peripheral pulmonary artery stenosis. This finding is particularly true in complex forms of tetralogy of Fallot (such as those patients with major aortopulmonary collaterals) as well as those with Williams syndrome. Prior surgical palliation with aortic-to-pulmonary shunts (eg, Blalock-Taussig-Thomas or Potts shunt) can distort the pulmonary arteries, causing asymmetric pulmonary artery stenosis. In these circumstances, there are regional variations in pulmonary artery pressure, pulmonary blood flow, and resistance that can vary dramatically in different segments of lung. The evaluation of patients with segmental PH is difficult. Echocardiographic measurements of RVSP gives misleading information about the health of the distal pulmonary vasculature, which may be protected by proximal stenosis and vary considerably throughout the lung. To calculate regional resistances requires information on local pressures and regional pulmonary blood flow. This information can be obtained through careful pressure measurements in multiple distal pulmonary beds at the time of catheterization combined with regional flow information obtained by cardiac MRI or quantitative lung perfusion imaging.

When possible, treatment of segmental PH is aimed at relieving obstruction with either balloon or surgical angioplasty done at an experienced congenital heart center. When complete relief of obstruction is not possible, there may be a role for pulmonary vasodilators. Small uncontrolled retrospective studies suggest that endothelial receptor antagonists or PDE5 inhibitors are effective in improving symptoms and 6-minute walk distances in patients with distal segmental PH due to CHD.[67,68] Segmental PH in CHD may be similar

to chronic thromboembolic PH, wherein medical therapy has been shown to be a useful adjuvant to surgery or angioplasty.[69,70]

SUMMARY

ACHD-PH is a complex and evolving field. There are an increasing number of medical options, but optimal medication selection and overall therapeutic approach depend on understanding the underlying phenotype of the patient. Compared with non-ACHD patients with PH, the ACHD patient is more likely to have physiology explained by multiple causes/WHO groups, and therefore, requires an even more holistic approach to evaluation and management.

REFERENCES

1. van Riel AC, Schuuring MJ, van Hessen ID, et al. Contemporary prevalence of pulmonary arterial hypertension in adult congenital heart disease following the updated clinical classification. Int J Cardiol 2014;174(2):299–305.
2. Lowe BS, Therrien J, Ionescu-Ittu R, et al. Diagnosis of pulmonary hypertension in the congenital heart disease adult population impact on outcomes. J Am Coll Cardiol 2011;58(5):538–46.
3. Engelfriet PM, Duffels MG, Moller T, et al. Pulmonary arterial hypertension in adults born with a heart septal defect: the Euro Heart Survey on adult congenital heart disease. Heart 2007;93(6):682–7.
4. Opotowsky AR, Siddiqi OK, Webb GD. Trends in hospitalizations for adults with congenital heart disease in the U.S. J Am Coll Cardiol 2009;54(5):460–7.
5. Marelli AJ, Mackie AS, Ionescu-Ittu R, et al. Congenital heart disease in the general population: changing prevalence and age distribution. Circulation 2007;115(2):163–72.
6. Duffels MG, Engelfriet PM, Berger RM, et al. Pulmonary arterial hypertension in congenital heart disease: an epidemiologic perspective from a Dutch registry. Int J Cardiol 2007;120(2):198–204.
7. Diller GP, Dimopoulos K, Okonko D, et al. Exercise intolerance in adult congenital heart disease: comparative severity, correlates, and prognostic implication. Circulation 2005;112(6):828–35.
8. McLaughlin VV, Archer SL, Badesch DB, et al. ACCF/AHA 2009 expert consensus document on pulmonary hypertension: a report of the American College of Cardiology Foundation Task Force on expert Consensus Documents and the American Heart Association: developed in collaboration with the American College of Chest Physicians, American Thoracic Society, Inc., and the Pulmonary Hypertension Association. Circulation 2009;119(16):2250–94.

9. Simonneau G, Gatzoulis MA, Adatia I, et al. Updated clinical classification of pulmonary hypertension. J Am Coll Cardiol 2013;62(25 Suppl):D34–41.

10. Opotowsky AR. Clinical evaluation and management of pulmonary hypertension in the adult with congenital heart disease. Circulation 2015;131(2):200–10.

11. Braunwald E, Braunwald NS, Ross J Jr, et al. Effects of mitral-valve replacement on the pulmonary vascular dynamics of patients with pulmonary hypertension. N Engl J Med 1965;273:509–14.

12. Atz AM, Adatia I, Jonas RA, et al. Inhaled nitric oxide in children with pulmonary hypertension and congenital mitral stenosis. Am J Cardiol 1996;77(4):316–9.

13. Wood P, Besterman EM, Towers MK, et al. The effect of acetylcholine on pulmonary vascular resistance and left atrial pressure in mitral stenosis. Br Heart J 1957;19(2):279–86.

14. Masutani S, Senzaki H. Left ventricular function in adult patients with atrial septal defect: implication for development of heart failure after transcatheter closure. J Card Fail 2011;17(11):957–63.

15. Hoeper MM, Bogaard HJ, Condliffe R, et al. Definitions and diagnosis of pulmonary hypertension. J Am Coll Cardiol 2013;62(25 Suppl):D42–50.

16. Rich JD, Shah SJ, Swamy RS, et al. Inaccuracy of Doppler echocardiographic estimates of pulmonary artery pressures in patients with pulmonary hypertension: implications for clinical practice. Chest 2011;139(5):988–93.

17. Yoganathan AP, Valdes-Cruz LM, Schmidt-Dohna J, et al. Continuous-wave Doppler velocities and gradients across fixed tunnel obstructions: studies in vitro and in vivo. Circulation 1987;76(3):657–66.

18. Ge Z, Zhang Y, Kang W, et al. Noninvasive evaluation of interventricular pressure gradient across ventricular septal defect: a simultaneous study of Doppler echocardiography and cardiac catheterization. Am Heart J 1992;124(1):176–82.

19. Opotowsky AR, Ojeda J, Rogers F, et al. A simple echocardiographic prediction rule for hemodynamics in pulmonary hypertension. Circ Cardiovasc Imaging 2012;5(6):765–75.

20. Opotowsky AR, Clair M, Afilalo J, et al. A simple echocardiographic method to estimate pulmonary vascular resistance. Am J Cardiol 2013;112(6):873–82.

21. Abbas AE, Franey LM, Marwick T, et al. Noninvasive assessment of pulmonary vascular resistance by Doppler echocardiography. J Am Soc Echocardiogr 2013;26(10):1170–7.

22. St John Sutton MG, Tajik AJ, McGoon DC. Atrial septal defect in patients ages 60 years or older: operative results and long-term postoperative follow-up. Circulation 1981;64(2):402–9.

23. Attie F, Rosas M, Granados N, et al. Surgical treatment for secundum atrial septal defects in patients >40 years old. A randomized clinical trial. J Am Coll Cardiol 2001;38(7):2035–42.

24. Epstein SE, Beiser GD, Goldstein RE, et al. Hemodynamic abnormalities in response to mild and intense upright exercise following operative correction of an atrial septal defect or tetralogy of Fallot. Circulation 1973;47(5):1065–75.

25. Maron BJ, Redwood DR, Hirshfeld JW Jr, et al. Postoperative assessment of patients with ventricular septal defect and pulmonary hypertension. Response to intense upright exercise. Circulation 1973;48(4):864–74.

26. Kulik TJ, Bass JL, Fuhrman BP, et al. Exercise induced pulmonary vasoconstriction. Br Heart J 1983;50(1):59–64.

27. Santos M, Systrom D, Epstein SE, et al. Impaired exercise capacity following atrial septal defect closure: an invasive study of the right heart and pulmonary circulation. Pulm Circ 2014;4(4):630–7.

28. Van De Bruaene A, De Meester P, Buys R, et al. Right ventricular load and function during exercise in patients with open and closed atrial septal defect type secundum. Eur J Prev Cardiol 2013;20(4):597–604.

29. Ewert P, Berger F, Nagdyman N, et al. Masked left ventricular restriction in elderly patients with atrial septal defects: a contraindication for closure? Cathet Cardiovasc Interv 2001;52(2):177–80.

30. MacDonald ST, Arcidiacono C, Butera G. Fenestrated Amplatzer atrial septal defect occluder in an elderly patient with restrictive left ventricular physiology. Heart 2011;97(5):438.

31. Swan HJ, Zapata-Diaz J, Burchell HB, et al. Pulmonary hypertension in congenital heart disease. Am J Med 1954;16(1):12–22.

32. Vogel M, Berger F, Kramer A, et al. Incidence of secondary pulmonary hypertension in adults with atrial septal or sinus venosus defects. Heart 1999;82(1):30–3.

33. Steele PM, Fuster V, Cohen M, et al. Isolated atrial septal defect with pulmonary vascular obstructive disease–long-term follow-up and prediction of outcome after surgical correction. Circulation 1987;76(5):1037–42.

34. Sachweh JS, Daebritz SH, Hermanns B, et al. Hypertensive pulmonary vascular disease in adults with secundum or sinus venosus atrial septal defect. Ann Thorac Surg 2006;81(1):207–13.

35. Gabriels C, De Meester P, Pasquet A, et al. A different view on predictors of pulmonary hypertension in secundum atrial septal defect. Int J Cardiol 2014;176(3):833–40.

36. D'Alto M, Romeo E, Argiento P, et al. Hemodynamics of patients developing pulmonary arterial hypertension after shunt closure. Int J Cardiol 2013;168(4):3797–801.

37. Beghetti M, Galie N, Bonnet D. Can "inoperable" congenital heart defects become operable in patients with pulmonary arterial hypertension? Dream or reality? Congenit Heart Dis 2012;7(1):3–11.

38. Schwerzmann M, Zafar M, McLaughlin PR, et al. Atrial septal defect closure in a patient with "irreversible" pulmonary hypertensive arteriopathy. Int J Cardiol 2006;110(1):104–7.

39. Dimopoulos K, Peset A, Gatzoulis MA. Evaluating operability in adults with congenital heart disease and the role of pretreatment with targeted pulmonary arterial hypertension therapy. Int J Cardiol 2008;129(2):163–71.

40. Warnes CA, Williams RG, Bashore TM, et al. ACC/AHA 2008 guidelines for the management of adults with congenital heart disease: a report of the American College of Cardiology/American Heart Association Task Force on Practice Guidelines (Writing Committee to Develop Guidelines on the Management of Adults with Congenital Heart Disease). Circulation 2008;118(23):e714–833.

41. Baumgartner H, Bonhoeffer P, De Groot NM, et al. ESC guidelines for the management of grown-up congenital heart disease (new version 2010). Eur Heart J 2010;31(23):2915–57.

42. Rosenzweig EB, Barst RJ. Congenital heart disease and pulmonary hypertension: pharmacology and feasibility of late surgery. Prog Cardiovasc Dis 2012;55(2):128–33.

43. Balzer DT, Kort HW, Day RW, et al. Inhaled nitric oxide as a preoperative test (INOP Test I): the INOP Test Study Group. Circulation 2002;106(12 Suppl 1):I76–81.

44. Chakinala MM. Changing the prognosis of pulmonary arterial hypertension: impact of medical therapy. Semin Respir Crit Care Med 2005;26(4):409–16.

45. Hopkins WE. The remarkable right ventricle of patients with Eisenmenger syndrome. Coron Artery Dis 2005;16(1):19–25.

46. Opotowsky AR, Landzberg MJ, Beghetti M. The exceptional and far-flung manifestations of heart failure in Eisenmenger syndrome. Heart Fail Clin 2014; 10(1):91–104.

47. Rozkovec A, Montanes P, Oakley CM. Factors that influence the outcome of primary pulmonary hypertension. Br Heart J 1986;55(5):449–58.

48. Sandoval J, Gaspar J, Pulido T, et al. Graded balloon dilation atrial septostomy in severe primary pulmonary hypertension. A therapeutic alternative for patients nonresponsive to vasodilator treatment. J Am Coll Cardiol 1998;32(2):297–304.

49. Sandoval J, Gomez-Arroyo J, Gaspar J, et al. Interventional and surgical therapeutic strategies for pulmonary arterial hypertension: beyond palliative treatments. J Cardiol 2015. [Epub ahead of print].

50. Labombarda F, Maragnes P, Dupont-Chauvet P, et al. Potts anastomosis for children with idiopathic pulmonary hypertension. Pediatr Cardiol 2009; 30(8):1143–5.

51. Baruteau AE, Serraf A, Levy M, et al. Potts shunt in children with idiopathic pulmonary arterial hypertension: long-term results. Ann Thorac Surg 2012;94(3):817–24.

52. Esch JJ, Shah PB, Cockrill BA, et al. Transcatheter Potts shunt creation in patients with severe pulmonary arterial hypertension: initial clinical experience. J Heart Lung Transplant 2013;32(4):381–7.

53. Wood P. The Eisenmenger syndrome or pulmonary hypertension with reversed central shunt. I. Br Med J 1958;2(5098):701–9.

54. Reitz BA, Wallwork JL, Hunt SA, et al. Heart-lung transplantation: successful therapy for patients with pulmonary vascular disease. N Engl J Med 1982; 306(10):557–64.

55. Adriaenssens T, Delcroix M, Van Deyk K, et al. Advanced therapy may delay the need for transplantation in patients with the Eisenmenger syndrome. Eur Heart J 2006;27(12):1472–7.

56. Senzaki H, Masutani S, Ishido H, et al. Cardiac rest and reserve function in patients with Fontan circulation. J Am Coll Cardiol 2006;47(12):2528–35.

57. Giardini A, Hager A, Pace Napoleone C, et al. Natural history of exercise capacity after the Fontan operation: a longitudinal study. Ann Thorac Surg 2008; 85(3):818–21.

58. Paridon SM, Mitchell PD, Colan SD, et al. A cross-sectional study of exercise performance during the first 2 decades of life after the Fontan operation. J Am Coll Cardiol 2008;52(2):99–107.

59. Mitchell MB, Campbell DN, Ivy D, et al. Evidence of pulmonary vascular disease after heart transplantation for Fontan circulation failure. J Thorac Cardiovasc Surg 2004;128(5):693–702.

60. Khambadkone S, Li J, de Leval MR, et al. Basal pulmonary vascular resistance and nitric oxide responsiveness late after Fontan-type operation. Circulation 2003;107(25):3204–8.

61. Morchi GS, Ivy DD, Duster MC, et al. Sildenafil increases systemic saturation and reduces pulmonary artery pressure in patients with failing Fontan physiology. Congenit Heart Dis 2009;4(2):107–11.

62. Giardini A, Balducci A, Specchia S, et al. Effect of sildenafil on haemodynamic response to exercise and exercise capacity in Fontan patients. Eur Heart J 2008;29(13):1681–7.

63. Goldberg DJ, French B, McBride MG, et al. Impact of oral sildenafil on exercise performance in children and young adults after the Fontan operation: a randomized, double-blind, placebo-controlled, crossover trial. Circulation 2011;123(11):1185–93.

64. Van De Bruaene A, La Gerche A, Claessen G, et al. Sildenafil improves exercise hemodynamics in Fontan patients. Circ Cardiovasc Imaging 2014;7(2): 265–73.

65. Opotowsky AR, Halpern D, Kulik TJ, et al. Inadequate venous return as a primary cause for Fontan circulatory limitation. J Heart Lung Transplant 2014;33(11):1194–6.

66. Krishnan US, Taneja I, Gewitz M, et al. Peripheral vascular adaptation and orthostatic tolerance in Fontan physiology. Circulation 2009;120(18):1775–83.

67. Schuuring MJ, Bouma BJ, Cordina R, et al. Treatment of segmental pulmonary artery hypertension in adults with congenital heart disease. Int J Cardiol 2013;164(1):106–10.

68. Lim ZS, Vettukattill JJ, Salmon AP, et al. Sildenafil therapy in complex pulmonary atresia with pulmonary arterial hypertension. Int J Cardiol 2008; 129(3):339–43.

69. Ghofrani HA, D'Armini AM, Grimminger F, et al. Riociguat for the treatment of chronic thromboembolic pulmonary hypertension. N Engl J Med 2013; 369(4):319–29.

70. Jais X, D'Armini AM, Jansa P, et al. Bosentan for treatment of inoperable chronic thromboembolic pulmonary hypertension: BENEFiT (Bosentan Effects in iNopErable Forms of chronIc Thromboembolic pulmonary hypertension), a randomized, placebo-controlled trial. J Am Coll Cardiol 2008; 52(25):2127–34.

Pregnancy and Adult Congenital Heart Disease

Ami B. Bhatt, MD[a,b,*], Doreen DeFaria Yeh, MD[a,b]

KEYWORDS

- Adult congenital heart disease • Pregnancy • Heart failure • Obstetrics • Obstetric anesthesia
- Congenital heart disease • Arrhythmia • Preconception counseling

KEY POINTS

- Best practice in the care of the pregnant patient with congenital heart disease (CHD) includes multidisciplinary cardiology/obstetric/anesthesiology preconception evaluation and planning.
- Heart failure and arrhythmias remain the primary complications in pregnant individuals with heart disease.
- Recommendations for pregnancy and delivery should be individualized according to congenital anatomy, current physiology, and the effects of superimposed pregnancy-related physiology.
- Many CHD patients are lost to follow-up in adulthood, and pregnancy is an opportunity to re-establish longitudinal adult congenital cardiac care.

INTRODUCTION

The population of adults with congenital heart disease (ACHD) continues to grow at an impressive rate because these individuals are now surviving beyond childhood as a result of medical and surgical advances. These medical and surgical advances result in an expanding number of women of childbearing age with congenital heart disease (CHD) with a significant increase in number of deliveries among women with CHD in recent years.[1] Importantly, with the high loss to follow-up rates in the ACHD population, many of these individuals only return to the health care system when contemplating pregnancy or already pregnant. This time is an opportunity to aid these women in resuming lifelong cardiac care, recognizing that, ideally, preconception counseling is paramount. In this review, general issues applicable to the ACHD population are addressed, including preconception counseling, risk assessment, lesion-based review of pregnancy physiology, and clinical management of potential complications for the general cardiologist (**Table 1**). Pregnancy in the ACHD population requires a multidisciplinary team, and therefore, the primary cardiologist, local (or remote but consulting) ACHD center, high-risk obstetrics or maternal fetal medicine, and obstetric anesthesia should all be involved in pregnancy planning, including patient selection and intrapartum and delivery planning. The entire care team, including the nurses who will spend the most time at the bedside during labor and delivery, should be included in the planning and education process. Individuals with ACHD can increasingly have successful pregnancies when planned with their team and with close communication throughout the process.

Disclosure Statement: The authors have nothing to disclose.

[a] Adult Congenital Heart Disease Program, Massachusetts General Hospital Heart Center, Boston, MA, USA;
[b] Cardiovascular Disease and Pregnancy Service, Massachusetts General Hospital Heart Center, Boston, MA, USA
* Corresponding author. Adult Congenital Heart Disease Program, Cardiology Division, Massachusetts General Hospital, 55 Fruit Street, Yawkey 5700, Boston, MA 02114.
E-mail address: abhatt@mgh.harvard.edu

cardiology.theclinics.com

Table 1
Adult congenital heart disease disease-specific risks and recommendations for pregnancy management

	Evaluate/Exclude	Potential Risks	Recommendations
VSD	PAH Ventricular dysfunction	Arrhythmia Endocarditis	Antibiotics if unrepaired

ASD (unrepaired)	PAH
	Ventricular dysfunction
		Arrhythmia
		Paradoxic embolism
			Low-dose aspirin
			  thromboembolic
			  prophylaxis (if bed rest)

Coarctation
  (repaired)
	Re-coarctation
	Aortic/brain aneurysm
		Pre-eclampsia/HTN
		Aortic dissection
		Left heart failure
			β-Blocker if HTN
			Avoid placental hypotension
			Consider C-section if
			  aneurysm

TOF (repaired)	Severe RVOT
	  obstruction
	Severe PR
	RV dysfunction
	DiGeorge syndrome
		Arrhythmia/VT
		Right heart failure
		Endocarditis
			Volume control
			Peridelivery
			Consider preterm delivery if
			  RHF
			Antibiotic prophylaxis

Mitral stenosis	Severe MS Pulmonary venous HTN	Atrial fibrillation Thromboembolic event Pulmonary edema	β–Blockers Diuresis 3rd-trimester bed rest Antibiotic prophylaxis

AS	Severe AS (peak
	  >80 mm Hg)
	Symptoms
	ST depressions
	LV dysfunction
		Arrhythmia
		Angina
		Heart failure/shock
		Endocarditis
			± 3rd-trimester bed rest
			Diuretics as needed
			If HF: valvotomy or preterm
			  C-section
			Antibiotic prophylaxis

Systemic RV	Ventricular dysfunction Severe systemic TR Arrhythmia Symptoms Venous pathway obstruction	Heart failure Arrhythmia Thromboembolic event	Restore NSR if needed Aspirin 81 mg daily ± Rhythm monitoring
Cyanotic lesions without PAH	Ventricular dysfunction Saturation <85%	Hemorrhage Thromboembolic events Increased cyanosis Heart failure Endocarditis	Bed rest and O_2 Thromboembolic prophylaxis

Fontan
  circulation
	Ventricular dysfunction
	Arrhythmia
	Prior heart failure
		Thromboembolic events
		Increased cyanosis
		Heart failure
		Endocarditis
			Anticoagulation or aspirin
			Avoid dehydration during
			  delivery
			Restore NSR quickly
			Avoid calcium channel
			  blockers
			Antibiotic prophylaxis

Marfan syndrome	Aortic root >4.0	Type A dissection	β–Blocker C-section if root >4.0–4.5 cm

Eisenmenger
  syndrome
	Ventricular dysfunction
	Arrhythmia
		30%–50% risk of death	Discuss termination
			If late for termination:
			• O_2
			• Bed rest
			• Thromboembolic
			  prophylaxis
			• Prolonged postpartum stay
			• Permanent contraception

Abbreviations: HTN, hypertension; MS, mitral stenosis; NSR, normal sinus rhythm; PAH, pulmonary arterial hypertension; PR, pulmonic regurgitation; RHF, rheumatic heart failure; VT, ventricular tachycardia.

NORMAL PREGNANCY PHYSIOLOGY

A multitude of maternal physiologic adaptions must take place to accommodate placental and fetal growth and development during pregnancy. Normal physiology of pregnancy includes a progressive increase in cardiac output, sodium and water retention, reduction in the systemic vascular resistance (SVR), and systemic blood pressure.

Expansion of plasma volume coincides with an increase in erythropoietin and red blood cell mass, both peaking between 28 and 34 weeks' gestation before plateauing (**Fig. 1**). The increase in intravascular volume exceeds the increase in red cell mass, resulting in a physiologic anemia of pregnancy and decreased blood viscosity and is adaptive to reduce resistance to placental blood flow and improve placental perfusion. Physiologic sodium and water retention may challenge the cardiac reserve of a marginal ventricular system, such as may be present among patients with CHD or those predisposed to cardiomyopathy.

Hemodynamically, cardiac output increases approximately 30% to 50% above baseline for a single pregnancy, and more than 50% for a twin pregnancy. This increase in cardiac output is a result of increased stroke volume due to increased

plasma volume as well as an increase in heart rate (see **Fig. 1**). A decrease in systolic BP is also noted as a result of a reduction in SVR, and this reduction in SVR may be favorable for some women with physiology benefited by lower SVR, such as cardiomyopathy or regurgitant lesions.

Near delivery, the cardiac output increases by 15% above prelabor levels to approximately 25% in the active phase of labor, with an additional 50% increase while a woman is pushing, coinciding with an increase in heart rate in the context of pain and contraction. Autotransfusion occurs with contractions. The SVR quickly increases in the first 24 to 72 hours after delivery, and this rapid increase in afterload may precipitate clinical congestive heart failure among patients with a susceptible systemic ventricle. Fortunately, these predictable physiologic changes in pregnancy can be assessed in the context of an individual's ACHD anatomy and physiology during preconception counseling and evaluation.

PRECONCEPTION COUNSELING

Preconception counseling is essential for every CHD patient and begins with contraceptive counseling in the teenage years as well as educating

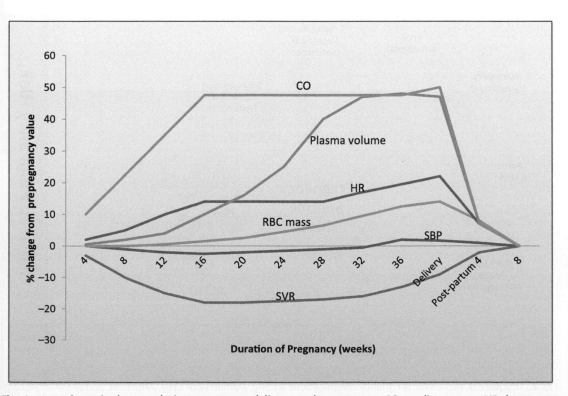

Fig. 1. Hemodynamic changes during pregnancy, delivery, and postpartum. CO, cardiac output; HR, heart rate; RBC, red blood cell; SBP, systolic blood pressure.

the individual on the anatomy and physiology of their CHD. Awareness of potential late complications is also important, because this foundation of knowledge will help the patient understand the importance of preconception risk stratification. Unfortunately, studies reveal that current counseling practice for pregnancy and contraception in women with CHD is inadequate[2] despite its clear potential benefits for maternal and fetal outcome.

PRECONCEPTION RISK PREDICTION

Most preconception visits will center on a discussion of maternal and fetal outcome assessment. In broad terms, a preconception history of an adverse cardiac event (arrhythmia, stroke, transient ischemic attack, pulmonary edema), poor functional capacity, pulmonary hypertension, aortic dilation, anticoagulation, mechanical valves, cyanosis, and impaired systemic ventricular function all increase the risk of a maternal event in pregnancy (**Fig. 2**).[3]

There are 3 commonly used risk scores for pregnancy and adverse events in individuals with

CHD: the ZAHARA, CARPREG, and WHO classification systems.[3–5] A recent study revealed the challenge with risk prediction, especially in the higher-risk ACHD individuals, because these risk scores seemed to sometimes overestimate the potential adverse cardiac event rate, were unable to reliably predict outcome in offspring, and often did not include other potential risk factors, thereby requiring practitioners to still rely on clinical acumen in advising these women regarding pregnancy risk and outcome.[6] In this analysis, the WHO classification seemed to be a reliable risk assessment model for estimating cardiovascular risk in pregnant women with CHD.

Cardiopulmonary exercise testing has been proven useful in risk stratification. Abnormal chronotropic response correlates strongly with adverse pregnancy outcomes in women with CHD.[7] A peak heart rate of 150 beats/min or more or maximal oxygen consumption greater than 25 mL/kg/min may predict a population at less risk for adverse pregnancy outcome, and better cardiopulmonary exercise parameters also strongly correlate with normal neonatal birth weight.[8] However, risk assessment must not be

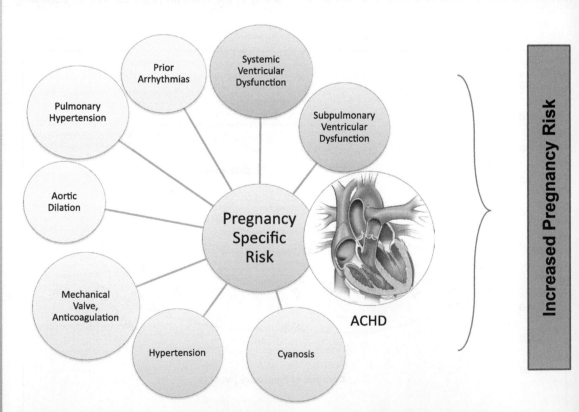

Fig. 2. Unique risk factors for pregnancy complications among women with CHD. Anatomic and physiologic complications combined with pregnancy physiology create a unique risk profile for each pregnant individual with ACHD.

based on single parameters, even quantitative ones, because there are many cases in practice and the literature that do not follow any currently established risk stratification model or cutoff.

Cardiac biomarkers may also hold value in assessing pregnancy risk in CHD. In a prospective multicenter cohort study with adverse cardiovascular events in 10.3% of the 213 pregnancies studied, the presence of a mechanical valve, subpulmonary ventricular dysfunction preconception, and N-terminal pro-B-type natriuretic peptide (NT-BNP) levels greater than 128 pg/mL at 20-weeks' gestation were independently associated with adverse cardiac events, with NT-BNP offering additive information even in the presence of other risk factors.[9]

For individuals with a known genetic syndrome, the inheritance pattern is often defined by the lesion (ie autosomal-dominant results in 50% risk of transmission to offspring such as Holt-Oram or Marfan syndrome). In the general population, the risk of CHD is ~0.8% with the risk in offspring anywhere from 3% to 7% based on family history, lesion, and maternal disease (more likely to be transmitted to offspring). Of note, the same congenital heart defect is not necessarily transmitted from generation to generation. Bicuspid aortic valve may be the most common genetically transmitted CHD seen by general adult cardiologists, and atrioventricular septal defects (AVSD; addressed in later discussion) may also demonstrate a strong familial tendency for CHD in offspring. In general, all women with CHD should be offered a fetal echocardiogram during pregnancy.

CONGENITAL HEART DIAGNOSES
Shunt Lesions

Shunt lesions include atrial level septal defects (ASD) or pre-tricuspid shunts (sinus venosus septal defect, partial anomalous pulmonary venous connection, secundum ASD, primum ASD as the most common lesions). The secundum ASD can vary in size and is usually an isolated lesion, although may involve mitral regurgitation in older age. The primum ASD can often be large if not previously diagnosed and addressed and presents with or without a VSD as well as with a cleft mitral valve with varying degrees of regurgitation, even after surgical repair. The sinus venosus defect is associated with partial anomalous pulmonary venous return and may demonstrate a low ectopic atrial rhythm on electrocardiogram (EKG) and dilated right ventricle (RV) on echocardiography without overt shunt detection on standard transthoracic echocardiogram, and therefore, should be suspected in right heart enlargement without other

identified cause. Fortunately, pregnancy and delivery are generally well tolerated in pre-tricuspid shunt lesions, especially if repaired. Newly diagnosed individuals may want to seek repair before pregnancy, especially to reduce the theoretic risk of paradoxic embolism during the hypercoagulable state of pregnancy and the risk of pre-eclampsia. If unrepaired individuals present pregnant, close blood pressure monitoring, filters on peripheral intravenous lines for procedures especially in individuals with large bidirectional shunts, consideration of aspirin, and education of the entire cardio-obstetric team is the foundation for their care. In any large septal defect, right ventricular systolic pressure on transthoracic echo may appear elevated as a result of increased pulmonary arterial flow; however, pulmonary vascular resistance may be normal. These individuals should have normal oxygen saturation and left-to-right flow through their atrial level defect. However, if any cyanosis, right-to-left shunt, or pulmonary hypertension is suggested, further ACHD evaluation is necessary for the safety of mother and fetus. Women with an unrepaired ASD are at increased risk of neonatal events in comparison with women with a repaired ASD. Compared with the general population, women with an unrepaired ASD are at increased risk for small-for-gestational-age (SGA) births and fetal mortality.[10]

Individuals with AVSD have a unique physiology, surgical repair, and residual defects when compared with simple ASD and ventricular septal defects (VSDs). Children with AVSDs are increasingly growing to healthy adult life, and therefore, pregnancy is a common occurrence; however, their risk may be underestimated if considered the same as any other repaired ASD or VSD. In the CONCOR registry, cardiovascular events complicated almost 40% of the completed pregnancies with more than 20% of patients having persistent postpartum New York Heart Association (NYHA) class deterioration and nearly 20% with progressive left atrioventricular-valvular regurgitation (17%).[11] In this cohort, offspring mortality was higher than expected as a result of complex CHD in the fetus.

Posttricuspid shunt lesions, including VSD and patient ductus arteriosus (PDA), if small, are generally well tolerated. On examination, a small restrictive VSD will present as a loud holosystolic murmur. Women with unrepaired VSD are at increased risk of pre-eclampsia similar to atrial level shunt patients. Women with repaired VSD are at increased risk of premature labor and intrauterine growth retardation as well.[12] A PDA, if small, will be silent or present as a soft continuous infraclavicular, left sternal border or left upper back murmur, which enhances with isometrics, while a moderate PDA may demonstrate ventricular enlargement and a displaced point of maximal impulse on palpation.

Large VSD or PDA lesions will have likely led to some degree of pulmonary hypertension by childbearing age; therefore, preconception counseling in unrepaired posttricuspid shunt lesions should include discussion of closure if feasible, and otherwise, an understanding of the high risk of adverse outcomes related to pulmonary hypertension in pregnancy as well as the significant risk of maternal and fetal mortality in individuals who have a diagnosis of Eisenmenger syndrome (increased pulmonary vascular resistance from long-term increased pulmonary flow, and reversal of the shunt flow from right to left with subsequent cyanosis).[13] A large PDA will create both left atrial and ventricular enlargement. If pulmonary hypertension exists, there will be a prominent pulmonic component to the second heart sound and RV heave with cyanosis and clubbing. An individual with Eisenmenger with PDA may have differential cyanosis: cyanosis of feet (clubbing of toes) and perhaps left hand with normal right hand pulse oximetry.

Maternal mortality is highest in the Eisenmenger population.[14] More than 60% of sudden cardiac deaths attributable to pulmonary hypertension in one pregnancy study were in individuals with CHD. Nearly half of those individuals had an isolated shunt lesion, which had been undiagnosed and progressed to develop pulmonary arterial hypertension.[15] Up to 33% of individuals with Eisenmenger syndrome had a cardiovascular event in pregnancy, with nearly 20% of individuals having thromboembolic complications, and more than half having premature delivery, with significant SGA births and the second highest rate of fetal deaths among the ACHD population (the highest rate in cyanotic CHD).[14]

Both cyanotic isolated shunts and more complex cyanotic heart diseases carry a significant pregnancy risk. Cyanotic CHD demonstrates one of the highest rates of maternal complication or adverse cardiac event as well as fetal complications of premature delivery, intrauterine growth retardation (IUGR), and mortality.[14] In general, individuals who are densely cyanotic should be counseled to avoid pregnancy. Cyanotic CHD, patients with Eisenmenger syndrome, and patients with pulmonary atresia/VSD all share considerable risk for developing heart failure and are among the highest-risk individuals to embark on pregnancy; therefore, contraceptive counseling beginning at a young age is essential, as is outlining options for family structure.

Left Heart Outflow Obstructions

Congenital mitral stenosis is rare but, unlike rheumatic mitral stenosis, which may be amenable to balloon dilation if women develop pulmonary edema or arrhythmias during pregnancy, congenital mitral variants (parachute mitral valve, supravalvular mitral ring) are not amenable to percutaneous balloon valvuloplasty and must be treated surgically. Surgical correction for congenital mitral stenosis must be addressed before pregnancy to avoid later pregnancy complications.

Congenital aortic valve disease is common (approximately 1%–2% of the general population) and bicuspid aortic valve disease is the most common cause of aortic stenosis (AS) in childbearing women. Most young nonpregnant women with AS, even when severe, are asymptomatic; therefore, careful prepregnancy cardiac evaluation and functional capacity assessment are critical. Women with AS who are symptomatic or have left ventricle (LV) dysfunction should be actively advised to avoid pregnancy and undergo evaluation for intervention before pregnancy consideration. Women who are asymptomatic with normal exercise capacity and normal LV function who desire pregnancy must be monitored closely by a physician trained in obstetric cardiology. Diuretics may be needed if fluid accumulation develops later in pregnancy. Preterm labor and hypertensive-related disorder are increased among women with severe AS. Fetal complications may also occur in up to 25% of mothers with severe stenosis, including IUGR, preterm birth, and low birth weight. Multidisciplinary discussion before delivery should include location of delivery (hospital with both cardiac interventional and surgical backup), anesthesia plan, need for telemetry (usually only if arrhythmia present), preferred method of delivery (vaginal unless significantly dilated aorta or obstetric indication), need for antibiotics, plan for postdelivery cardiac monitoring, and various emergency scenarios should also be reviewed with a documented plan. This multidisciplinary discussion should also involve cardiac interventionalists and cardiac surgeons. If a woman presents pregnant with severe symptoms or heart failure despite medical therapy, percutaneous balloon dilation could be considered if valve anatomy is appropriate[16] or if percutaneous valvuloplasty is not feasible; early delivery by C-section followed by urgent surgical valve replacement may be required for life-threatening circumstances. Women with aortopathies associated with congenital AS are at higher risk of aortic dissection. Women with an aorta greater than 4.5 cm should be advised to avoid pregnancy until correction.[17,18]

Coarctation of the aorta is defined as a discrete narrowing of the proximal descending aorta just distal to the left subclavian artery. Coarctation may be associated with congenitally abnormal aortic valves, subaortic membranes, VSDs, or arch anomalies such as arch hypoplasia or aberrant subclavian arteries. Although most women with well-repaired coarctation of the aorta and well-controlled blood pressure can do very well with pregnancy, patients with both operated and unoperated coarctation of the aorta carry a small risk of aortic dissection as well as an increased risk of pre-eclamspia and hypertension[14,19,20] as well as adverse cardiovascular complications related to hypertension, including stroke, arrhythmia, heart failure, and other embolic events.[21] Women with unrepaired coarctation and women with repaired coarctation with residual hypertension were at highest risk of aortic rupture and rupture of intracranial aneurysm.[5] Finally, physicians must remember that upper extremity blood pressure will overestimate placental perfusion pressure among women with unrepaired coarctation or residual or recurrent coarctation, and reduced placental perfusion pressure increases the risk of adverse fetal outcome. In the authors' practice, individuals with a coarctation gradient greater than 30 mm Hg, or less than 30 mm Hg with a significant drop in ankle brachial index in the preconception evaluation, are counseled to consider the risk and benefit of coarctation revision before pregnancy.

Tetralogy of Fallot

Tetralogy of Fallot (TOF) is the most common cyanotic congenital heart lesion. This anomaly is caused by the anterior and rightward deviation of the conal septum and results in development of a large conal VSD, an aorta that overrides the ventricular septum, RV outflow crowding and obstruction (valvular and infundibular), and subsequent RV hypertrophy. A proportion of cases may also have an associated ASD, a right aortic arch, coronary artery anomalies, absent left pulmonary artery, or aortic dilation. Older patients with TOF may have undergone a palliative systemic to pulmonary artery shunt (Blalock-Taussig-Thomas, or less commonly, Potts or Waterston shunts) in early childhood before a complete repair later in childhood (consisting of a right ventricular outflow tract [RVOT] augmentation and VSD patch); however, most younger patients of childbearing age underwent complete repair in earlier infancy obviating the palliative shunt. Complications that may develop in adulthood include pulmonic regurgitation (if a transannular patch was placed) with subsequent right ventricular dilation, dysfunction and clinical right heart failure, ventricular arrhythmias, residual VSDs or pulmonic stenosis (PS), and aortic dilation. Patients with well-repaired TOF without ventricular dysfunction, prior arrhythmias, or clinical right heart failure generally tolerate pregnancy very well, but involvement of high-risk obstetrics and congenital heart specialists is advised. History of ablation and the baseline cardiothoracic ratio on chest radiography are predictors of adverse events.[22] Risk of peridelivery right heart failure and arrhythmias is increased if severe pulmonic regurgitation with significant RV dilation or dysfunction is present or if LV dysfunction is present.[23] Right ventricular enlargement persists at least 6 months after delivery,[22] and long-term implications of pregnancy on RV performance of patients with TOF is unknown. TOF patients are at increased risk of fetal loss and their offspring are more likely to have congenital anomalies than offspring of the general population[23]; therefore, fetal imaging in experienced centers is indicated.

Ebstein Anomaly

Ebstein anomaly is a rare congenital heart diagnosis affecting approximately 1% of all CHDs. It is a genetically heterogeneous condition caused by failure of delamination of the tricuspid valve leaflets from the underlying myocardium and the interventricular septum, resulting in apical displacement of the attachments of the septal and posterior leaflets, variable degrees of tricuspid regurgitation, and a small true right ventricular cavity (**Fig. 3**). Associated anomalies include ASD or patent foramen ovales, Wolff-Parkinson-White syndrome, and pulmonic stenosis. Tachyarrhythmias are common, and patients may develop progressive right heart failure due to tricuspid regurgitation and poor compliance of the myopathic RV. They may develop desaturation from right-to-left shunting through an atrial defect if right heart pressures exceed left heart pressures (even in the absence of significant tricuspid regurgitation). Miscarriages are more frequent among mothers with Ebstein anomaly; however, among women with normal saturation, no arrhythmias, or symptoms before pregnancy (NYHA class I), the likelihood of normal full-term vaginal delivery is high.[24] The physiologic sodium and fluid retention of pregnancy may pose a challenge for some and may precipitate complications of tachycardia or right heart failure. Mothers with significant cyanosis (saturation <85%) or with symptomatic heart failure should be advised against pregnancy.[25]

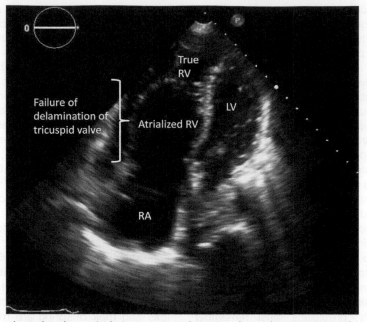

Fig. 3. Ebstein anomaly, 4-chamber apical view on transthoracic echocardiogram. RA, right atrium.

Transposition of the Great Arteries

D transposition of the great arteries (d-TGA) is a cyanotic CHD whose original surgical correction involved the atrial switch operation (**Fig. 4**), resulting in correction of the directionality of blood flow, however leaving the RV in the systemic position. Atrial arrhythmias and systemic tricuspid valve regurgitation and systemic right ventricular dysfunction can follow. Each of these complications has an increased risk during pregnancy and the post-partum period. In one study following women with d-TGA atrial switch over a decade, the preterm birth rate was 50%, with 20% maternal complication rate and serial echocardiography revealing intrapartum decline in right ventricular function with some improvement postpartum. Interestingly, intracardiac baffle obstruction that required postpartum

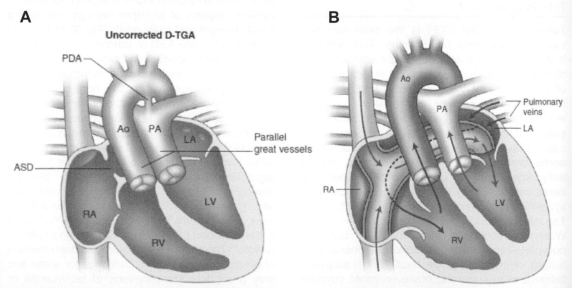

Fig. 4. D-TGA. (*A*) Uncorrected d-TGA and (*B*) D-TGA after the atrial switch operation. Atrial arrhythmias and systemic right ventricular dysfunction can both occur in pregnancy. Ao, aorta; LA, atrium; PA, pulmonary artery; RA, right atrium.

stenting occurred in 36% of the completed pregnancies.[26] An earlier study similarly revealed systemic right ventricular dilation, dysfunction, and systemic tricuspid valve regurgitation progression in one-quarter to one-half of pregnant individuals without postpartum recovery.[27] Pregnancy after atrial switch operation for repair of d-TGA therefore does carry risk and should be followed by a multidisciplinary team with expertise with an assumption that some clinical complications may arise even despite preconception optimization.[28]

Since the mid 1980s, individuals with d-TGA received a new surgical intervention, the Jatene arterial switch, which is now the repair of choice when feasible in d-TGA. Thus far, long-term complications include aortic dilation, neoaortic regurgitation, suprapulmonic and AS, and coronary ostial narrowing. As these patients are young, pregnancy outcomes data are limited; however, management at this time centers on assessing preconception anatomy and physiology, including regurgitation, stenoses, and coronary and aortic dimensions.

Congenitally corrected transposition of the great arteries (CC-TGA, L-TGA) is rare; however, it has unique examination and imaging findings and can present with specific cardiac complications. The anatomy involves systemic venous flow (vena cavae) entering the right atrium, traversing the mitral valve, and exiting the pulmonary artery to the lungs. The pulmonary veins meanwhile enter the left atrium normally but traverse a tricuspid valve to the RV and then out the aorta; this makes the RV the systemic ventricle and can result in heart failure over time, especially in the presence of systemic tricuspid valve regurgitation. Importantly, L-TGA can be associated with VSD, pulmonic stenosis, and anomalies of the atrioventricular valves (Ebstein-like malformation of the systemic atrioventricular valve) and has a significant rate of the development of complete heart block. Those individuals with isolated L-TGA may be initially identified during adult life and can receive a diagnosis during pregnancy. On examination, these individuals will likely have a loud second heart sound, which reflects an anterior aortic valve and may have a holosystolic murmur of systemic tricuspid regurgitation. The classic EKG demonstrates Q waves in the right precordial leads and should be obtained to demonstrate normal sinus rhythm rather than complete heart block. The development of complete heart block in L-TGA may be well tolerated with a high junctional rhythm; however, Holter monitoring to ensure no significant bradycardia is helpful.

In the literature, cardiac arrest or death during pregnancy or the postpartum period has been described in 12.3% of all systemic RV pregnancies.[29] Supraventricular arrhythmias appear to be common, but significant decline in systemic ventricular function does not appear to occur in the short term related to pregnancy.[30] Successful pregnancy can be achieved in most women with TGA; however, the rate of fetal loss and maternal cardiovascular morbidity is increased.[31]

Fontan Circulation

The Fontan palliation has been performed since the 1970s for individuals with a functional single-ventricle physiology, so that systemic venous return can be directed to the pulmonary arteries, allowing separation of pulmonary and systemic venous flow (**Fig. 5**). Many long-term complications ensue, including systemic ventricular dysfunction, atrial arrhythmias, thromboembolic complications, hepatic and renal disease, and sometimes baffle leaks or systemic to pulmonary venovenous collaterals leading to cyanosis. Fontan and D-TGA atrial switch patients seem to be at highest risk for arrhythmia (near 16% risk) during pregnancy, likely secondary to atrial baffle material creating foci/pathways for atrial reentrant circuits. Of note, individuals with Fontan physiology can have gynecologic complications and menstrual cycle disorders, resulting in amenorrhea or late onset menarche. Contraceptive counseling can also be challenging, but is extremely important in this population, who often has an underlying thromboembolic risk profile. Although individuals with Fontan palliation can have normal and successful pregnancies, maternal NYHA class deterioration and atrial arrhythmias as well as fetal complications of premature delivery and IUGR are prevalent.[32-34] Maintaining sinus rhythm reduces the risk of heart failure, and electrical cardioversion may be necessary if arrhythmia develops (of note, calcium channel blockers with negative ionotropic activity can be detrimental). Patients with Fontan palliation should be referred to maternal fetal medicine with expertise in complex CHD as well as ACHD cardiologists for coordinated multidisciplinary care plan.

Marfan Syndrome

Marfan syndrome is an autosomal-dominant diagnosis with a fibrillin-1 mutation, and nearly 80% of individuals have some cardiac involvement. Aortic events remain the primary cause of death, and dissection most commonly occurs in the last trimester or postpartum, although first- and second-trimester events have been reported. With an aortic root diameter of less than 4.0 cm, there is a 1% risk of cardiovascular event; however,

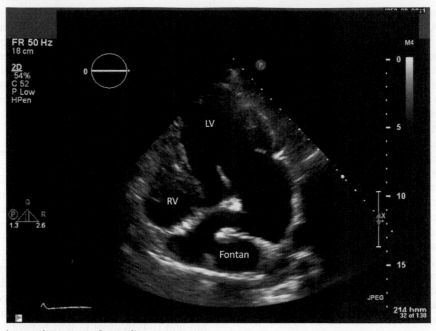

Fig. 5. Lateral tunnel Fontan echocardiogram.

at aortic root diameters greater than 4.0 cm, the dissection risk increases to 10%. In individuals with an aorta greater than 4.0 cm, nearly half of those individuals will need surgery, have aortic rupture, or have life-threatening dilation during pregnancy. Counseling in Marfan syndrome must begin preconception with genetic counseling regarding transmission, delineation of cardiac involvement, and a clear discussion as to maternal and fetal risk and outcomes.

ANESTHESIA AND DELIVERY

Anesthesia and the delivery period can be the most volatile physiologic time and stressor for the pregnant woman with CHD; however, with multidisciplinary planning, it can be accomplished safely. Delivery should ideally be planned. Vaginal delivery is generally preferred unless there is an obstetric indication for cesarean delivery. In high-risk cardiac patients, obstetric management of labor and delivery may be modified to accommodate the limitations imposed by cardiac dysfunction; however, cesarean delivery is rarely performed solely for a maternal cardiac indication. Individuals who with ideal preconception counseling would have been counseled against pregnancy may present the one group where a conversation regarding mode of delivery for maternal cardiac indications may arise. This group includes significant aortopathy (eg, chronic aortic dissection, dilated aortic root >4 cm, or

progressive root enlargement during gestation), severe pulmonary hypertension, or Eisenmenger syndrome.

Studies have revealed that, in most ACHD individuals, induction of labor is safe and not associated with higher cesarean rates. Even for most NYHA III and IV patients, a trial of labor is safe with expedited delivery under good analgesic control as dictated by obstetric needs.[35]

Other potential monitoring mechanisms include (1) continuous pulse oximetry throughout active labor for patients with cyanotic CHD or right-to-left vascular shunting, (2) telemetry for patients at increased risk of developing arrhythmias, (3) 5-lead EKG monitoring with computerized ST-segment trending capability in patients at risk for myocardial ischemia, (4) external defibrillator pads to achieve rapid cardioversion or defibrillation in patients with a history of poorly tolerated tachyarrhythmias, and (5) intra-arterial catheter to enable monitoring of moment-to-moment changes in blood pressure before induction of either regional or general anesthesia for cesarean delivery in high-risk patients and in laboring patients who are unstable. For most women with ACHD, a pulmonary artery catheter is not necessary for delivery unless the mother develops severe heart failure or cardiogenic shock, whereby tailored therapy to guide diuretic and ionotropic support may be useful.

Understanding the hemodynamic changes related to pregnancy, labor, and delivery allows the anesthesiologist to anticipate decompensation in the peripartum period in patients with cardiovascular lesions, and to select appropriate anesthetic monitoring and techniques to minimize this risk. The health care team, including the cardiology and obstetrics teams, anesthesiologist, and floor nursing staff, will determine the optimum location for delivery and monitoring plan for patients with high-risk cardiovascular lesions. These plans should be documented in the electronic medical record, with most recent assessment, ideal labor and delivery plan, and a premature labor and delivery plan outlined for all responding caregivers to access and use to deliver the best outcome for mother and child.

ANTIBIOTIC PROPHYLAXIS

Recommendations for antibiotic prophylaxis in various congenital heart lesions have evolved significantly over the past several years. Before the updated endocarditis guidelines in 2007,[36] almost all patients with congenital heart defects were advised antibiotics around the time of dental procedures and other procedures, including delivery. In 2007, the pendulum shifted to recommend antibiotic prophylaxis to patients only at the highest risk of morbidity or mortality if endocarditis were acquired. This antibiotic prophylaxis included patients with prior history of endocarditis, cyanosis, prior cardiac transplantation, or prosthetic material within the heart (including prior valve replacement). There were many patients with uncorrected CHD who were at that time advised against the use of prophylactic antibiotics, including patients with uncorrected bicuspid aortic valves and restrictive VSDs. Subsequent literature demonstrated that certain CHD lesions had increased risk of endocarditis.[37] As almost all patients who have undergone surgery for CHD have some residual disease, there are many who are at risk for infective endocarditis. Although the risk of infective endocarditis in pregnancy in general is quite low, the rates of maternal and fetal mortality once diagnosed with endocarditis are greater than 25% in some studies. As delay in diagnosis carries this risk of morbidity or mortality to the mother and the infant, a high index of suspicion is important in management, with close attention to fever in pregnancy or marked change in physical examination, not explained by pregnancy physiology. Maintaining oral health is also important in general in ACHD, and particularly in pregnancy. Considering the breadth of opinions and literature regarding endocarditis prophylaxis guidelines versus CHD-specific endocarditis patterns, risks and benefits in each case must be assessed

individually, and recommendation for prophylaxis must be tailored.

SUMMARY

Most women with known CHD can have successful pregnancy, labor, and delivery, an experience not significantly different from a non-CHD population. Preconception counseling and cardiac assessment are essential in understanding the woman's anatomy, repairs, and current physiology, all of which can influence risk in pregnancy. With that foundation, the cardio-obstetric team can predict and prepare for any complications that may occur with superimposed hemodynamic changes of pregnancy. Several risk estimation models have been established, along with individual tests and parameters that can aid the team in assessing and discussing risk with the patient and family. With a clear plan in place, including contingencies, most women with even moderately complex CHD anatomy or physiology will also be able to participate in a safe pregnancy and delivery. There are lesions, generally unrepaired, that carry prohibitively high risk for the mother and fetus, including Eisenmenger syndrome and cyanotic complex CHD. Individuals with significant ventricular dysfunction or pulmonary hypertension can be considered similarly high risk. Those individuals with reparable cardiac complications, including valvular disease, aortic dilation, and significant shunt lesions, should be counseled regarding unintervened versus intervened risk profile.

When counseling regarding risk, there are 3 major categories[14] to be considered:

1. Cardiac events: AVSD, d-TGA atrial switch, and Fontan carry the highest risk of arrhythmias. L-TGA and d-TGA, and aortic stenosis (AoS) carry a risk of heart failure (HF), but cyanotic CHD and Eisenmenger carry twice that risk. Eisenmenger carries the highest cardiac event rate in pregnancies that progress past 20 weeks.
2. Maternal obstetric complications: AoS and coarctation may develop pregnancy-induced hypertension, AVSD, PS, d-TGA; coarctation and PAVSD carry risk of preeclampsia, and ASD carries thromboembolic risk, however, one-third the risk that Eisenmenger carries.
3. Fetal outcomes: Premature delivery occurs across all diagnoses, with SGA and fetal mortality most notable in Eisemenger and cyanotic CHD.

Many ACHD patients are lost to follow-up in adulthood, and pregnancy may be the trigger that reintroduces them to medical care and re-establishes long-term adult congenital cardiac care.[38] With individualized assessment and a multidisciplinary management plan, pregnancy and delivery can be an empowering process for both the individual with ACHD and their family.

REFERENCES

1. Optowsky A, Siddiqi O, D'Zouza B, et al. Maternal cardiovascular events during childbirth among women with congenital heart disease. Heart 2011; 98:145–51.
2. Kaemmerer M, Vigl M, Seifert-Klauss V, et al. Counseling reproductive health issues in women with congenital heart disease. Clin Res Cardiol 2012; 101(11):901–7.
3. Siu SC, Sermer M, Colman JM, et al. Prospective multicenter study of pregnancy outcomes in women with heart disease. Circulation 2001;104:515–21.
4. Drenthen W, Boersma E, Balci A, et al. Predictors of pregnancy complications in women with congenital heart disease. Eur Heart J 2010;31:2124–32.
5. Regitz-Zagrosek V, Lundqvist CB, Borghi C, et al. ESC Guidelines on the management of cardiovascular diseases during pregnancy the Task Force on the Management of Cardiovascular Diseases during Pregnancy of the European Society of Cardiology (ESC). Eur Heart J 2011;32:3147–97.
6. Balci A, Sollie-Szarynska KM, van der Bijl AGL, et al. Prospective validation and assessment of cardiovascular and offspring risk models for pregnant women with congenital heart disease. Heart 2014; 100:1373–81.
7. Lui GK, Silversides C, Khairy P, et al. Heart rate response during exercise and pregnancy outcomes in women with congenital heart disease. Circulation 2011;123:242–8.
8. Ohuchi H, Tanabe Y, Kamiya C, et al. Cardiopulmonary variables during exercise predict pregnancy outcomes in women with congenital heart disease. Circ J 2013;77(2):470–6.
9. Kampman MA, Balci A, van Veldhuisen DJ, et al. N-terminal pro-B-type natriuretic peptide predicts cardiovascular complications in pregnant women with congenital heart disease. Eur Heart J 2014;35(11): 708–15.
10. Yap SC, Drenthen W, Meijiboom FJ, et al. Comparison of pregnancy outcomes in women with repaired versus unrepaired atrial septal defect. BJOG 2009; 116:1593–601.
11. Drenthen W, Pieper PG, van der Tuuk K, et al. Cardiac complications relating to pregnancy and recurrence of disease in the offspring of women with atrioventricular septal defect. Eur Heart J 2005;26: 2581–7.
12. Yap SC, Drenthen W, Pieper PG, et al. Pregnancy outcome in women with repaired versus unrepaired isolated ventricular septal defect. BJOG 2010;117: 683–9.
13. Uebing A, Steer PJ, Yentis SM, et al. Pregnancy and congenital heart disease. BMJ 2006;332:401–6.
14. Drenthen W, Pieper PG, Roos-Hesselink JW, et al. Outcome of pregnancy in women with congenital heart disease: a literature review. Am J Cardiol 2007;49:2303–11.
15. Krexi D, Sheppard MN. Pulmonary hypertensive vascular changes in lungs of patients with sudden unexpected death. Emphasis on congenital heart disease, Eisenmenger syndrome, postoperative deaths and death during pregnancy and postpartum. J Clin Pathol 2015;68(1):18–21.
16. Bhargava B, Agarwal R, Yadav R, et al. Percutaneous balloon aortic valvuloplasty during pregnancy: use of the Inoue balloon and the physiologic antegrade approach. Cathet Cardiovasc Diagn 1998;45:422–5.
17. Warnes CA, Williams RG, Bashore TM, et al. ACC/AHA 2008 guidelines for the management of adults with congenital heart disease: a report of the American College of Cardiology/American Heart Association Task Force on Practice Guidelines (Writing Committee to Develop Guidelines on the Management of Adults With Congenital Heart Disease). Developed in Collaboration with the American Society of Echocardiography, Heart Rhythm Society, International Society for Adult Congenital Heart Disease, Society for Cardiovascular Angiography and Interventions, and Society of Thoracic Surgeons. J Am Coll Cardiol 2008; 52:e143–263.
18. Hiratzka L, Bakris G, Beckman J, et al. Guidelines for the diagnosis and management of patients with thoracic aortic disease: a report of the American College of Cardiology Foundation/American Heart Association Task Force on Practice Guidelines, American Association for Thoracic Surgery, American College of Radiology, American Stroke Association, Society of Cardiovascular Anesthesiologists, Society for Cardiovascular Angiography and Intervention, Society of Interventional Radiology, Society of Thoracic Surgeons, and Society for Vascular Medicine. Circulation 2010;121:e266–369.
19. Vriend JW, Drenthen W, Pieper PG, et al. Outcome of pregnancy in patients after repair of aortic coarctation. Eur Heart J 2005;26:2173–8.
20. Beauchesne LM, Connolly HM, Ammash NM, et al. Coarctation of the aorta: outcome of pregnancy. Am J Cardiol 2001;38:1728–33.
21. Krieger EV, Landzberg MJ, Economy KE, et al. Comparison of risk of hypertensive complications of pregnancy among women with versus without coarctation of the aorta. Am J Cardiol 2011;107: 1529–34.
22. Kamiya CA, Iwamiya T, Neki R, et al. Outcome of pregnancy and effects on the right heart in women

with repaired tetralogy of fallot. Circulation 2012;76: 957–63.

23. Veldtman G, Connolly H, Grogan M, et al. Outcomes of pregnancy in women with tetralogy of Fallot. Am J Cardiol 2004;44:174–80.

24. Katsuragi S, Kamiya C, Yamanaka K, et al. Risk factors for maternal and fetal outcome in pregnancy complicated by Ebstein anomaly. Am J Obstet Gynecol 2013;209:452.e1–6.

25. Zhao W, Liu H, Feng R, et al. Pregnancy outcomes in women with Ebstein's anomaly. Arch Gynecol Obstet 2012;286:881–8.

26. Metz TD, Jackson GM, Yetman AT. Pregnancy outcomes in women who have undergone an atrial switch repair for congenital d-transposition of the great arteries. Am J Obstet Gynecol 2011;205(3):273.e1–5.

27. Guedes A, Mercier LA, Leduc L, et al. Impact of pregnancy on the systemic right ventricle after a Mustard operation for transposition of the great arteries. J Am Coll Cardiol 2004;44:433–7.

28. Canobbio MM, Morris CD, Graham TP, et al. Pregnancy outcomes after atrial repair for transposition of the great arteries. Am J Cardiol 2006;98:668–72.

29. Jain VD, Moghbeli N, Webb G, et al. Pregnancy in women with congenital heart disease: the impact of a systemic right ventricle. Congenit Heart Dis 2011;6(2):147–56.

30. Kowalik E, Klisiewicz A, Biernacka EK, et al. Pregnancy and long-term cardiovascular outcomes in women with congenitally corrected transposition of the great arteries. Int J Gynaecol Obstet 2014;125(2):154–7.

31. Connolly HM, Grogan M, Warnes CA. Pregnancy among women with congenitally corrected

transposition of great arteries. J Am Coll Cardiol 1999;33:1692–5.

32. Canobbio MM, Mair DD, van der Velde M, et al. Pregnancy outcomes after the Fontan repair. J Am Coll Cardiol 1996;28:763–7.

33. Hoare JV, Radford D. Pregnancy after Fontan repair of complex congenital heart disease. Aust N Z J Obstet Gynaecol 2001;41:464–8.

34. Drenthen W, Pieper PG, Ross-Hesselink JW, et al. Pregnancy and delivery in women after Fontan palliation. Heart 2006;92:1290–4.

35. Afour V, Murphy MO, Attia R. Is vaginal delivery or caesarean section the safer mode of delivery in patients with adult congenital heart disease? Interact Cardiovasc Thorac Surg 2013;17(1): 144–50.

36. Wilson W, Taubert KA, Gewitz M, et al. Prevention of infective endocarditis: guidelines from the American Heart Association Rheumatic Fever, Endocarditis and Kawasaki Disease Committee, Council on Cardiovascular Disease in the Young, and the Council on Clinical Cardiology, Council on Cardiovascular Surgery and Anesthesia, and the Quality of Care and Outcomes Research Interdisciplinary Working Group. Circulation 2007;116: 1736–54.

37. Rushani D, Kaufman JS, Onescu-Ittu R, et al. Infective endocarditis in children with congenital heart disease: cumulative incidence and predictors. Circulation 2013;128:1412–9.

38. Brickner ME. Cardiovascular management in pregnancy: congenital heart disease. Circulation 2014; 130(3):273–82.

More Than Just the Heart
Transition and Psychosocial Issues in Adult Congenital Heart Disease

 CrossMark

Adrienne H. Kovacs, PhD[a],*, Elisabeth M. Utens, PhD[b]

KEYWORDS

- Adult congenital heart disease • Transition • Depression • Anxiety • Psychosocial

KEY POINTS

- There is increasing recognition of the importance of a thoughtful and coordinated process of transition from pediatric to adult congenital heart disease (CHD) care.
- Approximately 1 in 3 North American adults with CHD face additional challenges associated with clinically significant depression or anxiety.
- Psychosocial outcomes of European studies seem more favorable, although reasons for international differences are currently unknown.
- It is time to move beyond description and begin developing and evaluating interventions targeting the psychosocial needs of adults living with CHD.

INTRODUCTION

As a result of significant advancements in the diagnosis and management of congenital heart disease (CHD), almost 90% are now expected to reach adulthood.[1] In North America, there are now more adults than children living with CHD.[2] Despite this success story of modern medicine, most adults with CHD of moderate or great complexity are not cured and are at significant risk of heart failure, arrhythmias, additional surgeries and interventional procedures, and premature mortality.[3–8] For these reasons, lifelong surveillance by CHD specialists is important.[9] Adults with CHD thus face 2 sets of challenges: (1) the transition from pediatric to adult care and (2) the psychosocial implications of coping with a chronic and often life-shortening medical condition. These challenges, along with proposed clinical management strategies, are the focus of this article.

TRANSITION FROM PEDIATRIC TO ADULT CARE

Among all subgroups of patients with pediatric-onset health conditions, there is growing recognition of the importance of addressing the unique needs of adolescents and young adults making the transition from pediatric to adult health care services. The Society of Adolescent Medicine defined transition as "a purposeful, planned process that addresses the medical, psychosocial, and educational/vocational needs of adolescents and young adults with chronic physical and medical conditions as they move from child-centered to adult-oriented health care systems."[10] Similarly, the American Academy of Pediatrics defined the goal of transition as "to maximize lifelong functioning and potential through the provision of high-quality, developmentally appropriate health care services that continue uninterrupted as the

Disclosures: No commercial or financial conflicts of interest or funding sources.
a Department of Psychiatry, Peter Munk Cardiac Centre, University Health Network, University of Toronto, 585 University Avenue, 5-NU-523, Toronto, Ontario M5G 2N2, Canada; b Department of Child and Adolescent Psychiatry/Psychology, Erasmus Medical Center-Sophia Children's Hospital, Wytemaweg 8, 3015 CN, Rotterdam, The Netherlands
* Corresponding author.
E-mail address: adrienne.kovacs@uhn.ca

cardiology.theclinics.com

individual moves from adolescence to adulthood."[11] Although young patients are the primary focus of transition, the list of key stakeholders also includes parents/guardians, pediatric care providers, and adult care providers.[12]

In 2011, the American Heart Association published a scientific statement describing best practices for the transition of adolescents with CHD from pediatric to adult care.[13] Guidelines recommend a flexible age of transfer between the ages of 18 and 21 years, although in some countries the age of transfer is mandated by the health care system (eg, at 18 years in Canada). The preparation of patients (and their parents) for the transfer from pediatric to adult CHD care should be a routine component of adolescent care. Unfortunately, a survey of almost 2000 young adults with a variety of health conditions revealed that only 55% recalled discussing with their health care providers how their needs would change as they aged.[14]

Absences from and lapses in specialized CHD care are unfortunately common. In a multisite American study that included almost 1000 adults with CHD, 42% of patients had a lapse in care of 3 years or longer.[15] A Canadian study revealed that only 47% of a cohort of 360 patients aged 19 to 21 years had received care in a specialized adult CHD center.[16] A German study of more than 10,500 patients revealed that 76% had not received specialized adult ACHD care within a 5-year period.[17] Findings were more positive in a Belgium study in which only 7% of adults with CHD were not receiving specialized CHD care, although this study occurred at a hospital in which the pediatric and adult CHD programs were physically colocated in the same building.[18] Absences from specialized care are not restricted to the adult care setting. Quebec researchers queried a provincial database to investigate the proportion of children and young adults with CHD receiving outpatient cardiology care.[19] Results indicated that 28% of patients had not received outpatient care after the age of 6 years; 47% had not received outpatient care after the age of 13 years, and 61% had not received outpatient care after turning 18.

When patients do re-establish specialized CHD care following a lapse in care, they are often found to be on suboptimal medication regimens,[20] to be less likely to have undergone surgical interventions expected for their form of CHD,[21] to be at high risk of late complications,[22] and to require urgent cardiac intervention.[23] The consistent finding, therefore, is that lapses in specialized CHD follow-up are associated with suboptimal medical care. Discussions regarding the importance of life-long care should be initiated with both patients and parents in the pediatric setting and emphasized before and after transfer of care.

Transition is not merely the transfer of patients and their medical records from pediatric to adult institutions. Rather, transition refers to an extended process that begins in early adolescence (ideally by the age of 12) and continues following transfer to adult care. Although transition is often focused on the needs of adolescents with special health care needs, young adults between the ages of 18 and 25 years are "emerging adults,"[24] who are taking increased responsibility and becoming independent decision-makers.[25] Both patient and parent reports suggest that many young people with CHD are insufficiently prepared for the transition to adult care and to assume control of their health care management.[26,27] Qualitative research has highlighted many challenges of transitional age youth with CHD, including managing interpersonal frustrations and learning how to develop strategies to coexist with the disease.[28] Unfortunately, a survey of European and American pediatric cardiology programs revealed that most programs do not provide structured preparation for transitioning patients and their family.[29]

Clinical Strategies to Optimize Transition

There are multiple review articles describing the importance of a thoughtful approach to transition as well as several empirical articles describing perspectives on transition according to the patients and other key stakeholders. What is most needed now is guidance for practical strategies to address the needs of transitioning patients, particularly in the context of health care systems with limited resources (both personnel and finances). Descriptions of an outpatient nurse-led transition clinic from Stockholm, Sweden and a transition task force from Toronto, Canada may provide guidance to other programs wishing to establish transition initiatives.[30,31] With regard to transfer from pediatric to adult care, pediatric CHD programs are encouraged to develop a policy by which their team's approach to transfer is clearly communicated to patients, parents, and other health care providers.[32]

Patient education and the fostering of self-management skills are hallmarks of the transition process and key components of a comprehensive transition program.[9,12,13,33] Not surprisingly, participation in a structured education program has been linked with improved knowledge among adolescents and adults with CHD.[34] In a clinical trial, a 1-hour nurse-led session significantly improved cardiac knowledge and self-management skills.[35] Education for adolescents and adults with CHD can be provided in inpatient and outpatient environments through verbal, written, and online formats and be comprehensive[12] to include

- Matters regarding cardiac health (eg, description of CHD, names and years of any major surgeries/interventions, names and purpose of medications, and whether endocarditis prophylaxis is required)
- The broader lifestyle implications of living with CHD (eg, any special considerations regarding physical activity, substance use, education, career planning, family planning)
- The importance of life-long care in order to optimize health outcomes
- Long-term health expectations

Patients should also be supported to develop the necessary self-management skills to gradually assume increasing responsibility for their health care management.[12] It is important for adolescents in the pretransfer phase to understand the differences between family-focused pediatric care and patient-centered adult care. Examples of self-management skills that are generally expected in the adult care system[12] include

- Knowing how to contact and independently communicate with health care providers
- Being able to schedule and attend outpatient appointments
- Knowing how and when to access emergency care
- Knowing how and when to access mental health care
- Managing medication regimens and prescription renewals
- Maintaining health records and a portable health summary

PSYCHOSOCIAL OUTCOMES
Biopsychosocial Challenges

One patient and their family may report minimal impact of living with CHD, whereas another patient with the same diagnosis may report multiple ways in which CHD has affected them and their family. Although there is certainly significant variability across individuals, the more common biopsychosocial challenges of living with CHD are well-documented and summarized in **Table 1**.[36–44] Although a 2015 meta-analysis of 22 studies concluded that patient emotional functioning of adolescents and adults with CHD was not different from that of normative data or healthy peers,[45] many studies that have reported poorer patient psychological functioning were excluded from the analysis.[44,46–48] Interestingly, there seems to

exist global variation with regard to psychosocial outcomes observed in samples of adults with CHD.[38,47,49] Specifically, psychological outcomes of North American samples of adults with CHD are generally less favorable than outcomes from certain European studies. An international multisite study is currently underway in order to understand global differences in CHD patient-reported outcomes.[50] These differences might reflect genuine variation in sociocultural factors or variability in study methodology (eg, different diagnostic groups, age ranges, sample sizes, response rates, and assessment instruments). Given that international variation in psychosocial adjustment is not currently understood, outcomes of adults with CHD living in North America and Europe are reviewed separately.

North American Psychosocial Outcomes
Psychological functioning
Within North America, adults with CHD seem to be at elevated risk of mood and anxiety disorders.[44,46,47] In a 2000 American study, interviews with 29 patients revealed that 14% met diagnostic criteria for major depressive disorder and 17% met criteria for panic disorder.[44] Three years later, standardized psychiatric interviews with 22 American adults with CHD revealed that 27% met criteria for a depressive episode and 9% met criteria for generalized anxiety disorder.[46] What was particularly interesting about this sample is that it was composed of patients who had been identified as well-adjusted by their health care providers, suggesting that psychological distress in adults with CHD may not be easily recognizable within routine clinical care. In a study published in 2009, the prevalence of mood and anxiety disorders among 58 adults with CHD recruited from outpatient clinics in Gainesville, Florida and Toronto, Ontario was investigated.[47] Across these 2 sites, 29% of patients met diagnostic criteria for a mood or anxiety disorder at the time of the assessment and 1 in 2 patients met criteria for a lifetime mood or anxiety disorder. Collectively, therefore, North American studies that used clinical interview methodology suggest that one-third of adults with CHD have low mood or anxiety of significance to warrant clinical diagnoses.

Social functioning
The term psychosocial reflects the important interplay between psychological and social adjustment and must be acknowledged when considering the experiences of adults with CHD. Fear of negative evaluation (ie, social anxiety) and loneliness have been shown to be strong predictors of symptoms of depression and generalized anxiety in this

Table 1
Potential biopsychosocial challenges faced by adults with congenital heart disease

Medical Challenges	Psychological Challenges	Social Challenges
Preparation for (repeated) surgical and percutaneous interventions	Low mood and anxiety	Feeling different
(Repeated) hospitalizations	Increased risk of neurocognitive difficulties	Difficulties with social interactions, loneliness, and isolation
(Repeated) diagnostic testing (including blood draws and diagnostic catheterization)	Self-esteem issues	Physical activity restrictions (eg, full participation in physical education classes)
Medical treatment decision-making	Body image concerns	Limitations in leisure time activities (clubs, sports)
Adjusting to implanted cardiac devices	Tolerating uncertainty	Managing social expectations
Undergoing evaluation and potentially being listed for heart and/or lung transplantation	Identity formation	Academic difficulties
Adherence to treatment recommendations	Developing resilience and coping skills	Deciding if, when, and how to disclose having CHD to others
Symptoms and treatment associated with heart failure, arrhythmias, and endocarditis	—	Comparing oneself to siblings and peers
First admission to adult inpatient ward following transfer	—	Educational and career limitations (eg, avoidance of physically demanding jobs)
(Often unexpected) decline in health status/physical functioning	—	Family planning concerns (sexual intimacy, fertility, contraception, pregnancy)
Shortened life expectancy and need for advance care planning earlier than healthier peers	—	Obtaining and maintaining employment

patient population.[47] Adults with CHD face both interpersonal and intrapersonal challenges; examples of interpersonal challenges included feeling different, social isolation, and conflicting social expectations.[40] Reports of parental overprotection are not uncommon[36] and have been linked with heart-focused anxiety in adulthood.[51]

European Psychosocial Outcomes

Psychological functioning
Results comparing the psychological adjustment of European adults with CHD to normative samples are more equivocal, with reports of negative outcomes,[48,52–54] neutral outcomes,[55] and even superior emotional outcomes.[56–59] Two Dutch studies indicated that patients received more favorable scores on select personality traits (neuroticism, social inadequacy, hostility, and self-esteem) than normative groups.[57,58] A German study compared symptoms of anxiety between adolescents and adults with CHD versus healthy controls and observed no difference in dispositional anxiety.[60]

Although these findings may indicate overcompensation and social desirability, they might also suggest a response shift by which patients with chronic health conditions may have different values and internal standards than healthy peers.[58]

Social functioning
Two Dutch studies have examined social outcomes in adults with CHD, specifically, a longitudinal 30- to 43-year follow-up study (n = 252) and a cross-sectional study of a national registry of adults with CHD (n = 1496).[58,61] Results demonstrated significant social impairments compared with healthy peers, particularly in the areas of educational and occupational attainment, unemployment, living conditions, romantic relationships, marital status, and offspring. Poorer social outcomes were observed even among subgroups of patients with milder forms of CHD.

Participants in the longitudinal 30- to 43-year follow-up study underwent their cardiac surgeries before 1980 and had previously undergone a psychological examination a decade earlier[57]; this allowed for a 10-year historical comparison of this cohort, the results of which demonstrated that certain characteristics (living conditions, marital status, and income) had significantly improved over time. These results were interpreted to suggest that by middle adulthood, many patients catch up with their peers. Another Dutch study compared educational outcomes of adults with tetralogy of Fallot and transposition of the great arteries in 2 cohorts: a historical cohort (patients operated on before 1980) versus a recent cohort (patients who underwent surgeries between 1980 and 1990).[62] Although the recent cohort had achieved higher educational attainment, the rate of learning difficulties was still higher than normative comparative data.

POTENTIAL CORRELATES OF PSYCHOLOGICAL DISTRESS
Demographic Factors

Sex and age
Few studies have investigated differences in psychosocial functioning between men and women with CHD.[52,53,55] This lack of studies between men and women is surprising given that sex differences are well known to exist in the general population and sex-specific normative data are available for many psychological questionnaires. Some studies have concluded that there is no link between sex and symptoms of depression or anxiety among adults with CHD[46,47,55,63,64]; however, a recent study from Portugal observed that women reported more psychological symptoms than men.[65] A Dutch cohort study showed that young women with CHD scored in the psychopathological range on the Young Adult Self-Report measure significantly more often than normative women (28% vs 10%).[53]

Results regarding the relationship between age and psychosocial outcomes among adults with CHD are inconclusive. Although there are data suggesting poorer psychological outcomes in older patients,[48,66] other studies have not observed this link.[46,47,63]

There is preliminary evidence of an interaction effect regarding sex and age on psychological outcomes in adults with CHD. In a German study, the Brief Symptom Inventory was administered to men and women and compared separately with same-sex normative peers.[52] The researchers found that younger women with CHD (aged 25–35 years) reported more interpersonal sensitivity, anxiety, and aggression compared with normative peers, whereas older women with CHD (aged 36–45 years) showed more obsessive-compulsive

thoughts and paranoid ideation compared with norms. Across all age categories, men with CHD also exhibited more somatization, depression, phobic anxiety, and psychoticism than healthy peers.

Education, employment, and marital status
Results are also inconsistent regarding education, employment, and marital status. For example, whereas some researchers have linked better psychological outcomes with higher education, employment, and being in a stable romantic relationship,[48,63] another study detected no differences based on education, employment status, marital status, or living arrangements.[46]

A Dutch cohort study investigated differences in the job participation of 1496 men versus women with CHD using the Dutch National CONCOR (Congenital Corvitia) registry.[67] Results showed that unemployment in men with CHD was more than twice as high as normative male data (16% vs 7%). In women, however, unemployment was only 1.4 times higher among patients with CHD compared with normative data. Proportionally, men with CHD were 1.6 times more likely than normative men data to work part-time, whereas women with CHD were only 1.2 times more likely than normative women to work on a part-time basis. The results indicate additional supports in identifying and maintaining suitable employment might target male adults with CHD. For both men and women with CHD, however, it is important to support the pursuit of higher education, employment, romantic relationships, and independent living, because these are important for the quality of life and well-being of most individuals with and without CHD.[68]

Medical Factors

Surgical scarring
Negative feelings regarding pediatric surgical scars may persist into adulthood. Even 20 years following cardiac surgery, 41% of female patients and 19% of male patients reported feeling restricted by their cardiac scars.[53] The scar may lead to uncertainty in sexual relationships, especially for female patients.[38] Scars have been documented to have a negative impact on self-confidence in 23% of women and 13% of men with CHD (n = 100).[37] Surprisingly, in this same study, the scars also had a positive impact for many patients because the scars served as reminders of the value of their health.

Disease complexity
Many studies have documented that there is no consistent relationship between medical factors

(eg, diagnosis, disease severity, age at first surgical procedure) and psychological distress,[46–48,53,56,64] although some studies have linked poorer psychological outcomes with more severe forms of CHD and surgical repair.[65,69] An emerging cohort consists of adults who have undergone a Fontan procedure for complex CHD and who often have limited exercise capacity. Two recent studies showed that these adults report a good (psychosocial) quality of life, irrespective of their disease severity.[70,71]

In fact, recent studies have shown that the perception of health status and cardiac disease severity are more closely associated with psychological well-being than actual CHD complexity.[47,72]

Early hospitalizations

The number of early hospitalizations has been shown to significantly predict long-term psychopathology, as reported by proxy (mostly parents) for adults with CHD, at both 20- and 30-year follow-ups following the first cardiac surgery.[73] This finding indicates that pediatric hospitalizations have an ongoing, long-lasting influence on the mental health of adults with CHD, even into middle adulthood.

Implanted cardiac devices

In 2004, having a pacemaker seemed to be associated with fewer externalizing problems (eg, less aggressive or delinquent behaviors) in adults with CHD.[73] However, more recent research has shown that adults with CHD with an implantable cardioverter defibrillator (ICD) had a lower quality of life and more anxiety and depressive symptoms compared with adults with CHD without ICDs.[74,75] Higher ICD shock-related anxiety among adults with CHD has been associated with higher depressive symptoms and poorer sexual functioning.[76]

CLINICAL STRATEGIES TO OPTIMIZE PSYCHOSOCIAL OUTCOMES

Admittedly, there exists variability between and within studies examining psychosocial outcomes of adults with CHD. However, given the elevated risk of mood and anxiety disorders detected in studies that used clinical interview methodologies, interventions targeting psychological distress are warranted. There is also preliminary evidence to suggest that elevated symptoms of depression among adolescents and adults with CHD are associated with a poorer prognosis.[54] Previous studies have documented that a minority of adults with CHD and mental health concerns receive appropriate mental health treatment.[44,47,77,78] At this time, there are no published randomized

controlled trials evaluating treatment of depression among adolescents or adults with CHD.[79] As the psychosocial phenotype is becoming better understood, the next challenge for CHD clinicians and researchers is to develop and evaluate psychosocial interventions targeting this unique group of cardiac patients.

As a group, adults with CHD value access to mental health services. In a study that surveyed 155 adults with CHD, 51% of patients reported significant interest in at least one area of psychological treatment, most commonly, stress management and coping with heart disease.[80] Within this study, there was a preference for psychotherapy over pharmacotherapy and one-third of patients were interested in receiving peer support. In a qualitative study, focus group participants (14 adults with CHD aged 19–67 years) expressed interest in (i) psychoeducation (learning about common psychological concerns and reactions to living with CHD), (ii) counseling, and (iii) opportunities to connect with other adults with CHD.[40]

Mental health services are ideally provided by professionals integrated within the adult CHD team[39] or by professionals working in the community with whom the CHD team has fostered a strong collaborative relationship. There are several options for mental health treatment, including both pharmacotherapy and psychotherapy. With regard to psychotherapy, cognitive behavioral therapy aims to challenge and modify maladaptive thought patterns and behaviors[81] and has proven effective at improving mood and reducing anxiety.[82–84] Mindfulness-based interventions, in which individuals develop a nonjudgmental awareness of their present state,[85] have also been shown to have mental health benefits for individuals with chronic medical conditions.[86,87] Interpersonal therapy, with a focus on symptom reduction and improving social and interpersonal functioning, has also been proposed for use with the adult CHD population.[88]

It is important to target psychological interventions to the needs of specific patients. For example, for patients with modifiable limitations in physical functioning, monitored physical training can be useful to realize both physical and psychological benefits. For patients for whom social relationships are problematic, social skills training can be provided. For patients facing the end of their lives, a more existential approach might be effective.

SUMMARY

Throughout their lives, adults with CHD potentially face multiple psychosocial challenges associated with coping with a chronic and often life-shortening medical condition. They might have struggled with the transition from pediatric to adult care, social interactions. It is thus perhaps not surprising that mood and anxiety disorders are not uncommon in the adult setting. Moving forward, clinicians and researchers are encouraged to design and trial interventions to optimize the psychosocial functioning and quality of life of this unique group of cardiac patients.

REFERENCES

1. Moons P, Bovijn L, Budts W, et al. Temporal trends in survival to adulthood among patients born with congenital heart disease from 1970 to 1992 in Belgium. Circulation 2010;122(22):2264–72.

2. Marelli AJ, Ionescu-Ittu R, Mackie AS, et al. Lifetime prevalence of congenital heart disease in the general population from 2000 to 2010. Circulation 2014;130(9):749–56.

3. Kaemmerer H, Bauer U, Pensl U, et al. Management of emergencies in adults with congenital cardiac disease. Am J Cardiol 2008;101(4):521–5.

4. Warnes CA. The adult with congenital heart disease: born to be bad? J Am Coll Cardiol 2005;46(1):1–8.

5. Kenny D, Stuart AG. Long-term outcome of the child with congenital heart disease. Paediatr Child Health 2009;19(1):37–42.

6. Verheugt CL, Uiterwaal CS, van der Velde ET, et al. Mortality in adult congenital heart disease. Eur Heart J 2010;31(10):1220–9.

7. Khairy P, Ionescu-Ittu R, Mackie AS, et al. Changing mortality in congenital heart disease. J Am Coll Cardiol 2010;56(14):1149–57.

8. Nasr VG, Kussman BD. Advances in the care of adults with congenital heart disease. Semin Cardiothorac Vasc Anesth 2014. [Epub ahead of print].

9. Warnes CA, Williams RG, Bashore TM, et al. ACC/AHA 2008 guidelines for the management of adults with congenital heart disease: a report of the American College of Cardiology/American Heart Association Task Force on Practice Guidelines (Writing Committee to Develop Guidelines on the Management of Adults With Congenital Heart Disease). Developed in Collaboration With the American Society of Echocardiography, Heart Rhythm Society, International Society for Adult Congenital Heart Disease, Society for Cardiovascular Angiography and Interventions, and Society of Thoracic Surgeons. J Am Coll Cardiol 2008;52(23):e1–121.

10. Rosen DS, Blum RW, Britto M, et al. Transition to adult health care for adolescents and young adults with chronic conditions: position paper of the Society for Adolescent Medicine. J Adolesc Health 2003;33(4):309–11.

11. American Academy of Pediatrics, American Academy of Family Physicians, American College of Physicians-American Society of Internal Medicine. A consensus statement on health care transitions for young adults with special health care needs. Pediatrics 2002;110(6 Pt 2):1304–6.

12. Kovacs AH, McCrindle BW. So hard to say goodbye: transition from paediatric to adult cardiology care. Nat Rev Cardiol 2014;11(1):51–62.

13. Sable C, Foster E, Uzark K, et al. Best practices in managing transition to adulthood for adolescents with congenital heart disease: the transition process and medical and psychosocial issues: a scientific statement from the American Heart Association. Circulation 2011;123(13):1454–85.

14. Sawicki GS, Whitworth R, Gunn L, et al. Receipt of health care transition counseling in the national survey of adult transition and health. Pediatrics 2011; 128(3):e521–9.

15. Gurvitz M, Valente AM, Broberg C, et al. Prevalence and predictors of gaps in care among adult congenital heart disease patients: HEART-ACHD (The Health, Education, and Access Research Trial). J Am Coll Cardiol 2013;61(21):2180–4.

16. Reid GJ, Irvine MJ, McCrindle BW, et al. Prevalence and correlates of successful transfer from pediatric to adult health care among a cohort of young adults with complex congenital heart defects. Pediatrics 2004;113(3 Pt 1):e197–205.

17. Wacker A, Kaemmerer H, Hollweck R, et al. Outcome of operated and unoperated adults with congenital cardiac disease lost to follow-up for more than five years. Am J Cardiol 2005;95(6):776–9.

18. Goossens E, Stephani I, Hilderson D, et al. Transfer of adolescents with congenital heart disease from pediatric cardiology to adult health care: an analysis of transfer destinations. J Am Coll Cardiol 2011; 57(23):2368–74.

19. Mackie AS, Ionescu-Ittu R, Therrien J, et al. Children and adults with congenital heart disease lost to follow-up: who and when? Circulation 2009;120(4): 302–9.

20. de Bono J, Freeman LJ. Aortic coarctation repair– lost and found: the role of local long term specialised care. Int J Cardiol 2005;104(2):176–83.

21. Wray J, Frigiola A, Bull C. Loss to specialist follow-up in congenital heart disease; out of sight, out of mind. Heart 2013;99(7):485–90.

22. Iversen K, Vejlstrup NG, Sondergaard L, et al. Screening of adults with congenital cardiac disease lost for follow-up. Cardiol Young 2007;17(6):601–8.

23. Yeung E, Kay J, Roosevelt GE, et al. Lapse of care as a predictor for morbidity in adults with congenital heart disease. Int J Cardiol 2008;125(1):62–5.

24. Arnett JJ. Emerging adulthood. A theory of development from the late teens through the twenties. Am Psychol 2000;55(5):469–80.

25. Arnett JJ. Emerging adulthood: what is it, and what is it good for? Child Dev Perspect 2007;1(2):68–73.

26. Heery E, Sheehan AM, While AE, et al. Experiences and outcomes of transition from pediatric to adult health care services for young people with congenital heart disease: a systematic review. Congenit Heart Dis 2015. [Epub ahead of print].

27. Clarizia NA, Chahal N, Manlhiot C, et al. Transition to adult health care for adolescents and young adults with congenital heart disease: perspectives of the patient, parent and health care provider. Can J Cardiol 2009;25(9):e317–22.

28. Chiang YT, Chen CW, Su WJ, et al. Between invisible defects and visible impact: the life experiences of adolescents and young adults with congenital heart disease. J Adv Nurs 2015;71(3):599–608.

29. Hilderson D, Saidi AS, Van Deyk K, et al. Attitude toward and current practice of transfer and transition of adolescents with congenital heart disease in the United States of America and Europe. Pediatr Cardiol 2009;30(6):786–93.

30. Berg SK, Hertz PG. Outpatient nursing clinic for congenital heart disease patients: Copenhagen Transition Program. J Cardiovasc Nurs 2007;22(6):488–92.

31. Kovacs AH, Cullen-Dean G, Aiello S, et al. The Toronto congenital heart disease transition task force. Progr Pediatr Cardiol 2012;34:21–6.

32. Cooley WC, Sagerman PJ. Supporting the health care transition from adolescence to adulthood in the medical home. Pediatrics 2011;128(1):182–200.

33. Gurvitz M, Saidi A. Transition in congenital heart disease: it takes a village. Heart 2014;100(14):1075–6.

34. Goossens E, Van Deyk K, Zupancic N, et al. Effectiveness of structured patient education on the knowledge level of adolescents and adults with congenital heart disease. Eur J Cardiovasc Nurs 2014;13(1):63–70.

35. Mackie AS, Islam S, Magill-Evans J, et al. Healthcare transition for youth with heart disease: a clinical trial. Heart 2014;100(14):1113–8.

36. Gantt LT. Growing up heartsick: the experiences of young women with congenital heart disease. Health Care Women Int 1992;13(3):241–8.

37. Kantoch MJ, Eustace J, Collins-Nakai RL, et al. The significance of cardiac surgery scars in adult patients with congenital heart disease. Kardiol Pol 2006;64(1):51–6 [discussion: 57–58].

38. Kovacs AH, Sears SF, Saidi AS. Biopsychosocial experiences of adults with congenital heart disease: review of the literature. Am Heart J 2005;150(2):193–201.

39. Kovacs AH, Silversides C, Saidi A, et al. The role of the psychologist in adult congenital heart disease. Cardiol Clin 2006;24(4):607–18, vi.

40. Pagé MG, Kovacs AH, Irvine J. How do psychosocial challenges associated with living with congenital heart disease translate into treatment interests and preferences? A qualitative approach. Psychol Health 2012;27(11):1260–70.

41. Claessens P, Moons P, de Casterle BD, et al. What does it mean to live with a congenital heart disease? A qualitative study on the lived experiences of adult patients. Eur J Cardiovasc Nurs 2005;4(1):3–10.

42. Oechslin EN, Harrison DA, Connelly MS, et al. Mode of death in adults with congenital heart disease. Am J Cardiol 2000;86(10):1111–6.

43. Marino BS, Lipkin PH, Newburger JW, et al. Neurodevelopmental outcomes in children with congenital heart disease: evaluation and management: a scientific statement from the American Heart Association. Circulation 2012;126(9):1143–72.

44. Horner T, Liberthson R, Jellinek MS. Psychosocial profile of adults with complex congenital heart disease. Mayo Clin Proc 2000;75(1):31–6.

45. Jackson JL, Misiti B, Bridge JA, et al. Emotional functioning of adolescents and adults with congenital heart disease: a meta-analysis. Congenit Heart Dis 2015;10(1):2–12.

46. Bromberg JI, Beasley PJ, D'Angelo EJ, et al. Depression and anxiety in adults with congenital heart disease: a pilot study. Heart Lung 2003;32(2):105–10.

47. Kovacs AH, Saidi AS, Kuhl EA, et al. Depression and anxiety in adult congenital heart disease: predictors and prevalence. Int J Cardiol 2009;137(2):158–64.

48. Popelova J, Slavik Z, Skovranek J. Are cyanosed adults with congenital cardiac malformations depressed? Cardiol Young 2001;11(4):379–84.

49. Callus E, Quadri E, Ricci C, et al. Update on psychological functioning in adults with congenital heart disease: a systematic review. Expert Rev Cardiovasc Ther 2013;11(6):785–91.

50. Apers S, Kovacs AH, Luyckx K, et al. Assessment of patterns of patient-reported outcomes in adults with congenital heart disease—International Study (APPROACH-IS): rationale, design, and methods. Int J Cardiol 2015;179:334–42.

51. Ong L, Nolan RP, Irvine J, et al. Parental overprotection and heart-focused anxiety in adults with congenital heart disease. Int J Behav Med 2011;18(3):260–7.

52. Geyer S, Hessel A, Kempa A, et al. Psychological symptoms and body image in patients after surgery of congenital heart disease. Psychother Psychosom Med Psychol 2006;56(11):425–31.

53. van Rijen EH, Utens EM, Roos-Hesselink JW, et al. Longitudinal development of psychopathology in an adult congenital heart disease cohort. Int J Cardiol 2005;99(2):315–23.

54. Kourkoveli P, Rammos S, Parissis J, et al. Depressive symptoms in patients with congenital heart disease: incidence and prognostic value of self-rating depression scales. Congenit Heart Dis 2015;10(3):240–7.

55. van der Rijken RE, Maassen BA, Walk TL, et al. Outcome after surgical repair of congenital cardiac malformations at school age. Cardiol Young 2007; 17(1):64–71.

56. Cox D, Lewis G, Stuart G, et al. A cross-sectional study of the prevalence of psychopathology in adults with congenital heart disease. J Psychosom Res 2002;52(2):65–8.

57. van Rijen EH, Utens EM, Roos-Hesselink JW, et al. Psychosocial functioning of the adult with congenital heart disease: a 20-33 years follow-up. Eur Heart J 2003;24(7):673–83.

58. Opic P, Roos-Hesselink JW, Cuypers JA, et al. Psychosocial functioning of adults with congenital heart disease: outcomes of a 30-43 year longitudinal follow-up. Clin Res Cardiol 2015;104(5):388–400.

59. Opic P, Roos-Hesselink JW, Cuypers JA, et al. Longitudinal development of psychopathology and subjective health status in congenital heart disease adults: a 30-43 year follow-up in a unique cohort. Cardiol Young 2015. [Epub ahead of print].

60. Muller J, Hess J, Hager A. General anxiety of adolescents and adults with congenital heart disease is comparable with that in healthy controls. Int J Cardiol 2013;165(1):142–5.

61. Zomer AC, Vaartjes I, Uiterwaal CS, et al. Social burden and lifestyle in adults with congenital heart disease. Am J Cardiol 2012;109(11):1657–63.

62. Opic P, Utens EM, Ruys TP, et al. Long-term psychosocial outcome of adults with tetralogy of Fallot and transposition of the great arteries: a historical comparison. Cardiol Young 2014;24(4):593–604.

63. Balon YE, Then KL, Rankin JA, et al. Looking beyond the biophysical realm to optimize health: results of a survey of psychological well-being in adults with congenital cardiac disease. Cardiol Young 2008; 18(5):494–501.

64. Utens EM, Bieman HJ, Verhulst FC, et al. Psychopathology in young adults with congenital heart disease. Follow-up results. Eur Heart J 1998;19(4): 647–51.

65. Freitas IR, Castro M, Sarmento SL, et al. A cohort study on psychosocial adjustment and psychopathology in adolescents and young adults with congenital heart disease. BMJ Open 2013;3(1).

66. Enomoto J, Nakazawa M. Negative effect of aging on psychosocial functioning of adults with congenital heart disease. Circ J 2015;79(1):185–92.

67. Sluman MA, Apers S, Bouma BJ, et al. Uncertainties in insurances for adults with congenital heart disease. Int J Cardiol 2015;186:93–5.

68. Moons P, Van Deyk K, Marquet K, et al. Individual quality of life in adults with congenital heart disease: a paradigm shift. Eur Heart J 2005;26(3):298–307.

69. Latal B, Helfricht S, Fischer JE, et al. Psychological adjustment and quality of life in children and adolescents following open-heart surgery for congenital heart disease: a systematic review. BMC Pediatr 2009;9:6.

70. Bordin G, Padalino MA, Perentaler S, et al. Clinical profile and quality of life of adult patients after the Fontan procedure. Pediatr Cardiol 2015;36(6): 1261–9.

71. Idorn L, Jensen AS, Juul K, et al. Quality of life and cognitive function in Fontan patients, a population-based study. Int J Cardiol 2013;168(4):3230–5.

72. Callus E, Utens EM, Quadri E, et al. The impact of actual and perceived disease severity on preoperative psychological well-being and illness behaviour in adult congenital heart disease patients. Cardiol Young 2014;24(2):275–82.

73. van Rijen EH, Utens EM, Roos-Hesselink JW, et al. Medical predictors for psychopathology in adults with operated congenital heart disease. Eur Heart J 2004;25(18):1605–13.

74. Opic P, Utens EM, Moons P, et al. Psychosocial impact of implantable cardioverter defibrillators (ICD) in young adults with Tetralogy of Fallot. Clin Res Cardiol 2012;101(7):509–19.

75. Bedair R, Babu-Narayan SV, Dimopoulos K, et al. Acceptance and psychological impact of implantable defibrillators amongst adults with congenital heart disease. Int J Cardiol 2015;181:218–24.

76. Cook SC, Valente AM, Maul TM, et al. Shock-related anxiety and sexual function in adults with congenital heart disease and implantable cardioverter-defibrillators. Heart Rhythm 2013;10(6):805–10.

77. Schoormans D, Sprangers MA, van Melle JP, et al. Clinical and psychological characteristics predict future healthcare use in adults with congenital heart disease. Eur J Cardiovasc Nurs 2014. [Epub ahead of print].

78. Saidi A, Kovacs AH. Developing a transition program from pediatric- to adult-focused cardiology care: practical considerations. Congenit Heart Dis 2009;4(4):204–15.

79. Lane DA, Millane TA, Lip GY. Psychological interventions for depression in adolescent and adult congenital heart disease. Cochrane Database Syst Rev 2013;(10):CD004372.

80. Kovacs AH, Bendell KL, Colman J, et al. Adults with congenital heart disease: psychological needs and treatment preferences. Congenit Heart Dis 2009; 4(3):139–46.

81. Beck JS. Cognitive behavior therapy: basics and beyond. 2nd edition. New York: Guilford Press; 2011.

82. Butler AC, Chapman JE, Forman EM, et al. The empirical status of cognitive-behavioral therapy: a review of meta-analyses. Clin Psychol Rev 2006; 26(1):17–31.

83. Hofmann SG, Smits JAJ. Cognitive-behavioral therapy for adult anxiety disorders: a meta-analysis of randomized placebo-controlled trials. J Clin Psychiatry 2008;69(4):621–32.

84. Osborn RL, Demoncada AC, Feuerstein M. Psycho-social interventions for depression, anxiety, and quality of life in cancer survivors: meta-analyses. Int J Psychiatry Med 2006;36(1):13–34.

85. Kabat-Zinn J. Full catastrophe living: using the wisdom of your body and mind to face stress, pain, and illness (15th anniversary edition). New York: Delta Trade Paperback/Bantam Dell; 2005.

86. Abbott RA, Whear R, Rodgers LR, et al. Effectiveness of mindfulness-based stress reduction and mindfulness based cognitive therapy in vascular disease: a systematic review and meta-analysis of randomised controlled trials. J Psychosom Res 2014;76(5):341–51.

87. Bohlmeijer E, Prenger R, Taal E, et al. The effects of mindfulness-based stress reduction therapy on mental health of adults with a chronic medical disease: a meta-analysis. J Psychosom Res 2010; 68(6):539–44.

88. Morton L. Can interpersonal psychotherapy (IPT) meet the psychosocial cost of life gifted by medical intervention. Couns Psych Rev 2011;26(3):75–86.

Evaluation of Health Care Quality in Adults with Congenital Heart Disease

Keri Shafer, MD[a,b,c], Michelle Gurvitz, MD, MS[a,b,c],*

KEYWORDS

- Adult congenital heart disease • Quality of care • Quality improvement

KEY POINTS

- To develop an understanding of quality assessment models and their application to the diverse population of adults with congenital heart disease (CHD).
- The design and implementation of quality assessment methods in acquired adult cardiovascular disease and general pediatrics can be used as a foundation for building quality assessment in adult CHD.
- Examples of current quality efforts in CHD are described.

> *Quality is a term that is used in many senses. One sort of quality let us call 'habit' or 'disposition.'*
>
> —*Aristotle[1]*

Providing medical care for adults with CHD is a complex endeavor requiring an understanding of all aspects of the health system. Adult patients with CHD often have multiple medical issues related to the underlying CHD, the sequelae of surgical or catheter interventions, and the addition of typical conditions of adulthood superimposed on the CHD. The complexity of care is compounded by the need to find physicians trained in adult medicine with understanding of CHD, its potential long-term care issues, and the interaction of the CHD with other conditions of adulthood. Pediatric cardiology care is more centralized among a limited number of providers and hospitals with congenital cardiac expertise, whereas care for adults with CHD is diversified among adult congenital cardiologists, pediatric cardiologists, and a larger number of general cardiology providers and institutions that do not necessarily have expertise in congenital

conditions.[2] In addition, the literature lacks comprehensive population studies of adults with CHD to understand the long-term medical and psychosocial issues associated with CHD. As a result of all these limitations in addition to other factors, medical care for patients with CHD can become fractionated and inconsistent in adulthood. In fact, patients with CHD start falling out of cardiology care in the preteen years, and as adults, over 40% have experienced a gap in care of more than 3 years at some point in their lives.[3,4] Unfortunately, there is no simple solution. Therefore, improving quality of care is not only difficult but also tremendously important to try to ensure the best outcomes for adult patients with CHD. In this article, the authors first frame the assessment of quality in the health care system as a whole and then focus on CHD and the unique approach required in the care of the adult with CHD.

WHAT IS QUALITY?

Quality of care has been defined as the effect of care on the health of the individual and the

---

Disclosure statement: the authors have nothing to disclose.
a Department of Cardiology, Boston Children's Hospital, 300 Longwood Avenue, Boston, MA 02115, USA;
b Department of Cardiology, Brigham and Women's Hospital, 75 Francis street, Boston, MA 02115, USA;
c Harvard Medical School, 25 Shattuck street, Boston, MA 02115, USA
* Corresponding author. Department of Cardiology, Boston Children's Hospital, 300 Longwood Avenue, Boston, MA 02115.
E-mail address: Michelle.Gurvitz@cardio.chboston.org

0733-8651/15/$ – see front matter © 2015 Elsevier Inc. All rights reserved.

cardiology.theclinics.com

population. Improvement in this quality should be reflected as improvement in health. Quality is differentiated from efficiency, which involves trying to streamline the steps and costs of medical care.[5] In 1990, the Institute of Medicine (IOM) further expounded on this idea to state that "quality of care is the degree to which health services for individuals and populations increase the likelihood of desired health outcomes and are consistent with current professional knowledge."[6] These definitions provide a framework and the goals for working to improve the quality of care for patients. Quality assessment can involve the individual provider, a practice or health care organization, or the entire health care system. Some measurements of quality may be universal for the general population, such as cancer screening, whereas others depend on the underlying health condition of the patient. Therefore evaluating quality of care for patient populations with chronic disease requires the development of condition-specific measures to evaluate and monitor quality of care. Once measures have been defined, areas of deficiency can be more easily identified and quality improvement initiatives can be designed and implemented.

Quality Measurement and Quality Improvement

In order to accurately and reproducibly evaluate the health care system, standards must be developed and agreed upon by which to measure quality. In further investigating this, the IOM developed a strategic direction for the redesign of health care by identifying aims to help focus efforts of improvement and innovation. The final report published in 2001 (*Crossing the Quality Chasm*) proposed 6 aims[7] outlining that health care should be:

- Safe
- Effective
- Patient centered
- Timely
- Efficient
- Equitable

Health care system changes are often required to ensure that each of the 6 aims is fully realized. In addition, health care should be constantly evaluated and improved to ensure that these aims are met to the fullest capacity. In many medical conditions, specific guidelines with identification of recommended care practices exist. Guidelines differ from quality measures in that guidelines are evidence- and/or consensus-based recommendations applied prospectively for care in a particular circumstance, whereas quality measures are designed to be applied retrospectively

to evaluate the type of care that was provided.[8] Guidelines can be highly beneficial in trying to provide consistency of care across settings but are not available for many medical conditions or may not be applicable for individual patients. At times, guidelines-based care can be incorporated into quality measures. However, ideal quality measures should focus on common occurrences that are fully within the individual's or system's ability to change or improve and not significantly influenced by rare, uncontrollable events. Selecting quality measures can be extremely difficult particularly in areas of medicine with heterogeneous populations.

Clinical quality measures generally fall into one of the following categories[9]:

- **Access:** assesses the patient's ability to obtain timely and appropriate health care.
- **Outcome:** measures the patient's health status after receiving health care services.
- **Patient experience:** aggregates reports of patients about their observations of and participation in health care.
- **Process:** assesses the actual health care service provided to, or on behalf of, a patient.
- **Structure:** describes a feature of a health care organization or clinician relevant to its capacity to provide health care (eg, nurse to patient ratio, number of beds).

Some types of measures are very difficult to accurately and reproducibly assess (eg, patient experience), whereas others are easier to assess, but may not reflect events that are clinically meaningful or modifiable (eg, structure measures). In order to accurately assess and evaluate the health care system as it relates to a particular disease or condition, disease-specific quality measures need to be developed. Once quality measures are proposed or developed, ensuring validity of the quality measures can be difficult because all methods have limitations. First, one must start with ensuring that the measures are relevant to those participating in and accessing the medical system (stakeholders) and have face validity. Then one should be sure that each measure is quantifiable and collectable in a consistent and reliable manner. Some aspects of care may be easy to measure but lack significant importance in relation to health outcomes and thus do not make adequate quality measures, even though the data can be easily obtained. Alternatively, some aspects of care may be highly important to improved health but cannot be measured in a reliable way and thus also do not make good measures of quality. Ideally, all patients in question should have equal eligibility of being evaluated by the selected quality measure. It is important to preemptively determine those at risk for exclusion and then determine additional measures to capture those groups. For example, if a quality measure involves receiving flu shots, patients with egg allergies would not be eligible to be counted for quality of care. Other times, subjects may be inadvertently excluded because of socioeconomic status, race, or region. Regardless of what measure is selected, sufficient details should be obtained to ensure that significant confounders can be eliminated or addressed; this is particularly useful with outcomes measures such as length of stay or mortality[10] (i.e. due to racial or ethnic difference).

Reporting of Quality Measures

The IOM recommends that health care systems work toward a culture of transparency. As a result, public reporting of health care system quality is a priority. With accurate public reporting, the quality of health care can make significant strides toward improvement by standardizing measures, providing feedback, and allowing for hospital comparison.[11] Therefore, in selecting and measuring quality, the goal should be toward making the data available to providers, patients, and the public so that health systems can improve. Outcome measures are the most appealing for reporting, but appropriate risk adjustment to accurately compare outcome rates is extremely difficult. In 2006, the American Heart Association (AHA) released a scientific statement outlining the approach to public reporting.[12] However, only about half of the states in the United States publicly report hospital quality.[11] Moreover, the reliability of the data to accurately describe comparable hospital quality has been questioned primarily with concerns of incomplete risk adjustment. Hospital infection rates, hospital mortality, and readmission rates are among the most commonly reported measures, but some have called into question the validity of these measures in certain populations.[11,13,14] Given the difficulty in determining accurate measures to report, it may be first appropriate to report at a group or institutional level rather than at the level of the individual provider. Further analyses can be performed to determine if the information used to assess the quality measures can be easily and consistently collected and if the measures reflect care delivery that would be considered high quality. Despite the proposed improvement in health care quality as a result of public reporting, the effects are not universally accepted as positive.[15]

Quality as Assessed in Acquired Cardiovascular Disease in Adults, General Pediatrics, and Adult Congenital Heart Disease

Acquired cardiovascular disease in adults
The care of adults with acquired heart disease has an ongoing focus on delivering timely, appropriate, and high-value care. However, even in diagnostic groups with high volumes of patients such as coronary artery disease and congestive heart failure, the variation among patients, providers, as well as health care systems has not been fully assessed. Standard quality metrics have been proposed, implemented, and then critiqued by national leaders. The AHA and American College of Cardiology (ACC) have put forth guidelines regarding health care quality specifically addressing performance measures for the diagnoses most frequently associated with hospitalization and mortality.[16–18] One commonly cited example is the door to balloon time in acute ST-elevation myocardial infarction (STEMI). After studies showed that prolonged ischemic time during STEMI resulted in worse outcomes, recommendations shifted and a metric of 90 minutes was set as the maximum time from presentation to the emergency room with STEMI to reperfusion.[19] The implementation of this metric has resulted in improved cardiovascular outcomes and mortality.[20] Another commonly cited quality measure is the 30-day readmission rate in patients admitted to the hospital for management of congestive heart failure. This outcome measure has the advantage of being relatively easily measured and relevant to most stakeholders. However, it has become an example of selection of an outcome that is disproportionately affected by socioeconomic factors and disease acuity, while being only partially modifiable. As a result, reimbursement based on readmissions rates penalizes safety net and teaching hospitals largely because of the diversity and acuity in their patient populations.[21]

Pediatrics
Concerted efforts have been made to understand and improve the quality of medical care for children. The issues are somewhat different in pediatrics than in adults owing to interactions of primary school education, parental involvement, and different medical conditions. Care guidelines do exist for certain aspects of general pediatric care, but comprehensive data have been limited in documenting the adherence to indicated care guidelines for children. To investigate this, a recent publication used the RAND-University of California Los Angeles (UCLA) modified Delphi method to simultaneously develop and evaluate metrics of

quality of care.[22,23] Mangione-Smith and colleagues identified significant gaps between delivered and recommended care, finding underuse of services most common. Preventative care was most frequently underused, a startling and concerning reality.[24]

Adult congenital heart disease

When coupled with the limited scientific data available and significant regional differences in care, establishing quality metrics in adult CHD is quite complex. The assessment and measurement of quality of care for adults with CHD differs from both general adult cardiology and pediatrics, but there are important parallels with both that can be helpful. Although adult CHD may have some similarities to other areas of adult cardiology, the size of the population and complexity of disease prevents significant overlap with conditions such as coronary artery disease and congestive heart failure. In addition, owing to few large population-based studies or randomized trials, the evidence base on which to set a gold standard or benchmarks to assess quality of care is limited and guidelines frequently rely on expert consensus.[25–27] Although guidelines are clearly different from quality measures, they can be used as a foundation for crafting quality measures to be tested and refined in relation to feasibility of data collection and relationship to outcomes. In CHD, published studies on quality of care in relation to outcomes are mostly limited to pediatric congenital heart surgery and catheter intervention.[28–32] As with the general pediatric study developing and evaluating a quality assessment strategy for pediatric care, the RAND-UCLA modified Delphi method has been used to develop pilot quality measures for adult CHD.[33] These measures are only for certain outpatient conditions and are still being evaluated, but they are a proposed method of measuring quality in adult CHD care.

CURRENT QUALITY EFFORTS IN CONGENITAL HEART DISEASE

In response to the increasing importance of providing, measuring, and improving quality of care at the national level, several efforts have been devised to measure and improve care for pediatric and adult patients with CHD. A summary of some of these efforts are listed in **Table 1**.

One effort in congenital cardiology quality measurement and improvement was the Congenital Cardiac Catheterization Project on Outcomes-Quality Improvement (C3PO-QI). This multicenter collaboration effort among 15 institutions was designed to reduce radiation exposure during catheterization procedures for the pediatric and adult CHD populations.[31] At present, there is a lack of standardization in catheterization techniques, including interoperator and intercenter variability. By comparing methods and techniques between the 15 centers, the collaborating institutions are improving patient care and are coming closer to establishing standardization in catheterization techniques.

Another national effort to improve and measure quality in pediatric cardiology is the National Pediatric Cardiology Quality Improvement Collaborative (NPC-QIC). This collaborative was established in 2009 and is a network of 57 pediatric cardiology care centers across the United States and the District of Columbia, including patients, families, clinicians, and researchers,

---

Table 1
Current efforts to evaluate quality of care in adults and children with CHD

Name	Organization	Date Started	Web Site
IMPACT registry	ACC/NCDR	2011	http://cvquality.acc.org/en/NCDR-Home/Registries/Hospital-Registries.aspx
SCAMPs	IRCDA	2010	http://www.scamps.org/
NPC-QIC	Collaborative; Cincinnati Children's Hospital	2009	https://jcchdqi.org/
C3PO	Collaborative, Boston Children's Hospital	2006	—
TPS	Collaborative, Boston Children's Hospital	2006	—

Abbreviations: C3PO, The Congenital Cardiac Catheterization Project on Outcomes; IMPACT, Improving Pediatric and Adult Congenital Treatment; IRCDA, Institute for Relevant Clinical Data Analytics; NCDR, National Cardiology Data Registry; NPC-QIC, National Pediatric Cardiology-Quality Improvement Collaborative; SCAMPs, Standardized Clinical Assessment and Management Program; TPS, Technical Performance Score.

working together to improve the outcomes for children with cardiovascular disease. As an initial project, the collaborative focused on improving care for one of the most complex patient populations, infants with hypoplastic left heart syndrome during the interstage period (between discharge from the initial open heart surgery and admission for a bidirectional Glenn procedure).[34–36]

The Improving Pediatric and Adult Congenital Treatment (IMPACT) registry was created in 2011 by the ACC as part of the National Cardiology Data Registry (NCDR) to improve patient care by promoting quality improvement at participating institutions. The registry seeks to assess the prevalence, demographics, management, and outcomes of patients undergoing diagnostic catheterization and catheter-based interventions for CHD. The data collected will facilitate performance measurement, benchmarking, and quality improvement for hospitals performing these procedures for patients with CHD.[37,38]

Standardized Clinical Assessment and Management Programs (SCAMPs) were first described in 2010 to bridge the gap between clinical care and best practices.[39] SCAMPs aim to take a heterogeneous patient population through assessment and management algorithms designed to capture clinical management and guide (but not mandate) the providers through appropriate care. The 3 main goals of SCAMPs are to improve patient outcomes with a reduction in practice variation and unnecessary resource use; they have the potential to be more useful than care guidelines in that they are iterative with prospective data collection, which allows for frequent analysis and algorithm revision as well as for evaluation of a real-world implementation and outcomes. Initial evaluations of this technique show promise for improving and standardizing care in small groups of patients.[32] However, additional study is needed.

The congenital heart surgical technical performance score (TPS) is an echocardiographic and clinical tool to assess the adequacy of surgical repair. Initially developed for 5 common congenital cardiac procedures, scores have now been expanded to assess over 90% of congenital cardiac procedures. Each congenital cardiac procedures is divided into its component subprocedure, and each subprocedure is categorized into 3 classes: Class 1(optimal with trivial or no residual defect), Class 2 (adequate with minor residual defect), and Class 3 (inadequate with major residual defect or unplanned surgical or catheter reintervention before discharge from index operation). The final TPS for each procedure depends on the subprocedure score. Work from a single institution has shown that TPS has a strong association not only with early outcomes such as mortality, occurrence of major adverse events, and resource use but also with midterm outcomes such as postdischarge mortality, unplanned midterm reinterventions, and neurodevelopmental outcomes.[28–30,40,41]

FUTURE DIRECTIONS

The need and desire to provide the highest possible quality of care is foundational to the practice of medicine. For the patient population of adults with CHD, measuring and improving quality is not a straightforward endeavor. Barriers encountered in measuring and improving quality include the diversity of underlying conditions and treatment strategies, difficulty transitioning from pediatric to adult-oriented health systems, and a lack of clinical registries with which to follow long-term outcomes. There is also a paucity of clinical trials and evidence-based strategies on which to base quality measures. Isolated efforts in quality measurement and improvement in CHD are beneficial but only some efforts include or relate specifically to adults. In addition, the current efforts are relatively recent and are without broad adaptation in clinical, particularly nonprocedural, care. Another hurdle is the lack of population-based data on long-term outcomes in adult CHD, leading to quality measurement focused on processes of care rather than on both processes and outcomes.

In order to learn more about providing, measuring, and improving quality of care for adults with CHD, large-scale changes in data recording and reporting are essential. As the adult CHD population has significant diversity not only among conditions but also in severity and models of care, the approach must be specific and rigorous but adaptable in multiple settings. Accomplishing this task will require a foundation of uniform systems of nomenclature and data collection across care sites and providers. Establishing this uniform platform among specialty centers for adult congenital care would be a tremendous advance in terms of case ascertainment and evaluation of outcomes, as well as resource use and care patterns. Once validated and established, this foundation could then be disseminated to all adult CHD care providers including general cardiologists and primary care providers. This basis could be used to evaluate multiple aspects of care and allow measurement of care processes and relationship to outcomes for the full adult CHD population as well as for different segments individually (eg, by diagnosis or age). Ideally, the measurement of quality of care will allow for increased numbers and implementation of quality improvement strategies. It is hoped that in the future, uniform data collection, quality measurement and improvement efforts, and expansion of current projects will provide the opportunity for continual improvement of the quality of care provided to adults with CHD.

REFERENCES

1. Aristotle. Categories. 350 BCE. Available at: http:// classics.mit.edu/Aristotle/categories.2.2.html. Accessed May 15, 2015.

2. Gurvitz MZ, Inkelas M, Lee M, et al. Changes in hospitalization patterns among patients with congenital heart disease during the transition from adolescence to adulthood. J Am Coll Cardiol 2007;49(8): 875–82.

3. Mackie AS, Ionescu-Ittu R, Pilote L, et al. Hospital readmissions in children with congenital heart disease: a population-based study. Am Heart J 2008; 155(3):577–84.

4. Gurvitz M, Valente AM, Broberg C, et al. Prevalence and predictors of gaps in care among adult congenital heart disease patients: HEART-ACHD (The Health, Education, and Access Research Trial). J Am Coll Cardiol 2013;61(21):2180–4.

5. Rutstein DD, Berenberg W, Chalmers TC, et al. Measuring the quality of medical care. A clinical method. N Engl J Med 1976;294(11):582–8.

6. America's Health in Transition: protecting and improving quality. In: Shine KI, editor. A statement of the council of the Institute of Medicine. Washington, DC: National Academy Press; 1994.

7. Institute of Medicine. Crossing the quality chasm: a new health system for the 21st Century. Washington, DC: National Academy Press; 2001.

8. Spertus JA, Eagle KA, Krumholz HM, et al. American College of Cardiology and American Heart Association methodology for the selection and creation of performance measures for quantifying the quality of cardiovascular care. Circulation 2005;111(13): 1703–12.

9. Varieties of Measures in NQMC. 2015. Available at: http://www.qualitymeasures.ahrq.gov/tutorial/varieties. aspx. Accessed April 15, 2015.

10. Mant J. Process versus outcome indicators in the assessment of quality of health care. Int J Qual Health Care 2001;13(6):475–80.

11. Ross JS, Sheth S, Krumholz HM. State-sponsored public reporting of hospital quality: results are hard to find and lack uniformity. Health Aff (Millwood) 2010;29(12):2317–22.

12. Krumholz HM, Brindis RG, Brush JE, et al. Standards for statistical models used for public reporting of health outcomes: an American Heart Association Scientific Statement from the Quality of Care and Outcomes Research Interdisciplinary Writing Group: cosponsored by the Council on Epidemiology and Prevention and the Stroke Council. Endorsed by the American College of Cardiology Foundation. Circulation 2006;113(3):456–62.

13. Backes CH, Bergersen L, Rome JJ, et al. Quality metrics in cardiac catheterization for congenital heart disease: utility of 30-day mortality. Catheter Cardiovasc Interv 2015;85(1):104–10.

14. Gheorghiade M, Vaduganathan M, Fonarow GC, et al. Rehospitalization for heart failure: problems and perspectives. J Am Coll Cardiol 2013;61(4): 391–403.

15. Werner RM, Asch DA. The unintended consequences of publicly reporting quality information. JAMA 2005;293(10):1239–44.

16. Yancy CW, Jessup M, Bozkurt B, et al. 2013 ACCF/ AHA guideline for the management of heart failure: a report of the American College of Cardiology Foundation/American Heart Association Task Force on practice guidelines. Circulation 2013;128(16): e240–327.

17. Anderson JL, Heidenreich PA, Barnett PG, et al. ACC/AHA statement on cost/value methodology in clinical practice guidelines and performance measures: a report of the American College of Cardiology/American Heart Association Task Force on Performance Measures and Task Force on Practice Guidelines. J Am Coll Cardiol 2014;63(21):2304–22.

18. Bonow RO, Ganiats TG, Beam CT, et al. ACCF/AHA/ AMA-PCPI 2011 performance measures for adults with heart failure: a report of the American College of Cardiology Foundation/American Heart Association Task Force on Performance Measures and the American Medical Association-Physician Consortium for Performance Improvement. Circulation 2012;125(19):2382–401.

19. O'Gara PT, Kushner FG, Ascheim DD, et al. 2013 ACCF/AHA guideline for the management of ST-elevation myocardial infarction: executive summary: a report of the American College of Cardiology Foundation/American Heart Association Task Force on Practice Guidelines. J Am Coll Cardiol 2013; 61(4):485–510.

20. Chen HL, Liu K. Effect of door-to-balloon time on in-hospital mortality in patients with myocardial infarction: a meta-analysis. Int J Cardiol 2015;187:130–3.

21. Joynt KE, Jha AK. Characteristics of hospitals receiving penalties under the Hospital Readmissions Reduction Program. JAMA 2013;309(4): 342–3.

22. Mangione-Smith R, DeCristofaro AH, Setodji CM, et al. The quality of ambulatory care delivered to children in the United States. N Engl J Med 2007; 357(15):1515–23.

23. Brook RH. The RAND/UCLA appropriateness method. In: McCormack K, Moore S, Siegel RA, editors. Clinical practice guideline development:

methodology perspectives. Rockville (MD): Agency for Healthcare Research and Policy; 1994. p. 59–70.

24. Corum J, Keller J, Park H, et al. Facts about the measles outbreak, in 2015. New York: The New York Times Company; 2015. Accessed May 29, 2015.

25. Warnes CA, Williams RG, Bashore TM, et al. ACC/AHA 2008 guidelines for the management of adults with congenital heart disease: executive summary. Circulation 2008;118:2395–451.

26. Baumgartner H, Bonhoeffer P, De Groot NM, et al. ESC guidelines for the management of grown-up congenital heart disease (new version 2010). Eur Heart J 2010;31(23):2915–57.

27. Silversides CK, Marelli A, Beauchesne L, et al. Canadian Cardiovascular Society 2009 consensus conference on the management of adults with congenital heart disease: executive summary. Can J Cardiol 2010;26(3):143–50.

28. Nathan M, Karamichalis J, Liu H, et al. Technical performance scores are strongly associated with early mortality, postoperative adverse events, and intensive care unit length of stay-analysis of consecutive discharges for 2 years. J Thorac Cardiovasc Surg 2014;147(1):389–94, 396.e1–3.

29. Nathan M, Karamichalis JM, Liu H, et al. Surgical technical performance scores are predictors of late mortality and unplanned reinterventions in infants after cardiac surgery. J Thorac Cardiovasc Surg 2012; 144(5):1095–101.e7.

30. Nathan M, Sadhwani A, Gauvreau K, et al. Association between technical performance scores and neurodevelopmental outcomes after congenital cardiac surgery. J Thorac Cardiovasc Surg 2014; 148(1):232–7.e3.

31. Chaudhry-Waterman N, Coombs S, Porras D, et al. Developing tools to measure quality in congenital catheterization and interventions: the Congenital Cardiac Catheterization Project on Outcomes (C3PO). Methodist Debakey Cardiovasc J 2014; 10(2):63–7.

32. Porras D, Brown DW, Rathod R, et al. Acute outcomes after introduction of a Standardized Clinical Assessment and Management Plan (SCAMP) for balloon aortic valvuloplasty in congenital aortic stenosis. Congenit Heart Dis 2014;9(4):316–25.

33. Gurvitz M, Marelli A, Mangione-Smith R, et al. Building quality indicators to improve care for adults with congenital heart disease. J Am Coll Cardiol 2013; 62(23):2244–53.

34. Brown DW, Cohen KE, O'Brien P, et al. Impact of prenatal diagnosis in survivors of initial palliation of single ventricle heart disease: analysis of the National Pediatric Cardiology Quality Improvement Collaborative database. Pediatr Cardiol 2015;36(2): 314–21.

35. Schidlow DN, Gauvreau K, Patel M, et al. Site of interstage care, resource utilization, and interstage mortality: a report from the NPC-QIC registry. Pediatr Cardiol 2015;36(1):126–31.

36. Hurst DM, Oster ME, Smith S, et al. Is clinic visit frequency associated with weight gain during the interstage period? A report from the Joint Council on Congenital Heart Disease National Pediatric Cardiology Quality Improvement Collaborative (JCCHD-NPCQIC). Pediatr Cardiol 2015. [Epub ahead of print].

37. IMPACT registry [Internet]. Available at: https://www.ncdr.com/webncdr/impact.

38. Vincent RN, Moore J, Beekman RH, et al. Procedural characteristics and adverse events in diagnostic and interventional catheterisations in paediatric and adult CHD: initial report from the IMPACT registry. Cardiol Young 2015;1–9.

39. Rathod RH, Farias M, Friedman KG, et al. A novel approach to gathering and acting on relevant clinical information: SCAMPs. Congenit Heart Dis 2010;5(4):343–53.

40. Karamichalis JM, Colan SD, Nathan M, et al. Technical performance scores in congenital cardiac operations: a quality assessment initiative. Ann Thorac Surg 2012;94(4):1317–23 [discussion: 1323].

41. Nathan M, Sleeper LA, Ohye RG, et al. Technical performance score is associated with outcomes after the Norwood procedure. J Thorac Cardiovasc Surg 2014;148(5):2208–13, 2214.e1–6.

Index

Note: Page numbers of article titles are in **boldface** type.

A

ACHD. *See* Adult congenital heart disease (ACHD)

Adult congenital heart disease (ACHD), **503–512**
- across life span
  - prevalence of, 504–506
- arrhythmias in, **571–588** (*See also* Arrhythmia(s), in ACHD)
- burden of, 506–507
- distribution of
  - gender differences in, 504–505
- future directions in, 510
- health care quality in
  - current efforts, 638–639
  - evaluation of, **635–641**
  - future directions in, 639–640
- heart failure in, **589–598** (*See also* Heart failure, in ACHD)
- impact on health services utilization, 507–508
- incidence of, 504
- introduction, 503, 625
- management of
  - specialized care in, 508–509
    - delivering of, 509–510
- mortality data, 505–506, 508
- outcomes of
  - gender differences in, 504–505
- population size of, 506
- pregnancy and, **611–623** (*See also* Pregnancy, ACHD and)
- prevalence of, 506
  - across life span, 504–506
  - birth-related, 504
- psychosocial issues related to, **625–634**
  - biopsychosocial challenges, 627
  - clinical strategies in optimizing, 630
  - demographic factors, 629
  - European outcomes, 628–629
  - medical factors, 629–630
  - psychological distress, 629–630
  - psychologic functioning, 627, 628
  - social functioning, 627–629
- quality of life effects of, 508
- survival shifts in, 505–506
- transition to, **625–634**
  - from pediatric to adult care, 625–627

AF. *See* Atrial fibrillation (AF)

Anesthesia/anesthetics
- in pregnancy-related ACHD, 620–621

Aneurysm(s)
- after CoA management, 527

Antibiotics
- in ACHD prevention during pregnancy, 621

Aorta
- coarctation of, **521–530** (*See also* Coarctation of aorta (CoA))

Aortic root dilation
- TOF and, 537

Arrhythmia(s)
- in ACHD, **571–588**
  - ICDs-related sudden cardiac death and risk stratification for, 581–582
  - introduction, 571–572
  - management of, 575–582
    - atrial arrhythmias, 575–577
    - catheter ablation in, 578–580
    - device therapy in, 580–581
    - surgical, 580
    - ventricular arrhythmias, 577
  - tachycardia, 572–575 (*See also* Tachycardia(s), in ACHD)
- decreased cardiac output and, 561–563
- D-TGA and, 548–549
- TOF and, 536–537

Arterial switch
- in D-TGA evaluation, 551–553
- in D-TGA management, 550, 554–556
  - anatomic complications of, 550–551
  - long-term outcomes of, 547–549

Arterial switch operation (ASO)
- defined, 544
- in D-TGA palliation, 545

ASD. *See* Atrial septal defect (ASD)

ASO. *See* Arterial switch operation (ASO)

Atrial arrhythmias
- in ACHD
  - management of, 575–577
    - catheter ablation in, 579–580
    - thromboprophylaxis of, 577–578

Atrial fibrillation (AF)
- in ACHD, 574
  - management of
    - catheter ablation in, 580

Atrial septal defect (ASD), 513–516
- clinical presentation of, 514–515
- described, 513–514
- management of

http://dx.doi.org/10.1016/S0733-8651(15)00100-9
0733-8651/15/$ – see front matter © 2015 Elsevier Inc. All rights reserved.

United States Postal Service

Statement of Ownership, Management, and Circulation
(All Periodicals Publications Except Requestor Publications)

1. Publication Title	2. Publication Number	3. Filing Date
Cardiology Clinics	0 0 0 - 7 0 0 1	9/18/15

4. Issue Frequency	5. Number of Issues Published Annually	6. Annual Subscription Price
Feb, May, Aug, Nov	4	$320.00

7. Complete Mailing Address of Known Office of Publication (Not printer) (Street, city, county, state, and ZIP+4®)

Elsevier Inc.
360 Park Avenue South
New York, NY 10010-1710

Contact Person
Stephen R. Bushing

Telephone (Include area code)
215-239-3688

8. Complete Mailing Address of Headquarters or General Business Office of Publisher (Not printer)

Elsevier Inc., 360 Park Avenue South, New York, NY 10010-1710

9. Full Names and Complete Mailing Addresses of Publisher, Editor, and Managing Editor (Do not leave blank)

Publisher (Name and complete mailing address)

Linda Belfus, Elsevier Inc., 1600 John F. Kennedy Blvd., Suite 1800, Philadelphia, PA 19103

Editor (Name and complete mailing address)

Lauren Boyle, Elsevier Inc., 1600 John F. Kennedy Blvd., Suite 1800, Philadelphia, PA 19103-2899

Managing Editor (Name and complete mailing address)

Adrianne Brigido, Elsevier Inc., 1600 John F. Kennedy Blvd., Suite 1800, Philadelphia, PA 19103-2899

10. Owner (Do not leave blank. If the publication is owned by a corporation, give the name and address of the corporation immediately followed by the names and addresses of all stockholders owning or holding 1 percent or more of the total amount of stock. If not owned by a corporation, give the names and addresses of the individual owners. If owned by a partnership or other unincorporated firm, give its name and address as well as those of each individual owner. If the publication is published by a nonprofit organization, give its name and address.)

Full Name	Complete Mailing Address
Wholly owned subsidiary of	1600 John F. Kennedy Blvd, Ste. 1800
Reed/Elsevier, US holdings	Philadelphia, PA 19103-2899

11. Known Bondholders, Mortgagees, and Other Security Holders Owning or Holding 1 Percent or More of Total Amount of Bonds, Mortgages, or Other Securities. If none, check box ☐ None

Full Name	Complete Mailing Address
N/A	

12. Tax Status (For completion by nonprofit organizations authorized to mail at nonprofit rates) (Check one)
The purpose, function, and nonprofit status of this organization and the exempt status for federal income tax purposes:
☐ Has Not Changed During Preceding 12 Months
☐ Has Changed During Preceding 12 Months (Publisher must submit explanation of change with this statement)

13. Publication Title	14. Issue Date for Circulation Data Below
Cardiology Clinics	August 2015

15.	Extent and Nature of Circulation		Average No. Copies Each Issue During Preceding 12 Months	No. Copies of Single Issue Published Nearest to Filing Date
a.	Total Number of Copies (Net press run)		600	453
b. Legitimate Paid and Or Requested Distribution (By Mail and Outside the Mail)	(1)	Mailed Outside County Paid/Requested Mail Subscriptions stated on PS Form 3541. (Include paid distribution above nominal rate, advertiser's proof copies and exchange copies)	257	187
	(2)	Mailed In-County Paid/Requested Mail Subscriptions stated on PS Form 3541. (Include paid distribution above nominal rate, advertiser's proof copies and exchange copies)		
	(3)	Paid Distribution Outside the Mails Including Sales Through Dealers And Carriers, Street Vendors, Counter Sales, and Other Paid Distribution Outside USPS®	106	107
	(4)	Paid Distribution by Other Classes of Mail Through the USPS (e.g. First-Class Mail®)		
c.	Total Paid or Requested Circulation (Sum of 15b (1), (2), (3), and (4))		363	294
d. Free or Nominal Rate Distribution (By Mail and Outside the Mail)	(1)	Free or Nominal Rate Outside-County Copies included on PS Form 3541	34	35
	(2)	Free or Nominal Rate In-County Copies included on PS Form 3541		
	(3)	Free or Nominal Rate Copies mailed at Other classes Through the USPS (e.g. First-Class Mail®)		
	(4)	Free or Nominal Rate Distribution Outside the Mail (Carriers or Other means)		
e.	Total Nonrequested Distribution (Sum of 15d (1), (2), (3) and (4))		34	35
f.	Total Distribution (Sum of 15c and 15e)		397	329
g.	Copies not Distributed (See instructions to publishers #4 (page 63))		203	124
h.	Total (Sum of 15f and g)		600	453
i.	Percent Paid and/or Requested Circulation (15c divided by 15f times 100)		91.44%	89.36%

* If you are claiming electronic copies go to line 16 on page 3. If you are not claiming Electronic copies, skip to line 17 on page 3

16. Electronic Copy Circulation	Average No. Copies Each Issue During Preceding 12 Months	No. Copies of Single Issue Published Nearest to Filing Date
a. Paid Electronic Copies		
b. Total paid Print Copies (Line 15c) + Paid Electronic copies (Line 16a)		
c. Total Print Distribution (Line 15f) + Paid Electronic Copies (Line 16a)		
d. Percent Paid (Both Print & Electronic copies) (16b divided by 16c X 100)		

☐ I certify that 50% of all my distributed copies (electronic and print) are paid above a nominal price

17. Publication of Statement of Ownership
If the publication is a general publication, publication of this statement is required. Will be printed in the _November 2015_ issue of this publication.

18. Signature and Title of Editor, Publisher, Business Manager, or Owner

Stephen R. Bushing – Inventory Distribution Coordinator

Date
September 18, 2015

I certify that all information furnished on this form is true and complete. I understand that anyone who furnishes false or misleading information on this form or who omits material or information requested on the form may be subject to criminal sanctions (including fines and imprisonment) and/or civil sanctions (including civil penalties).

PS Form 3526, July 2014 (Page 3 of 3)

PS Form 3526, July 2014 (Page 1 of 3 (Instructions Page 3)) PSN 7530-01-000-9931 PRIVACY NOTICE: See our Privacy policy in www.usps.com

Moving?

Make sure your subscription moves with you!

To notify us of your new address, find your **Clinics Account Number** (located on your mailing label above your name), and contact customer service at:

Email: journalscustomerservice-usa@elsevier.com

800-654-2452 (subscribers in the U.S. & Canada)
314-447-8871 (subscribers outside of the U.S. & Canada)

Fax number: 314-447-8029

Elsevier Health Sciences Division
Subscription Customer Service
3251 Riverport Lane
Maryland Heights, MO 63043

*To ensure uninterrupted delivery of your subscription, please notify us at least 4 weeks in advance of move.

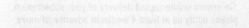